*The
Fundamentals of
Psychological
Medicine*

The Fundamentals of Psychological Medicine

R. R. TILLEARD-COLE
MA BM BCh MRC Psych DPM
Director, Oxford Institute of Psychiatry
Oxford

J. MARKS
MA MD FRCP FRC Path
Downing College
Cambridge

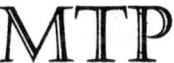

Medical and Technical Publishing Co. Ltd.

Published by
MTP
MEDICAL AND TECHNICAL PUBLISHING CO LTD
St Leonards House
Lancaster, England

ISBN-13: 978-94-011-7166-3   e-ISBN-13: 978-94-011-7164-9
DOI: 10.1007/978-94-011-7164-9

CONTENTS

1

INTRODUCTION AND GENERAL PRINCIPLES

During recent years, medical advancement within those scientific fields which serve the clinical speciality of psychiatry has occurred with breathtaking rapidity. The speed of this progress demands a continuous reformation of knowledge by which new and revolutionary concepts replace older and traditionally accepted ideas. Such rapid changes, which involve the substitution of controversial data for previously considered fact, frequently induce perplexity and bewilderment in those whose work lies in fields beyond the special limits of psychiatry.

This book has been written in response to many requests from both postgraduates and undergraduates whom it has been our pleasure to instruct in Psychological Medicine at Oxford and Physiology at Cambridge. Its style has been kept deliberately simple, though it is hoped that the dogmatic presentation which this sometimes involves has not reduced its fundamental accuracy.

We hope that the text will be of interest and value to doctors and others concerned in the problems of mental health care. The book is international in outlook and is not limited by the requirements of any specific syllabus, although its contents were originally formulated by the needs of postgraduate colleagues who have attended our courses at the Oxford Institute of Psychiatry. These doctors include not only psychiatrists-in-training but also Officers from the Prison Medical Services and Armed Forces, Medical Officers of Health and General

Practitioners, all of whom have recognized the importance of a basic knowledge of psychological medicine for their work and the necessity for this to be built upon a foundation of fundamental science.

In preparing the text, we have been mindful of the fact that the care of the mentally ill must now be an integrated team-effort requiring the professional skills of not only the medically qualified, but also those from the important groups of Clinical Psychologists, Psychiatric Nurses and Social Workers. In the belief that the training of these subsidiary groups should incorporate as far as is practicable the most comprehensive grounding in psychological medicine, we believe that this book will hold a special interest for the non-medically qualified members of the psychiatric team.

The importance of lucid and intelligible instruction on the anatomy and physiology of the nervous system during the early training of all medical workers cannot be overstated. Nor can the necessity for appropriate training in psychology. This vigorous, if relatively youthful, science finds daily application in all those fields of life where activity by the individual occurs. Psychology occupies a central position among the behavioural sciences, particularly those with a prime application to medicine. The medical worker in his search for meaningful symptoms and signs of illness in his patient, will spend a considerable time understanding and interpreting the behaviour pattern which confronts him. It is this understanding and interpretation of the patient's behaviour pattern, and its modification when indicated, that constitutes the medical science and art of the specialty of psychiatry.

It has been shown that approximately one person in three who consults his medical practitioner does so for psychological difficulties, even though the presenting symptom may be rationalized to masquerade as one from the vast range of physical complaints. The application of the fundamentals of psychological medicine will be found in all aspects of patient care, yet paradoxically until recently the teaching of psychology found little, if any place in the medical student's curriculum. It is our hope that this book will interest and assist you whichever may be the particular group in which you find yourself and whatever may constitute your specific needs for instruction and knowledge within the important field of psychiatry.

PSYCHOLOGICAL MEDICINE – SCIENCE AND ART

Mental illnesses are nothing new; their descriptions can be found in the earliest manuscripts. For thousands of years prior to the arrival of informed Greek and Roman thought, such illnesses were considered instances of demoniac possession. Systematized demonologies were available in all ancient civilizations of the world and each, quite independently, accounted for its mentally sick on the basis of supernatural possession.

The symptomatology of mental illness was equated with punishment – a form of retribution from the prevailing deities for sins both of omission and of commission. Forces of evil were unleashed accordingly and were despatched to enter and possess the soul of the afflicted person; there they wreaked the familiar havoc upon his or her cerebration.

It was these very concepts of mental illness which underlay the early practice of trephining, whereby holes were made in the wretched individual's skull to provide a portal of exit for those demons contained within. So also emerged the rationale for the more brutal therapies of whipping, beating, purging and the sudden immersion in icy water, designed not so much for the maltreatment of the patient in question but rather to render existence for the evil spirits within so intolerable that they might relinquish their hold and depart seeking a more hospitable domain elsewhere.

With the advent of Graeco-Roman civilization came an initial period of scientific thought with a surprisingly realistic insight into the true nature of mental illness. During this all too brief period of truth, the Pythagorean School identified the brain as the seat of intellectual activity and ascribed mental disorder to dysfunction of this organ. Hippocrates, in addition to his denunciation of the sacred concept of epilepsy, noted the role of heredity and predisposition in psychological disorders and again correlated insanity with disease of the brain. The tragedy of this era was that it proved all too short, for within a few hundred years the wisdom of its physicians and philosophers was already forgotten and the civilized world, as then known, relapsed to its earlier primitive and superstitious ignorance. Mental illness yet again was explained in terms of demoniac possession.

This totally unhappy situation prevailed throughout the whole of the Middle Ages, when mental illness was treated at best by holy men 'casting out the devils' (fig. 1) or at worst by torture and burning at the stake. The plight of the mentally ill until late in the eighteenth century

3

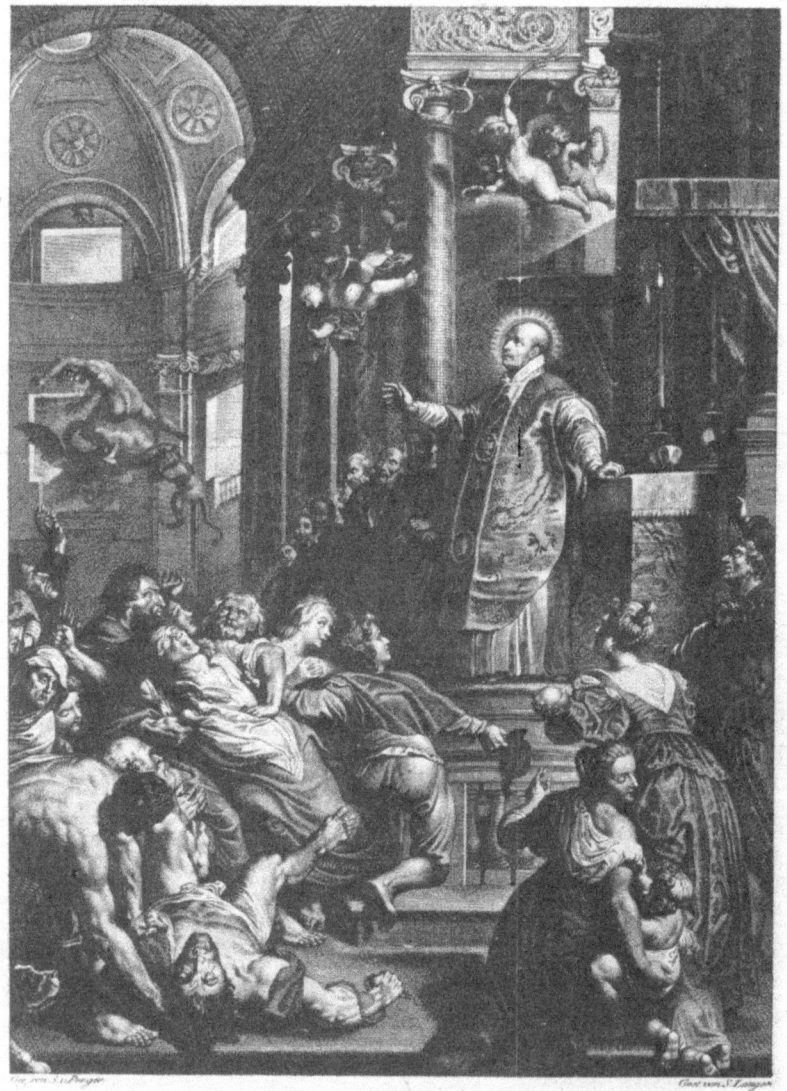

FIGURE 1 Saint Ignatius 'Casting out devils' (Mansell Collection).

defies any adequate description. Such patients were tethered by manacles, chained to the wall or restrained with iron bands encircling them. Since the normal excretory functions occurred *in situ*, the patients were nursed upon straw which served as their bedding. Depravities of all kinds were prevalent among their attendants, against whom the patients were powerless to protect themselves. Their so-called treatment was largely of an horrific kind and included such travesties as Reil's system of non-injurious torture.

With the French Revolution there came in 1793 an historic event in the annals of psychiatry, Philip Pinel, Physician Superintendent of the Bicêtre Hospital in Paris, most courageously threw off the shackles from his patients and ushered in an era of humanitarian consideration for the mentally sick in a setting of non-restraint. By the mid-nineteenth century, the earlier primitive practices had become replaced by incarceration in the unfortunate Victorian edifices, which so closely resembled the country's gaols and which, of necessity, are still used for the care and treatment of the mentally ill.

This heritage of the centuries still pervades the attitudes of many laymen towards mental illness and even today it is only in the most sophisticated communities that mental illness is looked upon, like physical illness, as a disease and not a cause for shame.

The psychoanalytical approach of the twentieth century gave tremendous impetus to the new considerations of mental illness, an impetus which gained further momentum from the era of physical treatments of the 1930s, and from the development during the last decade of specific chemotherapy for psychiatric abnormalities. Modern methods of treating mental ill-health have not only altered our attitudes to these diseases but have proved a powerful stimulus to the scientific study of the psyche. The wealth of current literature testifies to the effort which is being made to understand the normal mental processes and how abnormalities occur. Much is already known but far more is likely to emerge during the next decade as the science of psychological medicine develops further.

This book concerns itself *inter alia* with that scientific knowledge which exists today on the basic functions within the nervous system. The development of knowledge in psychological medicine is greatly dependent on an understanding of these normal processes within the brain. Little in this book could have been written some twenty years ago, since the advances which have occurred have done so most rapidly.

The Fundamentals of Psychological Medicine

The scientific aspects of psychological medicine concern themselves with the reactions of the nervous system during health and with their abnormalities in disease. The nervous system of an intact animal functions as a single integrated unit, within which a change in one part will produce change in most other parts. The description of such a complex structure *in toto* would produce a wholly indigestible mass. For the sake of clarity it is, therefore, necessary to make certain arbitrary and artificial divisions; such divisions by their very nature must inevitably involve disadvantages.

Before, however, we become too preoccupied with a scientific answer for all problems, it is important to stress that psychiatry, like any other form of medicine, will remain forever an art no less than a science. People are neither inanimate nor are they statistical units; each is an individual set in his own separate environment within which his behaviour is unique. Appropriate healing calls for the application of scientific knowledge, tempered by the art of the therapist to adapt such knowledge to those needs specific to the individual in question.

Part I
The scientific
basis

2

ANATOMY OF THE
NERVOUS SYSTEM

THE PURPOSE OF A NERVOUS SYSTEM AND ITS GENERAL FORM
Why do we possess a nervous system and why does it assume the curious form of a bulbous upper extremity with an attenuated tail which runs through most of the trunk? Such questions are of prime importance before examining the more detailed aspects of neuro-anatomy and neurophysiology, and raise important considerations of evolution, genetics and the embryology of the human nervous system.

In the progression of animal life from protozoon to the most complex multicellular forms, many structures become adapted for specialized function. In the unicellular amœba, control is simple, for all protoplasm can respond to an appropriate stimulus, and in the single cell this stimulus produces change throughout the protoplasm as a whole.

Differentiation necessitates specialization and with the evolution of multicellular animals came the need for an effective system of communication. One type of cell thus became specialized as an electric conductor and in the course of this process was so elongated that the length of the cell may be as much as 100,000 times its breadth. From such cells emerged the simplest nervous system, developed as a nerve net. The primitive animals which possessed such a nervous system, however, were capable of only a limited response to their environment and were incapable of mobility.

The development of more positive responses and of the power of mobility demanded a greater complexity within the nervous system. Purposeful mobility required a mechanism for movement itself, a mechanism for steering, receptors for the environment and an integration of cells within the nerve net for a limited interpretation of the

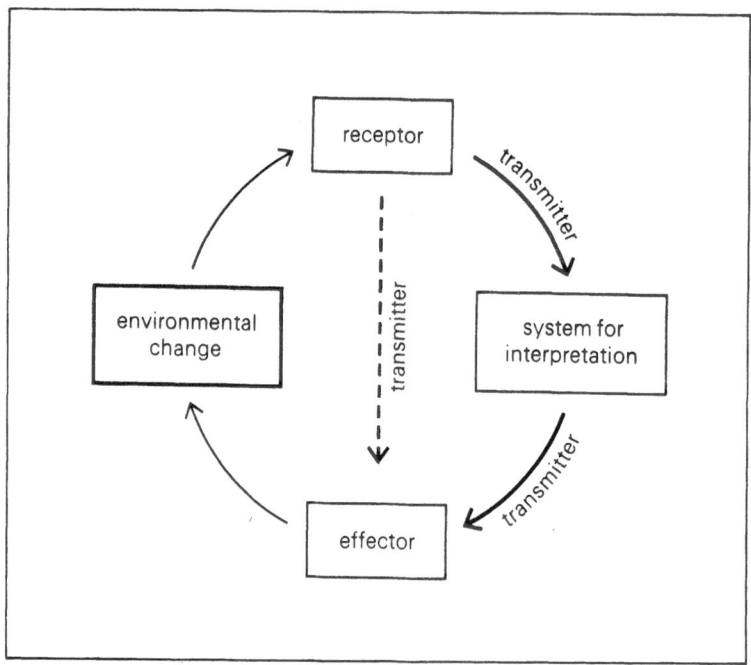

FIGURE 2 Schematic representation of a simple feed-back mechanism for control of response. At its simplest the response is fixed and automatic and the need for interpretation is removed.

sensory input to which would be coupled an appropriate output to the effector organs. This is the primitive feed-back mechanism with an input stimulus which can alter the response of the whole organism (fig. 2).

The nerve net then progressed to a more complicated form and became organized into specialized centres – the ganglia. A further evolutionary change of major importance was the inclusion of these ganglia into a neural cord through the length of the body. This neural cord was subsequently protected by a cartilaginous cage and later by a bony cage.

Creatures of this degree of development maintain a body temperature equal to that of the surroundings (poikilothermic). The rate of conduction of an impulse in specialized nerve tissue depends on the cell temperature. Thus in these animals with a cell temperature equal to their environment, nerve function, and hence activity by the animal, is largely lost when the external temperature becomes too low.

A most important change for further development was a modification to the fore-part of the neural tube, producing an area whose function was the maintenance of an internal body environment quite independent from that of the external environment. This independent control of the internal environment is termed homeostasis and the maintenance of a stable temperature, thermostasis.

At a still later stage, lateral ventricles developed from the fore-brain and around these grew the primitive cerebrum. Whilst the neural tube itself served mainly for the regulation of the internal environment, the cerebral hemispheres allowed a greater perception of the external environment and a more regulated response to it. In primitive animals the oldest part of the cerebrum and neighbouring structures, now designated the limbic system, served the function of response by the body to the external environment.

In all animals below *Homo sapiens*, the brain developed to a stage where perception of the surroundings was possible but evidence of original thought or imagination was lacking. Lower animals can learn (p. 115) and can unequivocally be shown to possess a memory (p. 112). The response to a stimulus is based directly upon past experience. It is only in man that we have the ability to predict response and to calculate probabilities. Man faced with an external stimulus is capable of imagining possible responses and postulating their end-result, then from these responses selecting the action which he believes to be appropriate. It is this ability to make calculations of the probable effects of a response which distinguishes man from all other animals.

EMBRYOLOGY

The nervous system, like the skin, is derived from the embryological germ-layer of ectoderm. In clinical medicine a close link can be found between many dermatoses and underlying psychological disorders. It is interesting to speculate to what extent this close association between psychiatric and dermatological illness may be attributable to the common embryological origin of both nervous system and skin.

The central nervous system first appears in the embryo as an early mid-line thickening of ectoderm, termed the neural plate. The edges of the neural plate rise up by a process of differential growth to form the neural folds, and these folds enclose between them the neural groove. The neural folds approach each other in the mid-line and fuse together – at first at a point approximately half-way along their length and then the process of fusion extends both cranially and caudally. By this means, the neural groove is converted to a hollow tube, open at both anterior and posterior ends – the neural tube. The openings constitute the anterior and posterior neuropores. It is from the neural tube that both brain and spinal cord develop (fig. 3).

Within the wall of the neural tube, the proliferating cells arrange themselves in three layers, innermost as the ependymal zone, next as the mantle zone and outermost as the marginal zone. It is from cells of the ependymal zone that both neuroblasts (forerunners of the neurones) and spongioblasts (forerunners of the neuroglial cells, with the exception of microglia) develop.

The fusion of both the anterior and posterior neuropores during the fourth week of foetal life converts the open-ended neural tube into a closed hollow structure. Anterior to the fourth somite of the embryo three major swellings appear, the fore-brain, mid-brain and hind-brain vesicles. From the fore-brain vesicle develop the telencephalon (cerebral hemispheres) and the diencephalon (thalamus, hypothalamus, epithalamus [pineal gland and adjoining structures] posterior pituitary). From the mid-brain vesicle develops the mesencephalon (mid-brain). From the hind-brain vesicle develop both the metencephalon (pons and cerebellum) and the myelencephalon (medulla oblongata).

Early in the development of the fore-brain vesicle, optic evaginations, forerunners of the retinae, appear and are obtruded one on either side to become the optic cups. At a later stage, a small vesicle of ectoderm appears at each side of the neck region (otocyst) and develops to form the cochlea and labyrinth of the inner ear.

Three main flexures, mid-brain, cervical and pontine, occur in the developing brain during the fourth, fifth and sixth weeks of embryonic life. These primary flexures re-align the growing portions of the brain to their definitive positions in adult life. The cavities within this hollow system provide the basis of the ventricular system. That of the fore-brain vesicle provides the lateral ventricles and third ventricle; that of the mid-brain vesicle provides the aqueduct of the mid-brain, that of the hind-brain vesicle provides the fourth ventricle.

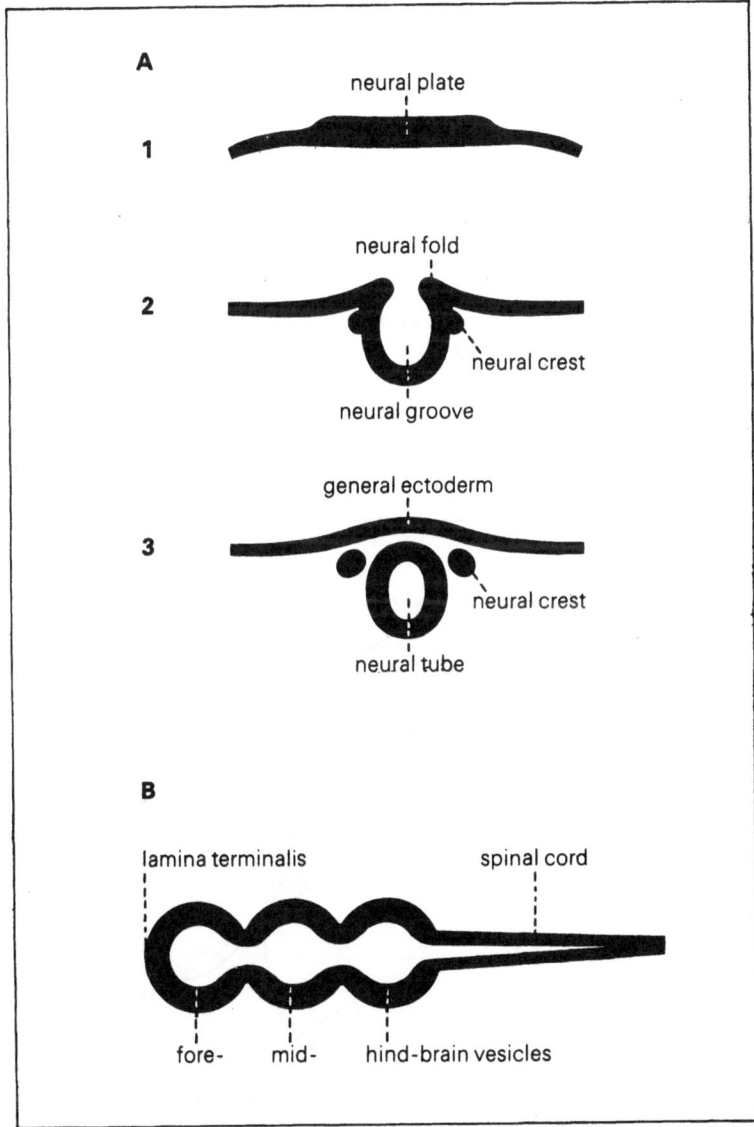

FIGURE 3 (A) Stages in the embryonic formation of neural tube and neural crest. (B) Development of fore-, mid- and hind-brain vesicles and spinal cord from embryonic neural tube.

During the sixth week of intra-uterine life a downgrowth from the floor of the diencephalon establishes the primordium of the posterior lobe and stalk of the pituitary gland (neurohypophysis). An earlier evagination (also ectodermal) from the primitive mouth region (Rathke's pouch) has established the primordium of the anterior lobe and pars intermedia (adenohypophysis).

The spinal cord develops from that portion of the neural tube which lies posteriorly to the fourth somite. Its cavity is finally reduced to the minute central canal found in the definitive spinal cord. Its cells are arranged in two basic groupings within the cord, an anterior motor group and a posterior sensory group. Fibres from the anterior horn cells grow outwards from the spinal cord to link up with their corresponding myotomes. Sensory fibres, in contrast, grow into the posterior horns of grey matter from the developing posterior root ganglia (fig. 4).

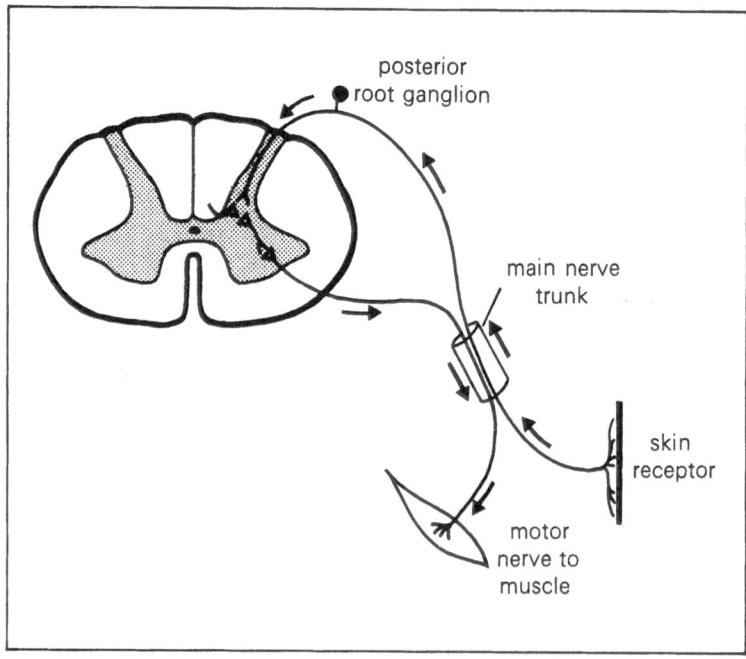

FIGURE 4 Schematic representation of anterior and posterior nerve roots.

At a time when by fusion the neural folds are forming the neural tube, ectodermal cells are budded off and form on either side an independent ridge of ectoderm. The two ridges so formed constitute the neural crest. It is from the neural crest that the sensory nerves with their posterior root ganglia, the neurilemmal sheaths of the peripheral nerves and the ganglia of the autonomic nervous system are all developed.

TOPOGRAPHY OF THE CENTRAL NERVOUS SYSTEM

The nervous system may be conveniently divided into the central nervous system (brain and spinal cord), the peripheral nervous system (cranial and spinal nerves with sensory function (p. 66) and motor function (p. 77)), and the special subdivision composed of the autonomic nervous system (parasympathetic and sympathetic p. 93).

The spinal cord (medulla spinalis) extends from the level of the foramen magnum of the skull, where it is continuous with the medulla oblongata of the brain. It passes through the vertebral foramina of the cervical and thoracic regions of the vertebral column and as far as the level of the upper lumbar vertebrae (L_1/L_2). At each segment of the cord, motor (efferent) fibres are despatched and sensory (afferent) fibres are received via the paired spinal nerves.

The brain. The brain of the adult can be conveniently subdivided into the following principal components: the cerebral hemispheres (p. 71); the brain-stem – which itself includes the thalamus (p. 16), the hypothalamus (p. 89), the mid-brain and the reticular formation (p. 84); the limbic system (p. 123); and the pons and cerebellum (p. 81).

Topographically, each cerebral hemisphere is composed of four lobes: frontal, temporal, occipital and parietal. Each lobe in turn, with the single exception of the parietal lobe, carries a corresponding pole of the cerebral hemisphere, frontal, temporal or occipital.

The two hemispheres are joined by the corpus callosum, a great commissure of transverse fibres which link identical points in the cerebral cortices of the hemispheres (p. 77).

Gyri and sulci convolute the surface of each cerebral hemisphere, and in so doing increase enormously the total number of neurones which may be packed within the cortex. Localized areas of cortex show complex degrees of specialization (fig. 32 p. 73), as for example the pre-central gyrus (motor cortex), the post-central gyrus (somatic sensory cortex), the calcarine sulcus (visual cortex), the superior temporal gyrus (auditory cortex), the superior operculum (gustatory cortex) and the uncus (olfactory cortex). The primary role of such specialized areas is supplemented by the diffuse association areas which surround them (p. 74).

The thalami are situated one on either side of the median third ventricle. Each thalamus is made up of a number of component nuclei which receive sensory impulses from lower levels and pass these to appropriate regions of the cerebral cortex. Impulses of pain, temperature and touch, of proprioception and muscle co-ordination, are relayed by the thalamic nuclei to the cerebral cortex. Primitive sensation and pain can be appreciated by the thalamus itself.

The special relay stations of the lateral geniculate body (sight) and medial geniculate body (sound) are best considered as outlying nuclei of the thalamic system (p. 69).

Below the thalamus, the hypothalamus (p. 89) provides an important link between the reticular and limbic systems. It is this linkage, together with the controlling influence of the hypothalamus upon the endocrine system and its further role as the highest centre for the control of the autonomic nervous system, which established this region of the diencephalon as chief in importance in the manifestations of emotion. In addition, the hypothalamus regulates temperature, water-balance and the intake of food.

The reticular system, confined to the brain-stem (p. 84), exists to adapt the state of the internal environment to those demands made on the body by the external environment. It does so by its composite effect of arousal upon the cortex, the limbic system, the spinal cord, the autonomic nervous system and the endocrine system.

Within the limbic system (p. 123) the affective (emotional) component of the response to an external stimulus is generated, and from this emerges the subjective component of mood. The complex anatomy of the limbic system encircles the attachment of the cerebral hemispheres to the brain-stem. It is richly supplied by fibres from the reticular system and despatches an equally rich supply of fibres to the hypothalamus.

The cerebellar hemispheres (p. 81) – joined to the pons by their massive middle peduncle – receive a continuous stream of proprioceptive impulses from muscle spindles and tendon organs. The function of the cerebellum is twofold: the regulation of balance and posture by the body, and the dynamic co-ordination of harmonious muscular movements.

The spinal cord. The spinal cord is approximately 18 inches (46 cm) long and extends from the medulla oblongata above (at the level of the foramen magnum) to the conus medullaris below (level of L_1/L_2). Macroscopically, it exhibits two swellings, the cervical and lumbar enlargements where those fibres involved in the brachial and lumbo-sacral plexuses respectively have their cells of origin.

In cross-section (fig. 5), the spinal cord can be seen to consist of white matter (nerve fibres) disposed about a central core of grey matter (nerve cell bodies). This grey matter – of characteristic 'H' appearance – is composed of two posterior horns (sensory), two anterior horns (motor) and a transverse bar (grey commissure) pierced by the minute central canal, a continuation of the ventricular system. Each posterior horn is tipped by the substantia gelatinosa. In thoracic segments of the spinal cord a third (lateral) horn will be found on each side, from which preganglionic fibres of the sympathetic nervous system take origin. The cell bodies of the motor neurones are situated within the spinal cord in the grey anterior horns. In marked contrast with this, the cell bodies of the sensory neurones are situated outside the cord in the posterior root ganglia of the corresponding spinal nerves.

Thirty-one pairs of spinal nerves are given off by the cord (8 cervical; 12 thoracic; 5 lumbar; 5 sacral; 1 coccygeal). Each spinal nerve carries both motor and sensory fibres. In the lower region of the cord, the anterior and posterior roots of the spinal nerves show special elongation. This is to accommodate that difference in level which exists between the segment of cord from which the spinal nerve originates and the intervertebral foramen of the vertebral column through which the spinal nerve passes. The system of elongated anterior and posterior roots of the sacral and coccygeal spinal nerves constitutes the cauda equina. The tip of the conus medullaris is tethered to the dorsum of the coccyx by the filum terminale.

Nerve fibres ascend (sensory) and descend (motor) in the columns of white matter of the spinal cord and are grouped as a number of designated tracts. The principal ascending tracts include on each side the gracile and cuneate (posterior columns) conveying impulses serving proprioception and some touch: the anterior and posterior spino-cerebellar tracts conveying reflex proprioceptive impulses to the cerebellum; the anterior spino-thalamic tract conveying some touch and

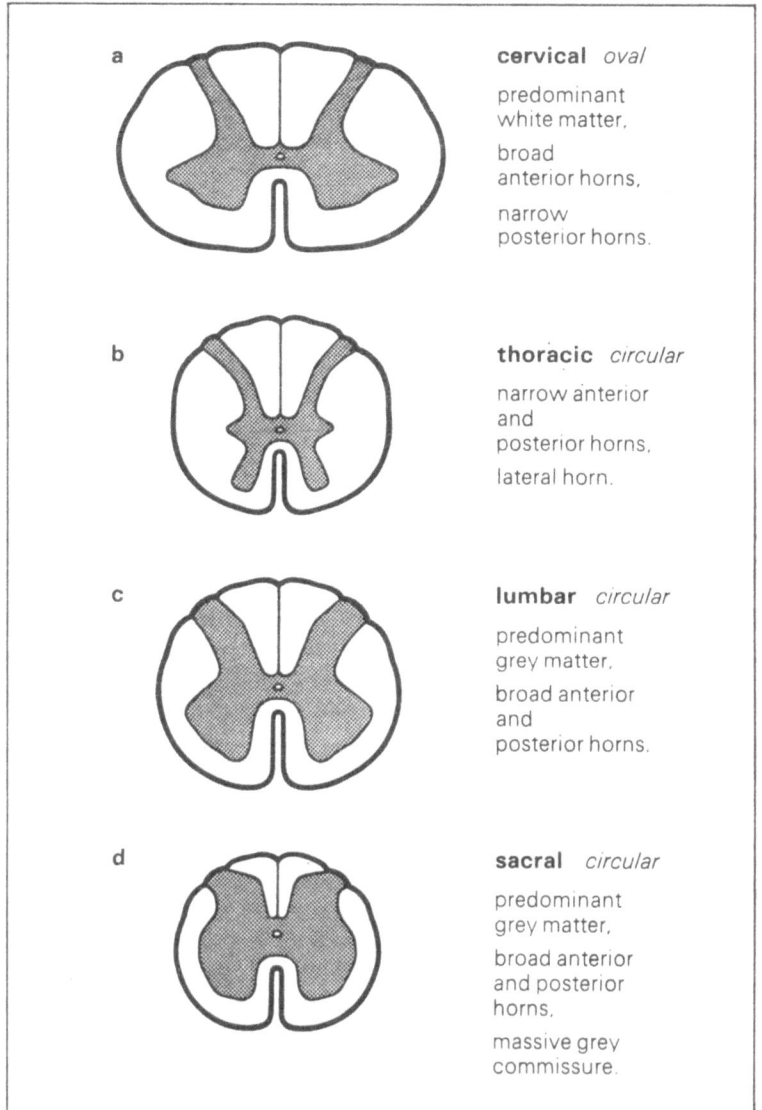

FIGURE 5 Transverse section of the spinal cord showing the general relationship of grey (hatched) and white matter. (*a*) Cervical region (*b*) Thoracic region (*c*) Lumbar region (*d*) Sacral region.

pressure, and the lateral spino-thalamic tract conveying impulses of pain and temperature (heat and cold).

The principal descending tracts include on each side the crossed pyramidal and 'uncrossed' pyramidal motor pathways for voluntary impulses (fig. 6); the vestibulo-spinal tract, serving postural and equilibration reflexes and the tecto-spinal tract (optic and auditory reflexes).

Over and above these pathways for particular nerve impulses, fibres of the important reticular system (p. 89) – spino-reticular and reticulo-spinal – ascend and descend in the anterior and lateral columns of white matter. Sensory impulses travel *en masse* via the ascending reticular system simultaneously, and in parallel as it were, with those impulses travelling via the orthodox sensory tracts.

Four features of neuronal arrangement within the spinal cord may, with advantage, be specially noted; the classical anterior horn cell (motor neurone) connects by a fast-conducting axon to somatic muscle via its motor unit composed of numerous motor end-plates. This is the α motor pathway (p. 78).

A second motor neurone of the anterior horn connects by a fine, slower-conducting axon to the intrafusal fibres of the muscle spindle. This is the γ motor pathway (p. 80).

The Renshaw cells are located near the antero-median border of the anterior horn. Their effect is that of inhibition of the α motor neurones to which their axons pass.

Sensory neurones for proprioception (of the second relay) are situated at the base of the posterior horn of the cord and compose the column of Clarke. To these neurones pass sensory impulses from the muscle spindles and tendon organs. From these neurones originate the high speed conduction fibres of the posterior spino-cerebellar tract (reflex proprioception). The physiological significance of these cells is considered on p. 81).

NEURONES AND NEUROGLIA

The elements of the nervous system are of two basic kinds – the nerve cells or neurones, supremely differentiated for their special function of conducting nerve impulses, and the neuroglial cells, providing that important supporting framework within which the nerve cells and their fibres may repose.

Each neurone (of which some ten thousand million – 10^{10} – exist

19

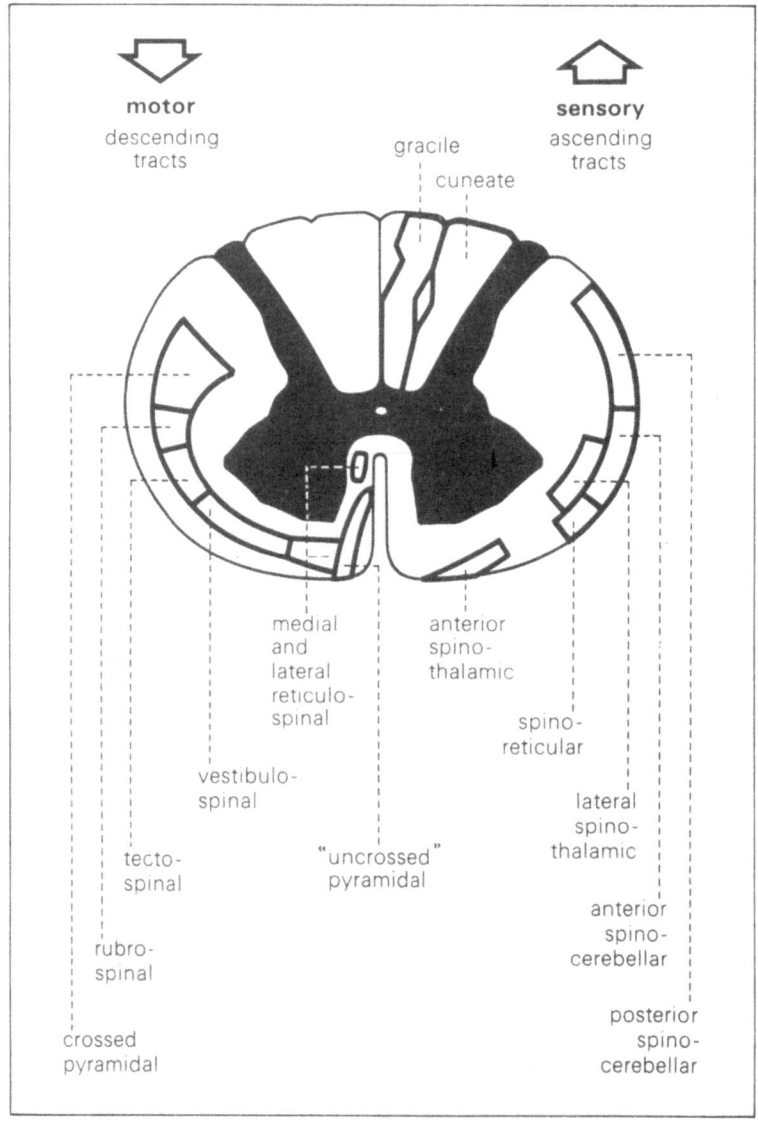

FIGURE 6 Diagram of spinal cord in transverse section showing main ascending tracts and descending tracts. An indication is given of the ascending and descending tracts of the reticular system.

within the brain) is a separate unit. Though it lies in the closest proximity to its fellow nerve cells, the neurone remains anatomically quite separate from them. Nerve impulses pass from neurone to neurone at the synapses – special contacts which occur between nerve process and nerve process, or between nerve process and nerve cell body. The nerve impulse is transferred across the synapse by means of chemical transmitters (p. 33).

Histologically (fig. 7), the neurone possesses a cell body with both nucleus and nucleolus. Within its cytoplasm are found Nissl granules which at times of stress will swell and disappear (chromatolysis); these granules then reappear as the nerve cell recuperates. A number of short, irregular and branched processes, the dendrites, conduct nerve impulses into the cell body (input), whereas one single, long, regular fibre, the axon, conducts the impulse from the cell to its ultimate destination (output). This axon may give off important collateral branches and of these one may return to the dendrites or body of its own nerve cell, a recurrent collateral. The axon ends by breaking into a number of terminal arborizations which may innervate other neurones, gland or muscle.

With voluntary muscle the axon of the motor neurone divides into many branches each one of which ends as a motor end plate (fig. 8). Each filament of the terminal arborization ends in a bulbous swelling; it is from here that the synaptic chemical transmitter is released.

Axons vary enormously in length, from a fraction of a millimetre to more than a metre. Their speeds of conduction vary with the transverse diameters of their fibres and the nerve impulse may travel at anything from one metre per second in axons of small diameter to approximately one hundred metres per second in those of large diameter. The diameter of the fibre is largely determined by the sheath of myelin which surrounds each axon. In many instances this myelin is obvious and the fibres have been termed 'myelinated fibres'. In other instances the myelin covering is scarcely appreciable and the fibres have been termed, erroneously but still conveniently, 'amyelinated fibres'. The thicker, myelinated fibres show constrictions of their myelin at intervals termed the nodes of Ranvier. The nerve fibres of the peripheral nervous system (but unfortunately not of the central nervous system) possess a nucleated sheath, the neurilemma (sheath of Schwann). The neurilemma plays a vital part in the regeneration which can occur in peripheral nerves. Hence, while regeneration can occur in peripheral nerves, damage to neurones in the central nervous system is permanent. The basic

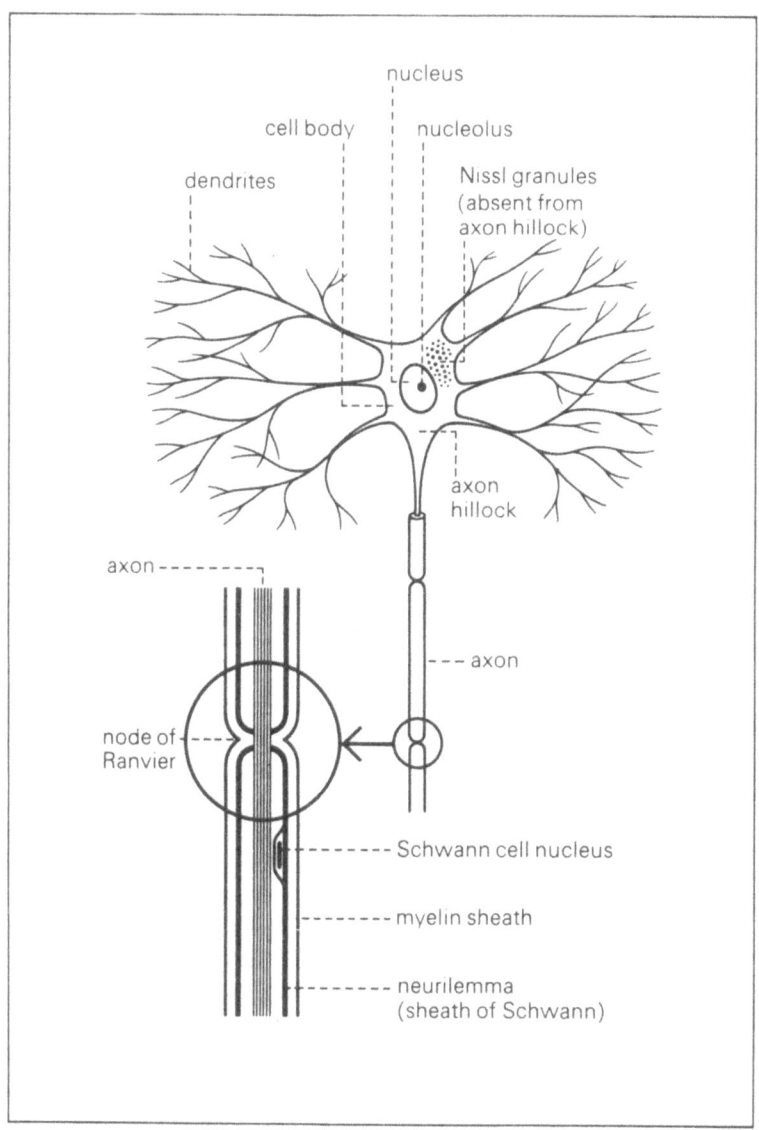

FIGURE 7 Diagram showing the main cytological features of the nerve cell and its processes.

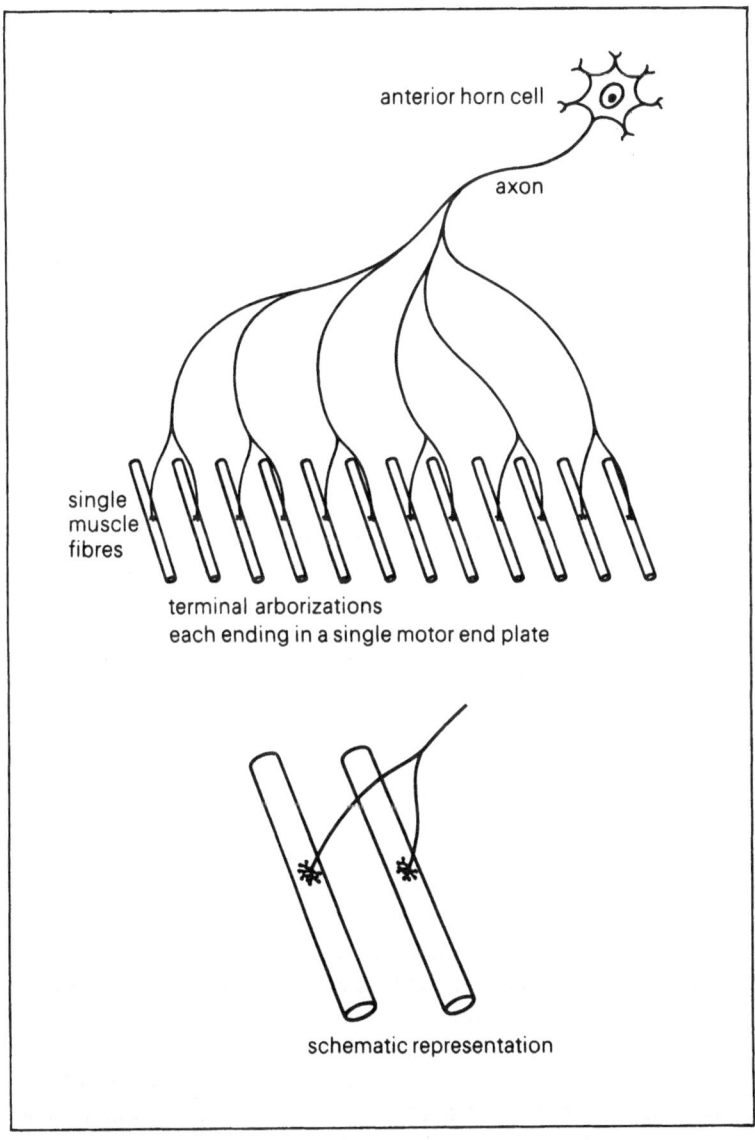

anterior horn cell

axon

single
muscle
fibres

terminal arborizations
each ending in a single motor end plate

schematic representation

FIGURE 8 Schematic representation of the terminal arborization of a motor nerve.

cytological features can be recognized in neurones throughout the central nervous system, though much individual variation will be found from cell to cell in special site or serving special function. As would be expected, the advanced degree of differentiation shown by the specialized neurone imposes upon it many limitations in terms of more primitive cellular function.

Perhaps less spectacular, yet of no less importance than the neurones, are the supporting cells of the nervous system, the neuroglia. These cells are classified as both protoplasmic and fibrous astrocytes (this latter type showing characteristic attached processes to blood vessels), oligodendrocytes (possible maintenance of myelin), microglia (mobile, phagocytic scavengers from the reticulo-endothelial system) and ependymal cells (lining the cavities of the ventricular system). The physiological roles of the neuroglial cells are not yet fully understood but pathologically their association with intracranial tumours is a common one.

BLOOD SUPPLY

Nervous tissue, more than any other tissue of the body, is wholly dependent for its normal function upon an adequate and efficient circulation of blood. A reduction in amount or in distribution of this critical blood-flow is liable, even though occurring for a brief interval of time, to be followed by permanent damage to underlying neurones. Approximately one-fifth of the heart's output of blood is pumped to the brain. It reaches this organ by two major pathways on each side of the body, the vertebral and internal carotid arteries (fig. 9).

The left and right vertebral arteries join at the lower border of the pons to form the median, unpaired, basilar artery. The basilar artery runs from the lower to the upper border of the pons, where it ends in a 'T' junction with its two terminal branches, the right and left posterior cerebral arteries.

The internal carotid artery of each side divides, lateral to the optic chiasma, into the anterior and middle cerebral arteries. Before doing so, it gives off its ophthalmic branch to supply the orbit and provide the important central artery of the retina.

Across the mid-line an anterior communicating artery connects both anterior cerebral arteries. On each side a posterior communicating artery connects the middle artery with the posterior cerebral artery. In this manner the three cerebral arteries from each side (anterior, middle and posterior) are linked together as an anastomotic ring – the circle

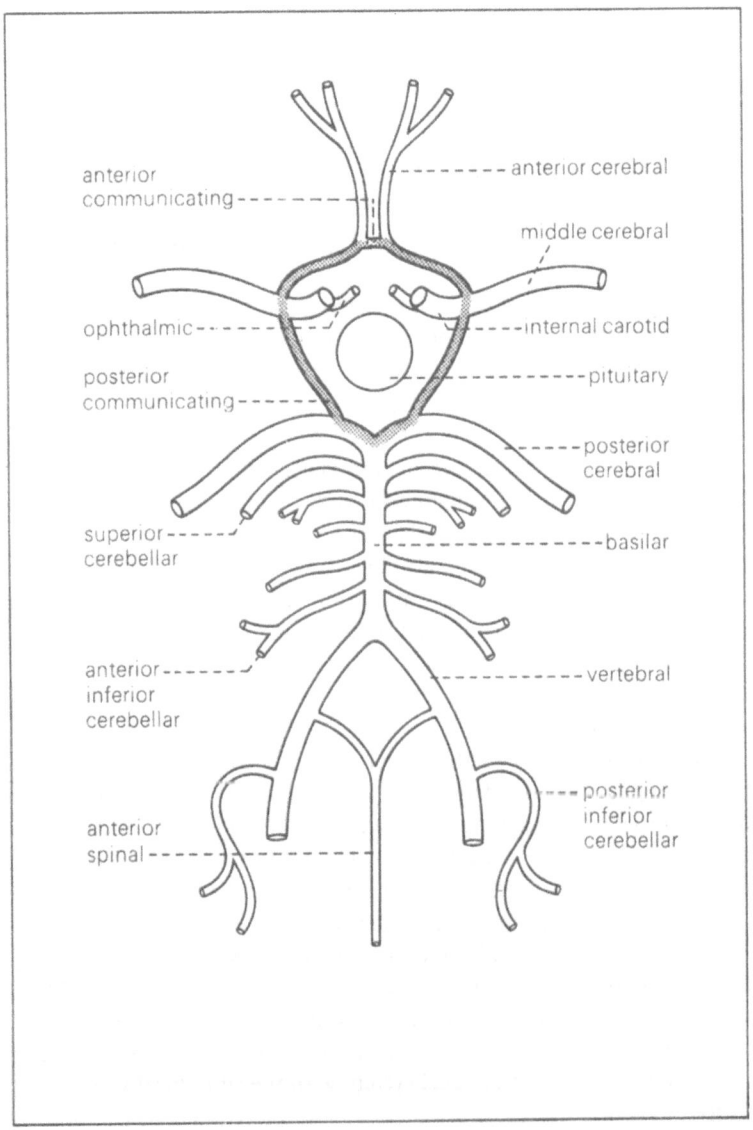

FIGURE 9 The principal arteries of the brain showing the anastomotic formation of the Circle of Willis.

of Willis (circulus arteriosus). The circle of Willis surrounds the pituitary stalk and adjacent structures. It is notorious for its variation in anatomical composition.

The middle cerebral artery supplies almost the whole of the lateral surface of the cerebral hemisphere (fig. 10). The medial surface is shared by the anterior and posterior cerebral arteries.

The generous anastomoses found between the main arteries of the brain provide an effective measure of safety in many instances of vascular occlusion. Collateral arterial pathways can be established via the circle of Willis or via the ophthalmic artery. The arterioles which supply the substance of the brain terminate with the minimum number of anastomoses. Occlusion of these arterioles will therefore result in ischaemic damage to the brain tissue. Deprived of their vital oxygen, the cerebral neurones cannot survive, and succumb within a matter of seconds.

Like the cerebrum, the cerebellum is served on each side by three main arteries of which one is superior and two are inferior. The superior cerebellar artery arises from the basilar artery shortly before its termination. The anterior inferior cerebellar artery arises from the commencement of the basilar artery. The posterior inferior cerebellar artery is a branch of the vertebral artery and, in addition to its cerebellar territory, supplies much of the medulla oblongata. Occlusion of this posterior inferior cerebellar artery may result in the dramatic clinical picture of 'cerebellar apoplexy'.

The principal artery of the spinal cord is the anterior spinal artery. Originating as a branch from each vertebral artery, it runs the length of the cord in the antero-median sulcus and supplies the greater part of the nervous tissue. It is assisted by two posterior spinal arteries, each running just medial to the posterior nerve roots and supplying only the tissues of their immediate neighbourhood.

The venous drainage of the brain is effected by superficial and deep cerebral veins which drain into the system of venous sinuses. These sinuses drain chiefly to the occipital confluence of the sinuses before discharging their blood into the internal jugular vein. Emissary veins connect veins of the intracranial system with the superficial veins of the scalp.

CEREBRO-SPINAL FLUID

Normal cerebro-spinal fluid (CSF) is a limpid, colourless and odourless fluid, aptly described by pathologists as 'gin-clear'.

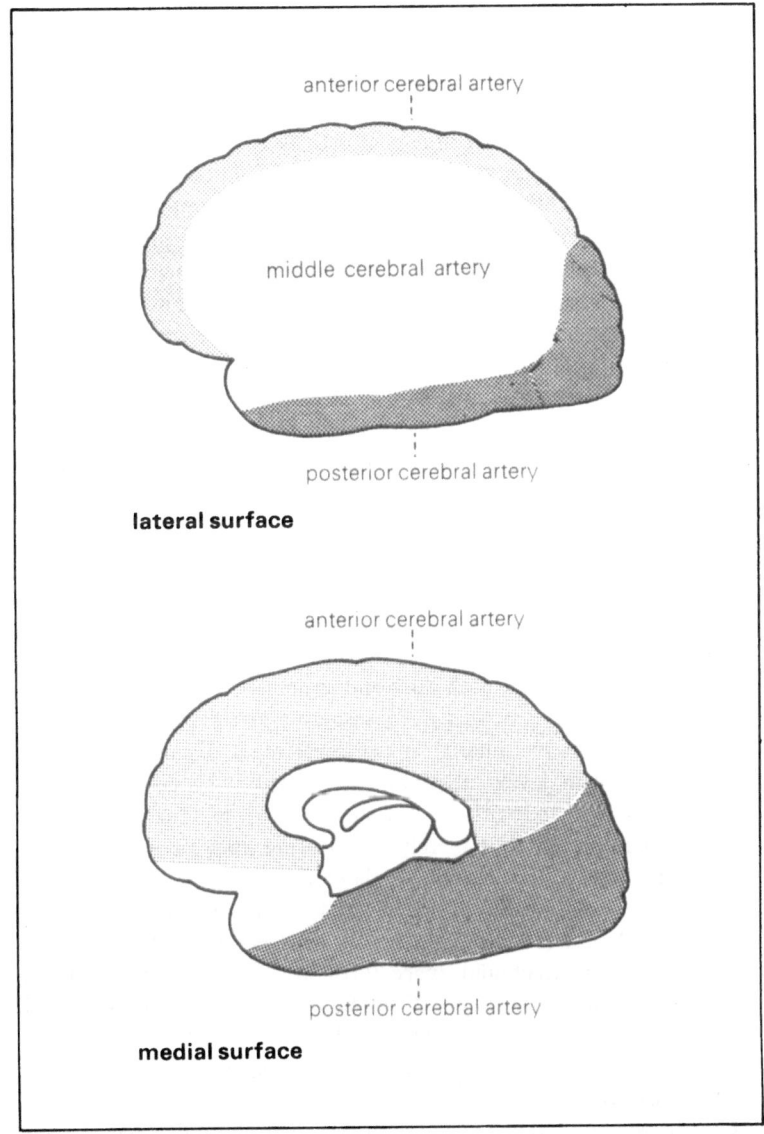

FIGURE 10 Lateral and medial surfaces of the cerebral hemisphere showing the distribution of the arterial supply.

Cerebro-spinal fluid fills the central cavities of the central nervous system – composed of the two lateral ventricles on the cerebral hemispheres and their interventricular foramina, the third ventricle of the diencephalon, the cerebral aqueduct of the mid-brain, the fourth ventricle of the medulla oblongata and the minute central canal of the spinal cord. From this seemingly closed system, the cerebro-spinal fluid escapes by way of three foramina in the fourth ventricle – the median foramen of Magendie and the two lateral foramina of Luschka – to enter the subarachnoid space enclosed within the meninges.

The subarachnoid space exists between the pia mater internally (a highly vascular membrane which intimately invests the nervous tissue) and the arachnoid mater externally (a cobweb-like membrane with fibro-elastic trabeculae traversing the subarachnoid space). External again to the arachnoid mater, and closely applied to it, lies the dura mater (a tough, fibrous, protective membrane). Within the skull, it should be noted, the endosteum of the cranial bones is, in turn, applied to the dura. This endosteum constitutes what is so often erroneously termed 'the outer layer of the dura' and explains why, on this basis, the brain appears to warrant two layers of so-called 'dura' whilst the spinal cord possesses merely one. Between arachnoid and dura a potential space exists, the subdural space and provides the site for the pathology of subdural haematoma.

In the vertebral canal, both dura and arachnoid descend to the level of S.2. The pia, for practical purposes, ends at the lowest tip of the spinal cord (conus medullaris) at the level of L_1/L_2. Between these lumbar and sacral levels, therefore, a test-tube shaped sac of subarachnoid space, filled with cerebro-spinal fluid, is situated. Here no spinal cord is present but merely the floating anterior and posterior roots of the lower spinal nerves (cauda equina).

This then is the favoured site for performing lumbar puncture. A needle passed between the vertebrae of this region (L_3/L_4 or L_4/L_5) can enter the subarachnoid space virtually with impunity and will enable the requisite specimen of cerebro-spinal fluid to be obtained. Cerebro-spinal fluid may be obtained by more advanced techniques from those dilatations of the subarachnoid space which form the cerebral cisterna.

Cerebro-spinal fluid is formed by the vascular choroid plexus present in each cerebral ventricle. The process is part diffusion and part an active secretion. It escapes via the foramina of the fourth ventricle to gain the subarachnoid space and then circulates freely about the brain and spinal cord. Ultimately, the cerebro-spinal fluid is returned by several different routes to the venous system. Most noted of these is the pathway via the arachnoid villi, which project into the venous sinuses. Substantial amounts are returned by the veins of the leptomeninges (pia and arachnoid) and some cerebro-spinal fluid drains into the lymphatic system via the sheaths of the cranial and spinal nerves. The cerebro-spinal fluid protects and supports the brain and spinal cord (water cushion). It compensates for alterations in intracranial volume. It may play a role in the transport of nutrient agents to the central nervous system and in the removal of metabolites from the nervous tissue.

An examination of the cerebro-spinal fluid provides one of the most important diagnostic investigations for disease of the central nervous system. Table I shows the normal findings for a sample of cerebro-spinal fluid. It will be remembered that although a maximum of 4 lymphocytes per cmm is allowable, the presence of polymorphs in cerebro-spinal fluid is incompatible with normality. In neurosyphilis, a Wassermann reaction may prove negative with blood yet show positive with cerebro-spinal fluid. The Lange (colloidal gold) test on cerebro-spinal fluid can yield paretic, luetic or meningeal reactions, and may include a paretic reaction in approximately 50 per cent of cases of disseminated sclerosis.

TABLE I

Appearance	'Gin-clear' fluid	Pressure	60–200 mm CSF
Total volume	100–150 ml	Protein	30 mg/100 ml approx
Specific gravity	1·005	Glucose	60 mg/100 ml approx
pH	7·4	Chlorides	730 mg/100 ml approx
Viscosity	1·03	Urea	30 mg/100 ml approx
		Cells	0–4 lymphocytes/cmm

3
PHYSIOLOGY AND BIOCHEMISTRY OF THE NERVOUS SYSTEM

The resting nerve cell may be visualized as a minute, fully-charged electrical battery. Its body and its processes are enclosed by a membrane of high resistance and its electrical charge is generated by the unequal distribution of sodium and potassium ions, inside and outside the cell on either side of the limiting membrane. This electrical charge is termed the resting potential. The interior of the neurone is negative to its exterior and a resting potential of some −70 millivolts may be recorded. The resting nerve cell is described as 'polarized'.

On excitation of the neurone, an action potential appears. The negative resting potential is abolished and a momentary swing to a positive electrical charge of approximately +40 millivolts occurs. This is followed, immediately and in sequence, by negative and positive after potentials before reverting to the *status quo ante* of the negative resting potential (−70 millivolts) once again.

The nerve impulse is accompanied by a wave of depolarization along the nerve fibre, electricity flowing from the active area to the inactive region ahead. With 'amyelinated' fibres this flow is a smooth one along the length of the fibre. With myelinated fibres, however, depolarization is restricted to the nodes of Ranvier. The nerve impulse therefore leaps from one node to the next (saltatory conduction) greatly increasing the speed of conduction.

Physiologically (fig. 11), the high resistance membrane of the neurone behaves as a selectively permeable structure with variable permeability. Potassium ions may pass freely through the membrane but passage to sodium ions is normally obstructed. In the fully-charged (resting or polarized) state, therefore, a high concentration of sodium ions is present on the outside of the membrane, whereas a high concentration of potassium ions will be found internally. Potassium ions will have permeated through into the extracellular fluid until the positive charge that results prevents further egress. On excitation of the neurone, the permeability of the membrane alters. Sodium ions now rush through from the outside to the inside of the neurone, carrying with them their positive electrical charges. In this manner is the negative resting potential of the inside of the cell suddenly abolished and replaced momentarily by the positive potential. The influx of sodium ions is immediately succeeded by an efflux of potassium ions from the inside to the outside of the cell – again restoring a negative intracellular potential. With this re-established, the neurone again may conduct a nervous impulse. The sodium ions and potassium ions are returned respectively to the outside and inside of the neurone by means of the 'sodium-potassium pump'. To do this work, energy is required. The energy for the sodium pump is obtained by the neurone from the breakdown of adenosine triphosphate to adenosine diphosphate and phosphate ($ATP = ADP + P + Energy$) (p. 43). It will be appreciated that the essential energy requirement of the nervous system is one necessitated by the restoration and maintenance of the resting (fully-charged) state of its neurones. The impulse is generated and transmitted without metabolic energy.

Excitation of the resting (polarized) neurone produces the characteristic action potential – initiated by the inrush of sodium ions into the cell. Should a second stimulus now be applied to the cell without intervening delay, no corresponding action potential can be recorded. The second stimulus has fallen at a time of depolarization and a measurable interval of time must elapse before repolarization is achieved. This interval constitutes the absolute refractory period for the neurone and lasts for 0·5 milliseconds. Immediately following this interval occurs the relative refractory period for the neurone, a period during which response may be obtained from the nerve cell but the stimulus required to elicit this must be of greater strength than normal.

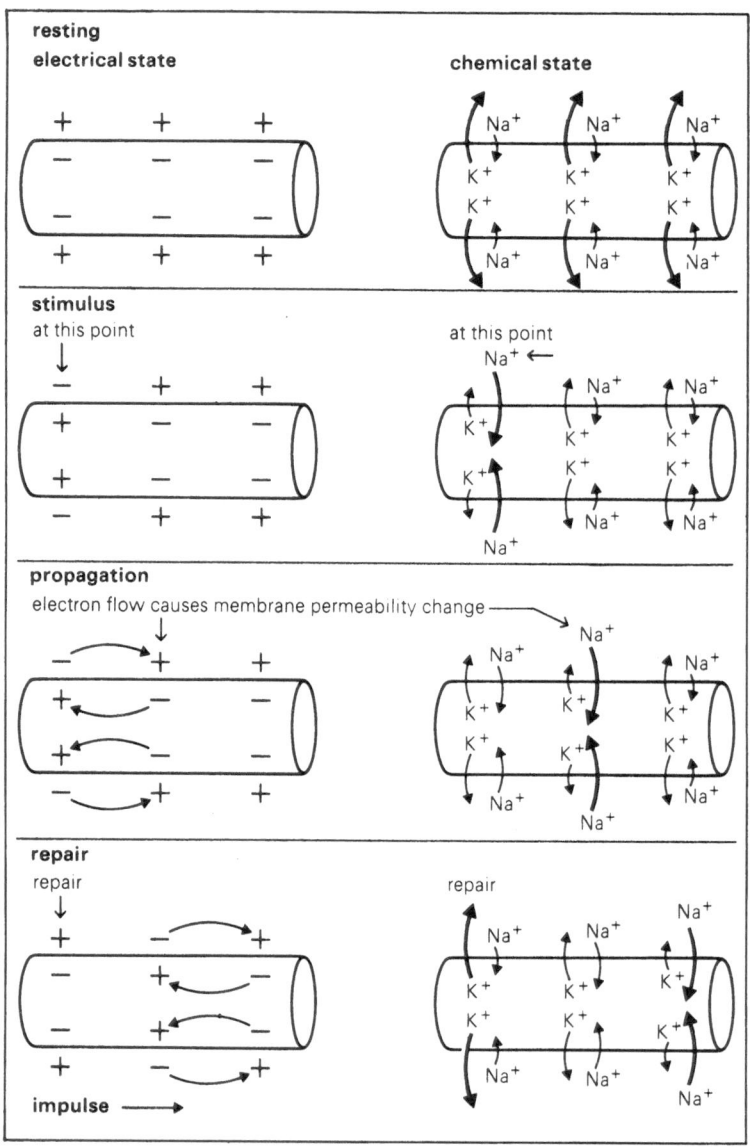

FIGURE 11 Electrical and ion changes in nerve conduction.

TRANSMISSION AT SYNAPSES

The synapse is that physiological junction or contact which exists between two nerve cells. Though such cells lie in the closest proximity to each other, no protoplasmic continuity extends from neurone to neurone and an infinitesimal gap of some 200 Å separates them. This gap is named the synaptic cleft.

Transmission of the nerve impulse from one nerve cell to the other occurs at the synapse and proceeds in one direction only. It passes from the presynaptic fibre, through the important presynaptic membrane found at its ending, across the synaptic cleft and on to the postsynaptic membrane of the second neurone.

On arrival at the termination of the presynaptic fibre of the first neurone, the nerve impulse as such is momentarily extinguished. In its stead a chemical transmitter is released from the presynaptic membrane. Minute synaptic vesicles representing quantitative units of transmitter are extruded, momentarily liberating their contents into the synaptic cleft (fig. 12).

The flow of transmitter into the synaptic cleft initiates ionic changes in the postsynaptic membrane. Excitatory and inhibitory synapses can be recognized. Excitatory synapses in which sodium inflow occurs at the postsynaptic membrane (fig. 13a) produce local depolarization. Inhibitory synapses depend on a further efflux of potassium ions to cause a local hyperpolarization (fig. 13b & c). In addition to the more usual postsynaptic inhibitory synapse (fig. 13b) presynaptic inhibition may be encountered (fig. 13c).

The effect on the receptor neurone is the summation of these potential changes. Once a threshold level of depolarization occurs in the cell, the nerve impulse is reinstigated at the axon hillock (fig. 7, p. 22) and is then propagated throughout the second neurone by the normal ionic migration. This total process of the transfer of the nerve impulse from one neurone to another takes a measurable interval of time. This interval is known as the synaptic delay and occupies just less than a millisecond.

In peripheral ganglia of both sympathetic and parasympathetic divisions of the autonomic nervous system, chemical transmission at the synapses involved has been well studied. The transmitter in question has been shown to be acetylcholine. This substance, moreover, is also liberated from nerve endings of the postganglionic fibres of the parasympathetic and from certain postganglionic fibres of the

33

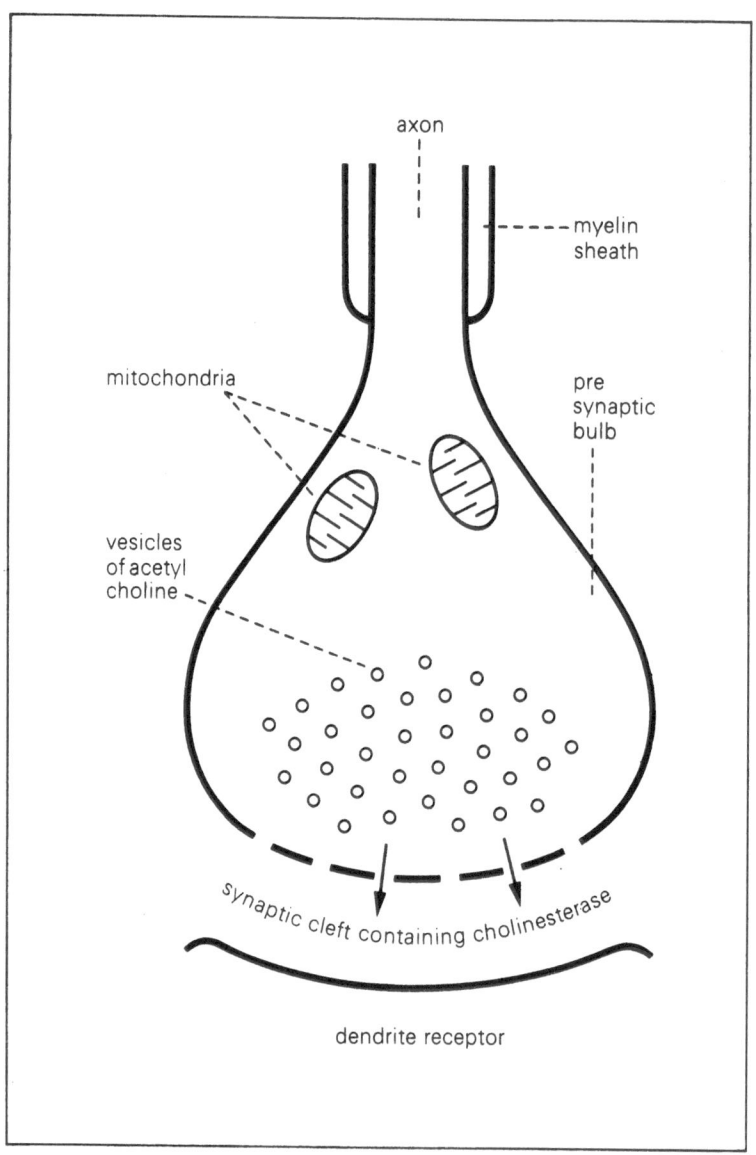

FIGURE 12 Transmission of an impulse through a cholinergic synapse.

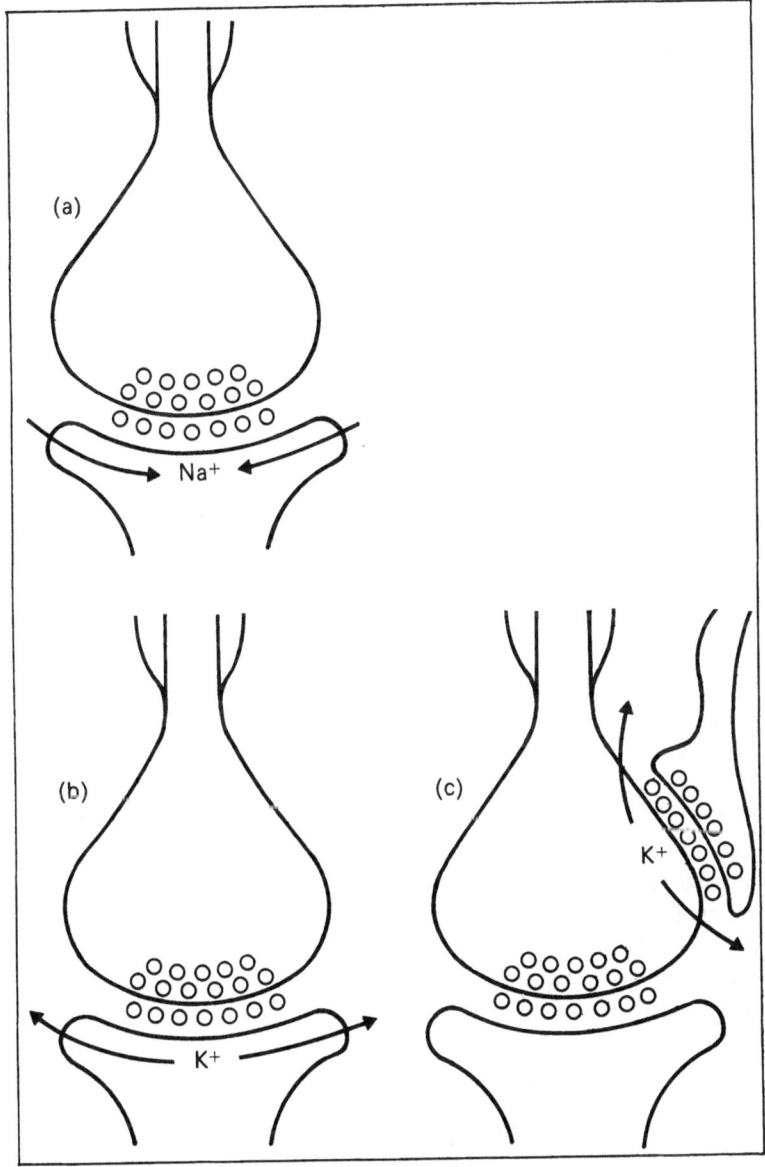

FIGURE 13 Forms of (a) excitatory (b) and (c) inhibitory synapse within the nervous system.

sympathetic, namely those innervating sweat glands and certain skeletal muscle vessels. In other instances, the substance liberated from postganglionic fibres of the sympathetic is noradrenaline. The nature of the chemical transmitter substance at various sites in the peripheral nervous system is shown in fig. 14.

Within the central nervous system the identity of transmitters at synapses is still uncertain. It has been shown – as might perhaps have been expected – that the transmitter released from the recurrent collateral fibre of the anterior horn cell at its synapse with the Renshaw cell within the central nervous system is, in fact, acetylcholine. Acetylcholine, noradrenaline, dopamine, serotonin (5-hydroxytryptamine), glutamine, glycine and GABA (γ-amino butyric acid) have all been postulated as transmitters at various sites throughout the brain and spinal cord. Our knowledge of their functions and sites of action are still incomplete. The metabolism of some of these transmitters is given below.

The myoneural junction, between nerve ending and somatic muscle fibre at the motor end-plate, behaves in many ways similarly to the synapse between neurones. At the myoneural junction, the chemical transmitter has again been shown to be acetylcholine. 'Quanta' of acetylcholine are released by vesicles from the motor nerve endings onto the muscle fibre membrane of the sarcolemma. Here depolarization occurs and, on reaching a critical threshold, an action potential is initiated with accompanying muscular contraction.

At both synapse and myoneural junction, the activity of acetylcholine is rigidly controlled by the enzyme cholinesterase. With extreme rapidity, cholinesterase inactivates the acetylcholine by hydrolysis to choline and acetic acid. The peripheral effect of acetylcholine may be enhanced by neostigmine. This drug, in common with other anticholinesterasees, inhibits the action of cholinesterase and delays therefore the destruction of acetylcholine. In adrenergic nerves (i.e. those with noradrenaline as transmitter) on the other hand, though an inactivating enzyme, catechol O-methyl transferase is present in the synapse, most of the unwanted transmitter is reabsorbed into the presynaptic vesicles (p. 41).

METABOLISM OF THE
CENTRAL NERVOUS SYSTEM SYNAPTIC TRANSMITTERS

Although the mechanism of transmission within the central nervous system is not yet established, certain substances play a significant role

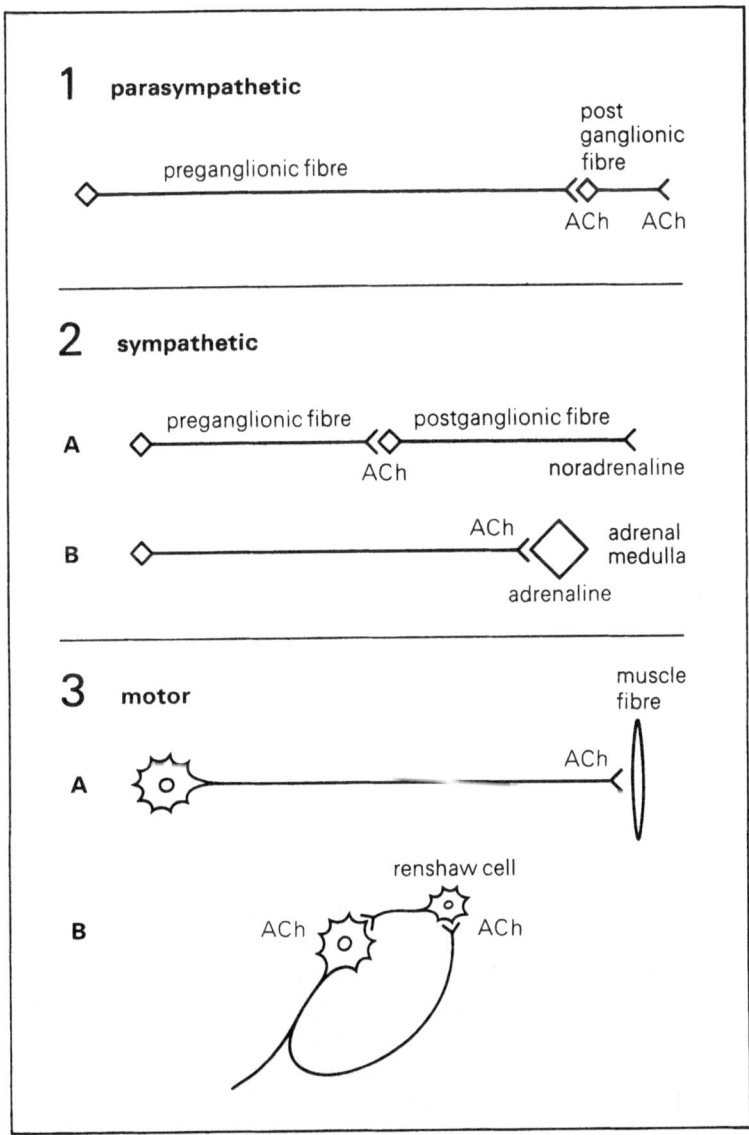

FIGURE 14 Arrangement of peripheral nerve fibres and the chemical transmitters at their synapses and endings.

in central nervous system activity. These include serotonin (5-hydroxy-tryptamine), the catechol amines – noradrenaline and adrenaline – together with the precursor dopamine and gamma-amino-butyric acid.

Serotonin. Serotonin is produced in the body from tryptophan (fig. 15). The process involves a hydroxylation followed by a decarboxy-

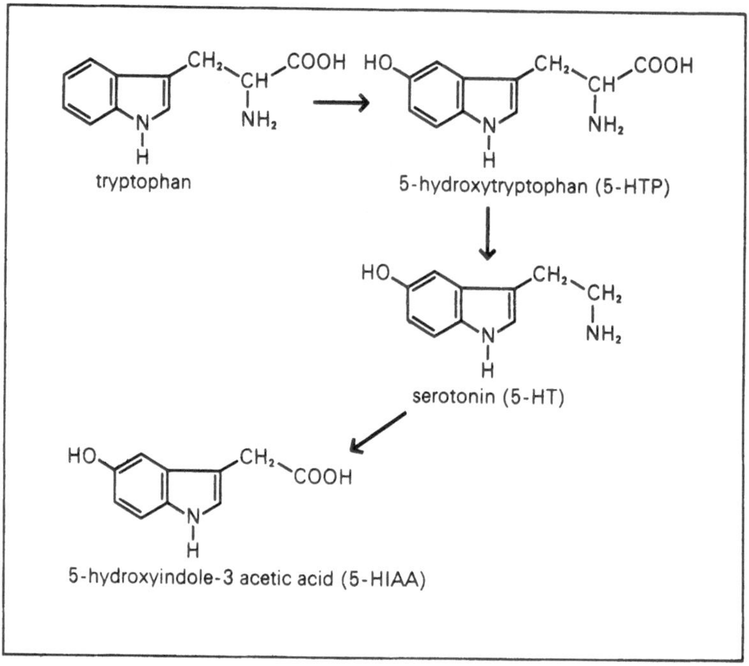

FIGURE 15 Biosynthesis and metabolism of 5-hydroxytryptamine (serotonin).

lation, the latter reaction being pyridoxal phosphate dependent. Serotonin is found not only in the central nervous system but in many body tissues, including the intestine and platelets.

Within the central nervous system, high concentrations are found in the hypothalamus and caudate nucleus with lower concentrations in other grey matter. Negligible amounts of serotonin are found in areas which consist predominantly of myelinated fibres.

The metabolism of serotonin is by an oxidative deamination, yielding as the main end-product 5-hydroxyindole-3 acetic acid (5 HIAA). The enzyme involved in this reaction is monoamine oxidase.

38

The administration of 5-hydroxytryptophan to animals increases the amount of serotonin in various tissues including the brain, particularly when monoamine oxidase inhibitors are given at the same time. Such elevation of serotonin produces behavioural changes similar to those resulting from the administration of lysergic acid diethylamide (LSD); indeed LSD blocks serotonin synapses at some concentrations.

These include autonomic changes and behavioural changes of apparent fear and sham rage. The physiological role of serotonin within the central nervous system is still not certain, but the available evidence suggests that it may be excitatory within the mid-brain area, concerned with sleep and behaviour, and in the hypothalamus regulating pituitary function.

Catechol amines. The three catechol amines are dopamine, noradrenaline, and adrenaline. Of these the catechol amines noradrenaline and adrenaline occur within the effector nerve endings of the sympathetic nervous system and within the adrenal medulla. Their function in these sites is now well understood. They are neuro-transmitters and neuro-hormones which produce the body response to an emergency.

High levels of the catechol amines, predominantly noradrenaline, are found in certain parts of the brain, mainly those of the hypothalamic and hind-brain structures.

Synthesis of the catechol amines occurs from the amino acid phenylalanine by a hydroxylation followed by a pyridoxal 5-phosphate dependent decarboxylation (fig. 16). Metabolism of the catechol amines occurs via methylation (using the enzyme catechol O-methyltransferase) and an oxidative deamination (using monoamine oxidase). The main final metabolite is vanyl mandelic acid (VMA).

The physiological action of noradrenaline within the central nervous system is poorly understood but like serotonin, alterations in noradrenaline produce behavioural changes. In particular, elevation of the total noradrenaline content of the central nervous system produces excitation.

The monoamines are thought to exist in the tissues in a stored and in a free form. The free amines show biological activity and are capable of being metabolized by O-methyltransferase. The stored amines occur in two storage sites within the neurone, the mobile and fixed amine pools. Here as special storage granules, they remain biologically inactive and are protected from metabolism by the granule covering. Part of the storage amines, located close to the nerve endings (mobile

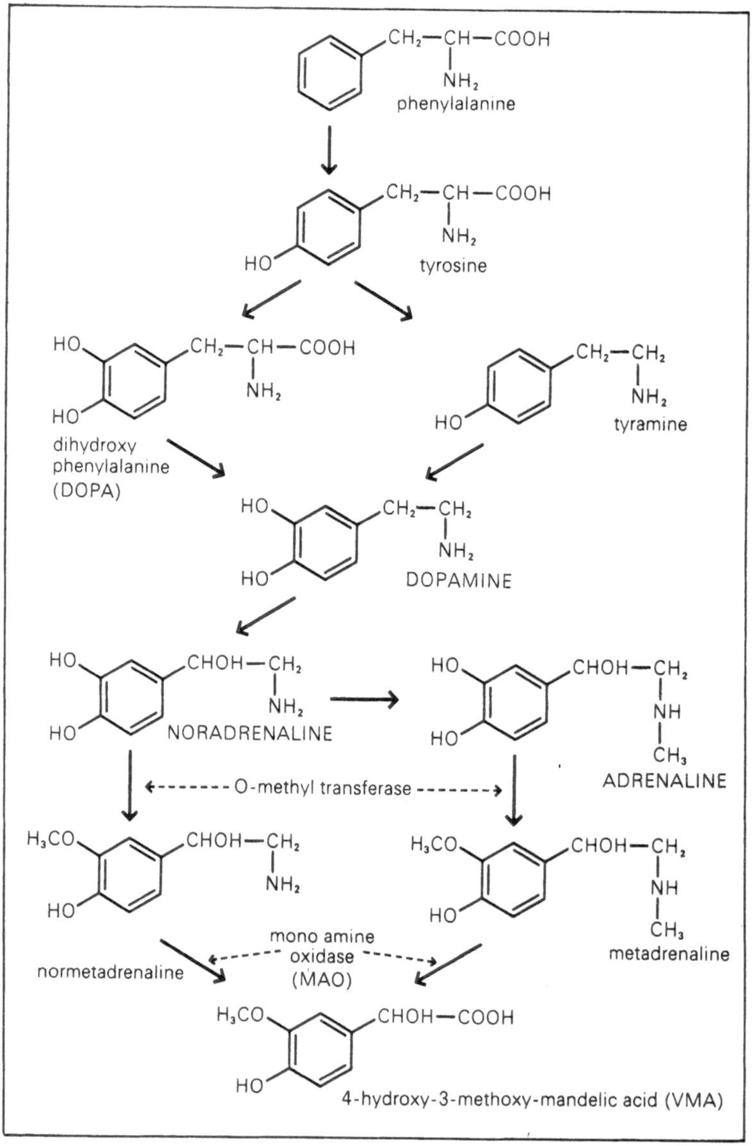

FIGURE 16 Biosynthesis and metabolism of catechol amines (dopamine, noradrenaline and adrenaline).

pool), is released into the synaptic space on nerve stimulation as free amine. There it stimulates the adrenergic receptor and is then inactivated. Some 95 per cent of this inactivation occurs by reabsorption into the granules and only a small fraction is metabolized by O-methyltransferase (fig. 17).

The second monoamine storage pool (fixed) is situated in the vicinity of structures containing monoamine oxidase (i.e. mitochondria). A dynamic equilibrium exists between the two intracellular storage areas (fixed and mobile), but any excess catechol amine released from the fixed storage area into the mobile pool is metabolized by monoamine oxidase before it exerts a physiological effect.

Experimental work in animals, and the results of drug studies in humans suggest, but do not prove, that these amines may be important transmitting substances or potentiators within the diencephalon. In particular they may be responsible for emotional reactions. A certain amount of evidence has been produced to suggest that some of the affective disorders may be directly related to alteration in brain monoamine levels (p. 205). The relationship of the monoamines to drug action is considered on p. 265.

The catechol amine, dopamine is the transmitter in the pathway leading from the substantia nigra to the corpus striatum. Degeneration of this pathway leads to Parkinsonism. Administration of levodopa, the precursor of dopamine produces improvement in some 60 per cent of patients. Dopamine is metabolized by monoamine oxidase and catechol O-methyltransferase. The butyrophenones are specific blockers of dopamine synapses and hence butyrophenones can produce Parkinsonism as a side effect (p. 269).

Gamma-amino-butyric acid. The formation of this amine is described on page 45. It is widely distributed through all parts of the central nervous system in rather similar concentrations. Recent experimental evidence suggests that it is an important synaptic transmitter, probably that released at most inhibitory synapses in the central nervous system.

Reduced levels of gamma-amino-butyric acid due to impaired synthesis is the probable explanation for the convulsions seen in pyridoxine deficiency, particularly those occurring in infancy (p. 48).

Glutamic acid. This amino acid is another brain neurotransmitter. Unlike gamma-amino-butyric acid which is inhibitory, glutamic acid is probably excitatory.

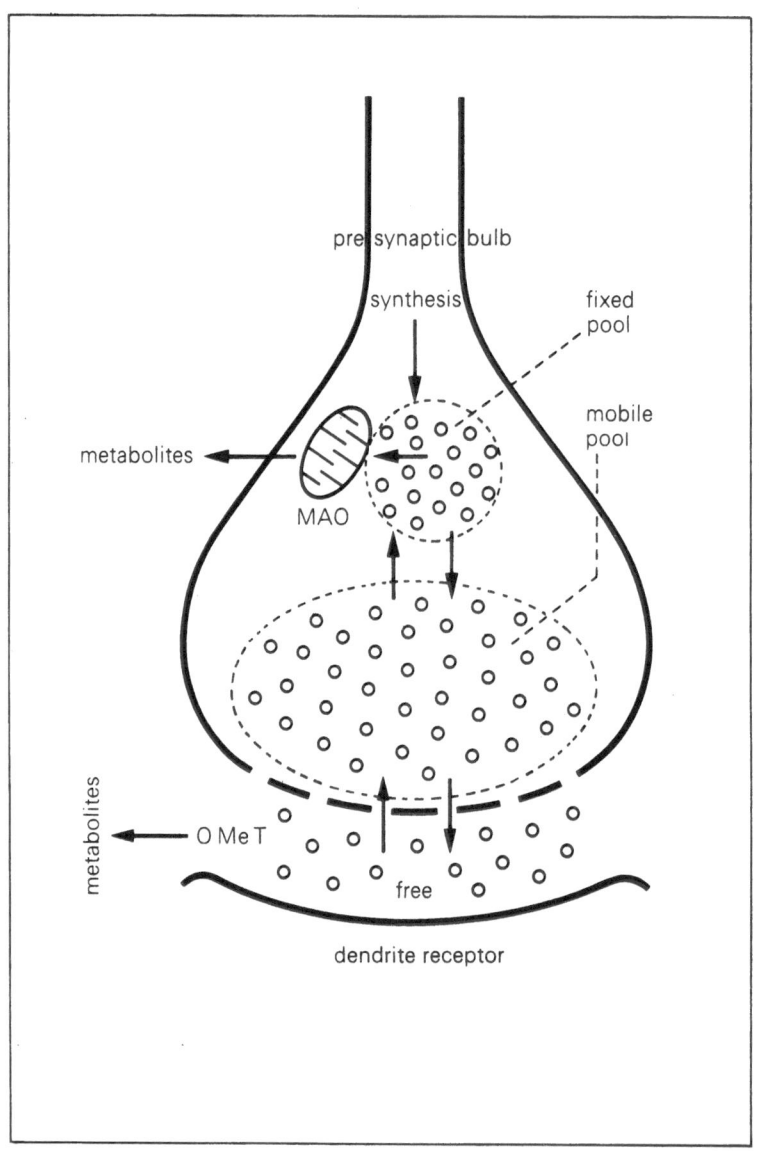

FIGURE 17 Representation of an adrenergic nerve ending. For details of the components see text.

Acetylcholine. Acetylcholine is the chemical transmitter of the parasympathetic system, of sympathetic ganglia, of sympathetic postganglionic cholinergic fibres (e.g. sweat glands and muscle blood vessels) and the neuro-muscular junction. It is the transmitter of Renshaw cells and is widely distributed in the brain. It is probably a transmitter in the cerebral cortex and in the reticular system. Imbalance of dopaminergic and cholinergic pathways may be important in Parkinsonism.

THE SUPPLY OF ENERGY

Conduction of impulses along neurones depends on ionic interchanges at the cell membrane which has a variable permeability (p. 30). Synaptic conduction occurs by chemical transmitters, either facilitatory or inhibitory (p. 33).

This nervous system communication takes place without energy expenditure. Energy is necessary for the maintenance of the membrane interface, for the 'sodium-potassium pump' mechanism (p. 31) and for the production of the chemical transmitters.

The respiratory quotient of nervous tissue is 1·0. Thus the main energy source must be carbohydrate. Glycogen stores within the central nervous system are minimal and energy is derived from the metabolism of blood-borne glucose. Energy production from glucose is only efficient under aerobic conditions. An adequate and uniform blood supply (p. 24) is therefore important for the supply of both glucose and oxygen. A reduction in glucose or oxygen produces successive depletion of central nervous system activity from cortex to lower medulla. Recovery takes place in the reverse order.

Energy formed during glucose catabolism is converted by oxidative phosphorylation into adenosine triphosphate (ATP). The energy can subsequently be released for use by breaking the high energy bond phosphate of ATP to reform adenosine diphosphate.

The metabolism of glucose takes place in two stages. In the first – a reaction known as glycolysis – the glucose is converted into two molecules of pyruvic acid (fig. 18). At one stage in this process, hydrogen is released and taken up by nicotinamide adenine dinucleotide (NAD) to form NADH. In the absence of oxygen NAD cannot be reformed and the two molecules of pyruvic acid are converted to lactic acid by the NADH.

43

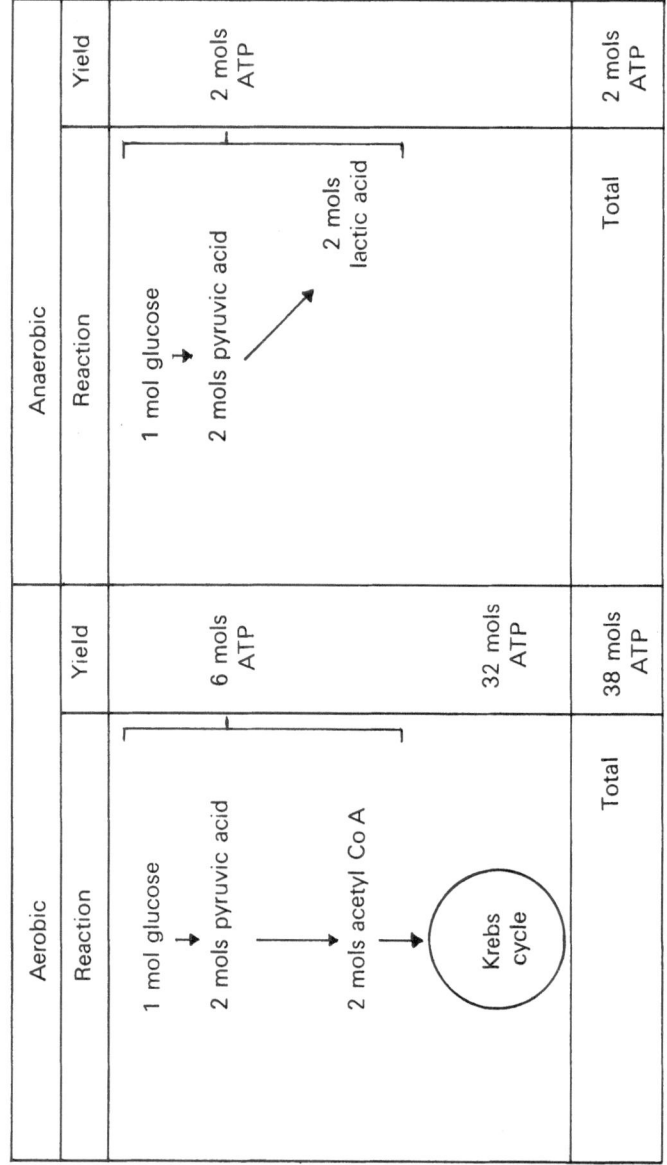

FIGURE 18 Aerobic and anaerobic metabolism of glucose.

Anaerobic glycolysis leads to a net synthesis of two molecules of ATP, but the net yield from aerobic glycolysis of one molecule of glucose is eight molecules of ATP (the 'oxidation' of each NADH molecule yields three molecules of ATP).

Under anaerobic conditions lactic acid cannot be metabolized further and the energy yield is low (two molecules of ATP per molecule glucose utilized). In the presence of oxygen, however, pyruvic acid can be further broken down to form carbon dioxide and water in the Krebs citric acid cycle (fig. 19). It enters the cycle via 'active acetate' which condenses with oxaloacetic to yield citric acid. This is then degraded through a series of decarboxylations and oxidations to reyield oxaloacetic acid. The oxidations which occur at reactions 4, 6 and 9 of the Krebs citric acid cycle occur by hydrogen acceptance by NAD: that at reaction 7 occurs by hydrogen acceptance by a flavoprotein coenzyme (FAD).

NADH and FADH are reoxidized through the respiratory enzyme chain (electron transport chain). The enzyme prosthetic groups are alternately reduced and oxidized as the hydrogen atoms or, more strictly, electrons are transmitted through the chain (fig. 20). The terminal step involves the combination with molecular oxygen to yield water. Some reactions in this chain are energy producing and this energy is utilized for the conversion of ADP to ATP. Oxidation of NADH yields three molecules of ATP while that of FADH yields only two ATP. A total of 15 molecules ATP is produced for each pyruvic acid molecule metabolized. Hence the overall energy production in the further oxidation of the two molecules of pyruvic acid derived from the glucose is 30 molecules ATP. With the eight molecules ATP during oxidative glycolysis, there is a total yield of 38 molecules ATP by the oxidative breakdown of one molecule of glucose (fig. 18). This can be compared with the two molecules of ATP derived during anaerobic breakdown of glucose. Thus oxidative metabolism is far more efficient for energy production.

Amino acid metabolism

Glutamic acid is the only amino acid metabolized by brain tissue in any quantity, although other amino acids related to the catecholamines (p. 39) are decarboxylated within brain tissue.

Glutamic acid serves as a precursor of γ-amino-butyric acid (p. 41).

45

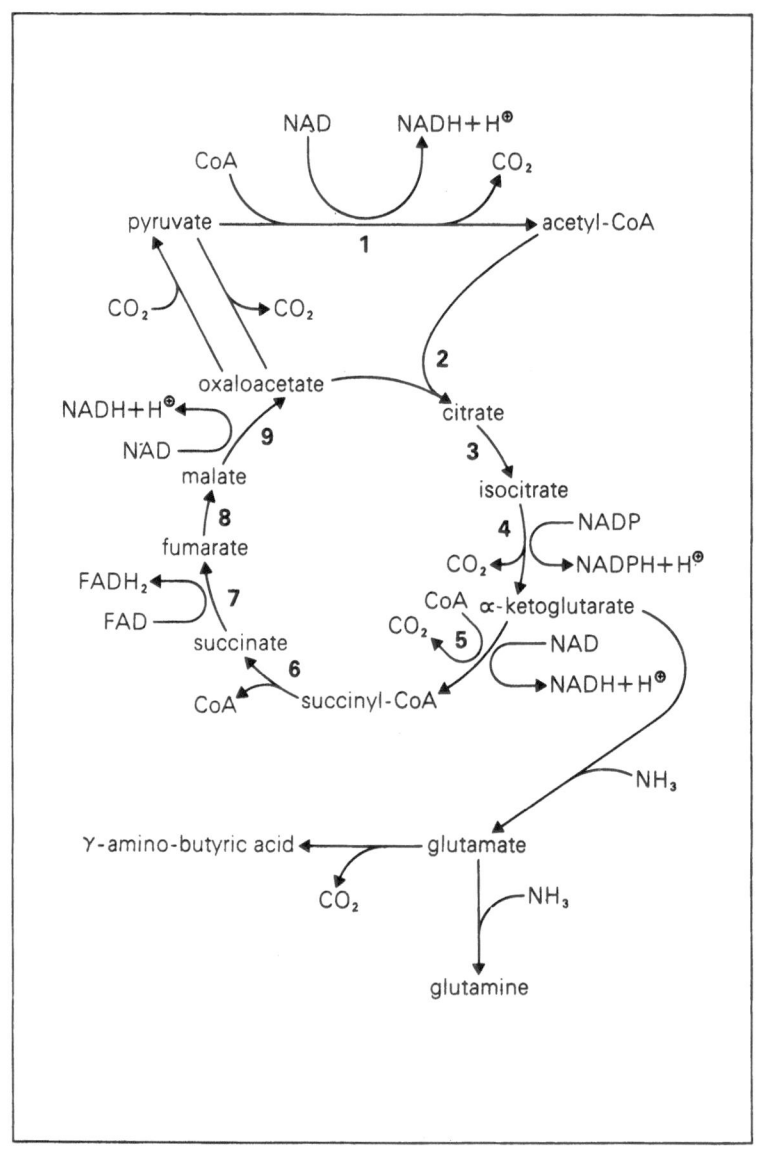

FIGURE 19 The Krebs citric acid cycle.

It is also an acceptor of ammonia in the blood. Glutamic acid may itself be utilized for this reaction, but the principal source is probably a precursor, ketoglutaric acid, derived from the Krebs citric acid cycle (fig. 19). Amination of ketoglutaric acid occurs within the brain. Each molecule of ketoglutaric acid reacts with two molecules during its

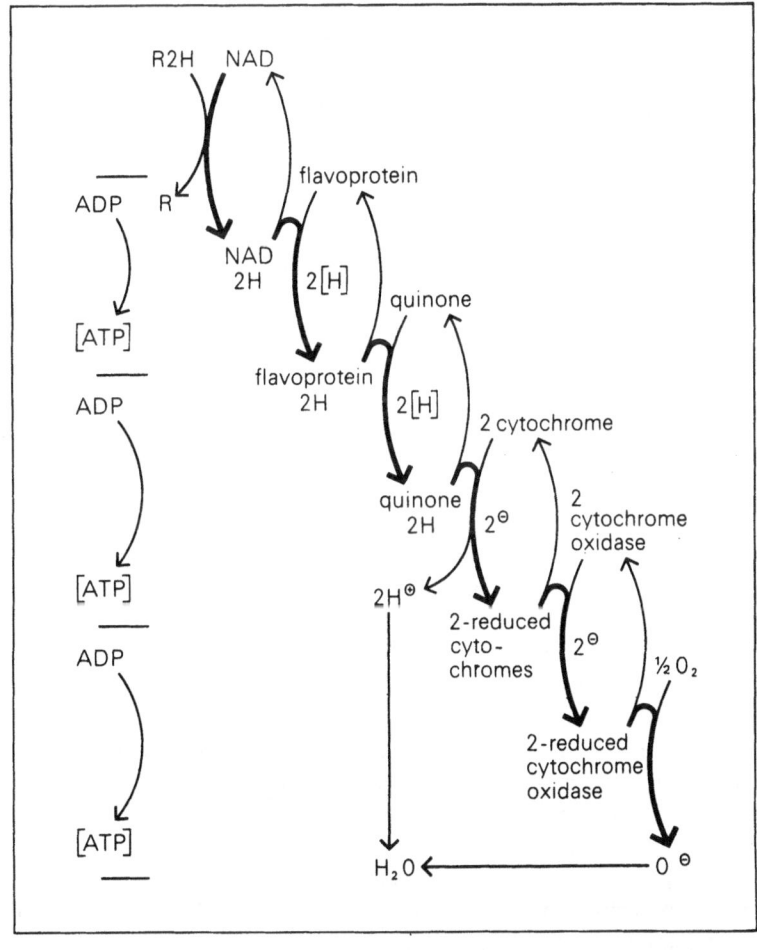

FIGURE 20 The respiratory enzyme chain (electron transport chain) showing stages of energy production.

complete amination to glutamine. Ketoglutaric acid can be formed by a carbon dioxide fixation involving pyruvate through malic acid to oxaloacetic acid (fig. 19) and hence to ketoglutaric acid. This reaction occurs in the brain as it does also in the liver.

Fatty acid metabolism

Enzyme preparations from animal brain are capable of the synthesis of long chain fatty acids and these reactions may also take place within the intact brain. This synthesis is necessary for the formation of the cerebrosides and the sphingomyelins of the nerve cell sheaths.

THE VITAMINS AND BRAIN METABOLISM

Many of the vitamins, and particularly those of the B-complex, form the prosthetic group of coenzymes. As such they are an essential component for normal cell metabolism, including the metabolism of the brain cells. It is therefore not surprising that vitamin deficiencies, particularly acute deficiencies, commonly manifest themselves by nervous system defects.

Thiamine (vitamin B_1 or aneurin), as the pyrophosphate, is an important co-factor in carbohydrate metabolism particularly on the alternative glycolysis pathway.

An acute thiamine deficiency leads to Wernicke's encephalopathy (cerebral beri-beri). In mild cases, nystagmus and mental confusion may be the only presenting signs. Some of the mental confusion in old age may be due to a mild thiamine deficiency.

Chronic thiamine deficiency (beri-beri) produces a peripheral neuritis, frequently irreversible, affecting first the sensory nerves and only later the motor nerves.

Thiamine deficiency is best confirmed by finding a raised blood pyruvate level or reduced transketolase activity.

Pyridoxine is a co-factor for transamination and decarboxylation of amino acids, and hence for the production of catechol amines (p. 39). Dietary pyridoxine deficiency in adults is rare, but interference with pyridoxine activity occurs with certain drugs (including isoniazid and penicillamine) producing a peripheral neuritis.

In infants with a genetic impairment of the pyridoxine binding site on the apoenzyme ('dependancy' state) convulsions may occur.

Pyridoxine deficiency is confirmed by a high urinary xanthurenic acid after a test dose of tryptophan.

Nicotinic acid and its derived amide, as nicotinamide adenine dinucleotide (NAD) and nicotinamide adenine dinucleotide phosphate (NADP), are essential hydrogen carrying co-enzymes for glucose metabolism (fig. 19).

One manifestation of nicotinic acid deficiency (pellagra) is a progressive dementia initially resembling a psychoneurosis which progresses to a Wernicke's syndrome and peripheral neuritis.

Pantothenic acid forms part of co-enzyme A which 'carries' acyl groups (e.g. 'acetate') within the body. It is therefore concerned with the acceptance of two carbon fragments into the citric acid cycle (fig. 19), the formation of acetyl choline and in certain drug detoxification reactions. Natural deficiency is rare but in some war prisoners a form of peripheral neuritis, the 'burning feet' syndrome, has been described.

Vitamin B_{12} (cobalamin) and folic acid are interrelated and concerned with the formation of nucleic acids. Vitamin B_{12} deficiency produces subacute combined degeneration of the cord due to demyelination of the posterior and lateral columns (fig. 21) with resulting sensory and motor loss. Some patients also show a mild dementia with impaired memory or a more advanced confusional psychosis.

Administration of folic acid to a patient who is deficient in vitamin B_{12} can precipitate a very severe subacute combined degeneration of the cord.

THE REFLEX

The reflex is the physiological unit of nervous activity and is manifest at all levels of the central nervous system.

The essentials of a spinal reflex, in its simplest or monosynaptic form, are in sequence, a sensory receptor, its afferent neurone, an efferent neurone and the effector organ. On appropriate stimulation of the receptor, a nerve impulse is sent the length of this restricted pathway (reflex arc) and an automatic response is elicited from the effector organ. Interruption of the pathway at any point will abolish the reflex response from the effector organ.

The interposition of additional neurones (intercalated neurones) between the afferent and efferent neurones of the reflex arc increases the number of synapses involved and, in so doing, makes possible

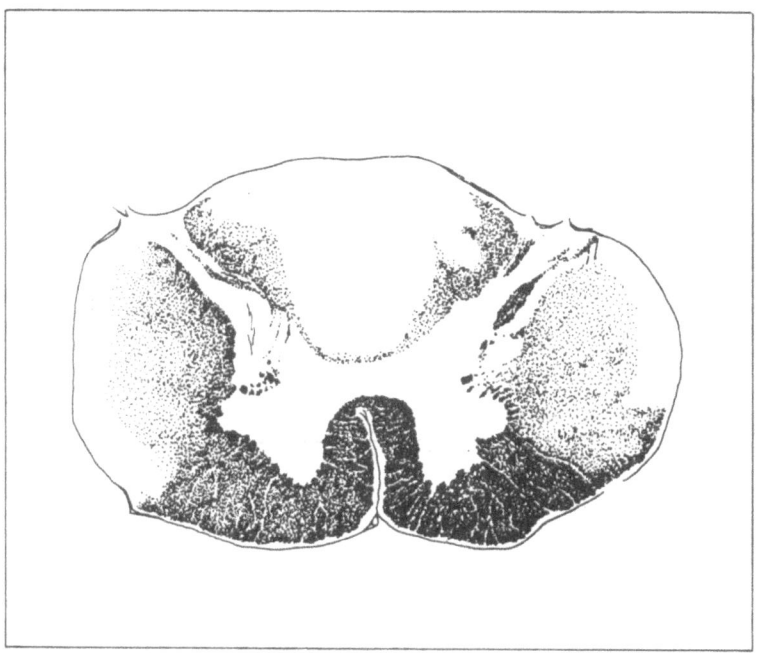

FIGURE 21 Subacute combined degeneration of the cord in cyanocobalamin deficiency (Weigert-Pal stain). Note degeneration of posterior and lateral columns (unstained).

that enormous complexity of reflex action of which the nervous system is capable. The individual neurones may be either excitatory or inhibitory in type and thus the synapses may liberate either excitatory or inhibitory transmitters (p. 33). The response of the next neurone depends upon the summation of the excitatory and inhibitory stimuli applied to its surface.

A localized stimulus can thus make widespread and complex activity by effector organs throughout the whole body. Reflex activity may be conscious, partly conscious or wholly unconscious. Many reflex responses may, furthermore, be modified by conscious control. Spinal reflexes are modified by higher centres in the brain, including those of the cerebral cortex and reticular formation (p. 87). Cord lesions which release the spinal reflexes from higher control produce various signs depending upon the pathways which are damaged.

Neurologically, reflexes may be conveniently classified:
(1) Superficial (e.g. upper and lower abdominal reflexes).
(2) Deep (e.g. knee jerk).
(3) Visceral (e.g. micturition).
Psychologically, the conditioned reflex is of profound importance in considerations both of learning and of behaviour. The conditioned reflex and its mode of production are considered in more detail on p. 115.

REVERBERATING CIRCUITS

Within the spinal cord, the reflex arc is the prime physiological unit for nerve activity. At higher levels of the brain, existing data suggest that the important functional units are modified reflex arcs termed 'reverberating circuits'. A nerve cell discharges through a number of synapses on to other nerve cells, each of which connects in turn with many more. At every synapse a balance is struck between facilitatory and inhibitory impulses. Circuits are completed by neurones which synapse back upon the original nerve cell. During its complicated passage the nerve impulse may be reduced by inhibition or potentiated by a process of spatial or temporal summation of facilitatory impulses (fig. 22). Other reverberating circuits can, moreover, be established via collateral pathways involving interrelated brain areas. Learning, memory and behaviour patterns may well be regarded as modifications of the patterns of reverberating circuits.

SLEEP

Sleep is a natural, recurrent and rhythmical loss of consciousness, concomitant with which is a greatly reduced mobility. Under normal circumstances sleep regularly follows periods of wakefulness and wakefulness, in its turn, follows upon a period of sleep.

Everyday life and psychological wellbeing demand this characteristic alternating pattern but the proportion of each twenty-four hours spent in either phase differs from one person to another. For adults the average period of sleep is from five to eight hours but in infants the proportion of the day spent asleep is considerably greater. A balance between the arousal reaction and rest reaction (p. 53) is responsible for the sleep-wake rhythm. It constitutes a regular cycle in which periods of wakefulness alternate with periods of sleep and this rhythm may be considered as a sleep-wake balance. During sleep, parasympathetic activity predominates; during wakefulness, sympathetic activity

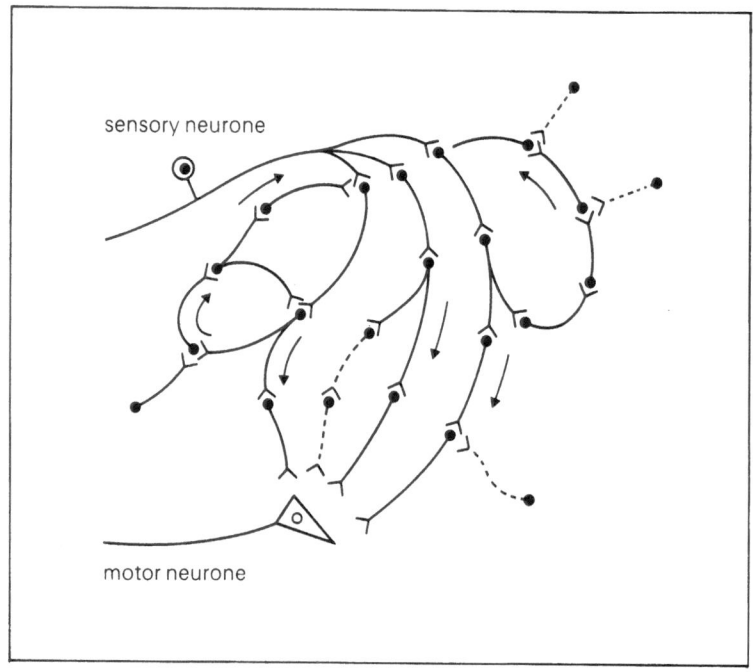

FIGURE 22 Polysynaptic paths in the nervous system illustrating reverberating circuits with positive reinforcement (on left), inhibition (dotted, on right) from other neurones, and inhibitory collaterals (dotted at centre). The motor neurone final situation is a balance of all the influences on it.

is greatest. Between these two extremes the mechanism of balance allows a variety of levels of alertness and consciousness dependent upon the requirements of the surroundings. Wakefulness results from a broad arousal outflow to all parts of the cerebral cortex from the 'wake' portion of the reticular formation, this portion also being termed the reticular activating system (fig. 39, p. 85).

In animal experiments, section or stimulation at various levels of the mid-brain recticular formation modifies the normal sleep pattern. The sleep-wake balance is maintained by two reciprocal inhibitory systems within the reticular formation. Each system has an inherent activity which is affected by various sensory impulses (Table 2). These impulses influence the balance and produce greater wakefulness or greater drowsiness. They may exert their influence directly or may form part of a conditioned reflex – hence, the problem of sleeping in a

TABLE 2

Sleep	Wake
Peripheral receptors	
Warmth	Visual stimuli
Minimum of external alerting stimuli	Pain
Higher centres	
Monotonous stimuli	Basic physiological drives
Conditioned reflex stimuli	Emotional circuit activity
Volitional desire	Volitional desire

strange bed. Natural sleep occurs when the outflow of these factors which stimulate the sleep system is increased sufficiently to inhibit the wake system. The period of sleep is not of uniform quality but shows considerable variation (stages) in depth. These are now designated by a numerical scale which ranges from I to IV, together with an additional stage referred to as 'paradoxical' or REM sleep. Each of these stages has its characteristic electroencephalographic wave pattern (p. 59).

The pattern of a normal night's sleep is provided by a reasonably rapid descent via Stages I to III to Stage IV. Stage I is characterized by drowsiness. Stage II represents early light sleep and electroencephalographically sleep spindles are seen together with K complexes in response to meaningful stimuli (p. 59). Stage III represents a deeper phase of sleep which then merges with Stage IV the deepest sleep of all. On reaching Stage IV, this phase of deep sleep is maintained for approximately 90 minutes. At the end of this time lightening of sleep occurs back through the preceding stages to Stage I. At this point (Emergent Stage I), rapid eye movements occur in conjugate deviation (REM). This phase is thus known as REM sleep – or by the synonyms paradoxical sleep, desynchronized sleep or dreaming sleep. The phases of REM sleep (lasting some 20–30 minutes) lengthen progressively in their duration as the night proceeds. The phase of REM sleep is succeeded by descent again to Stage III or IV sleep. Such sleep, during which the characteristic oscillations of the eyes are absent, is in contrast termed non-rapid eye movement (NREM) sleep, or by the synonyms orthodox sleep or slow wave sleep.

The pattern of descent and ascent through the stages of sleep continues throughout the night and some four periods of REM sleep will be interspersed with the periods of NREM sleep. In general terms towards the end of the night, the REM periods get longer and the depth of sleep gets less. Between the third and last period of REM it may well be that the depth does not go below Stage II and rarely, if ever, does it reach Stage IV (fig. 23). REM sleep or paradoxical sleep is a phase in which it seems that cortical activity becomes very much more intense. Paradoxically, however, the subject is very much more difficult to waken.

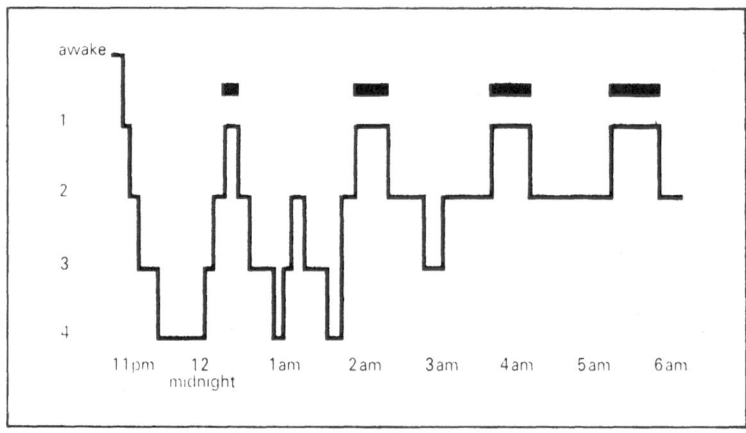

FIGURE 23 The stages of sleep during a normal night's sleep ▬ REM sleep.

The most dramatic feature of paradoxical sleep is provided by the rapid eye movements. These coincide with EEG cortical activity marking the commencement of Emergent Stage I sleep. The eye movements occur in short bursts and are quite distinct from eye movements which occur in the waking state. As many as fifty movements from side to side may occur in one burst of REM. Current studies point clearly to the pons as the centre responsible for paradoxical sleep. The normal pattern of paradoxical sleep or REM sleep in the human adult is cyclical and makes up 20–25 per cent of sleep during the night. In infants, however, 50–60 per cent of the sleeping time is occupied by REM sleep. It has been suggested that REM sleep is associated with protein synthesis in the brain and with brain regeneration. Hence the proportion of REM sleep is increased in neonates, after head injury or drug overdose, and is decreased in subnormality and old age. Suppression of REM sleep by certain drugs may induce a phenomenon of 'REM rebound'.

During the deeper stages of NREM (orthodox) sleep, the secretion of growth hormone by the anterior pituitary gland appears at its greatest. Governing not only the growing period of youth and adolescence, this hormone encourages growth in skin, liver and the blood-forming cells of the bone marrow as well as exerting an effect on carbohydrate and fat metabolism.

Fig. 24 shows the activity of different parts of the brain during paradoxical sleep and compares these with the situation during wake and slow wave sleep. The electro-oculograph (EOG) recording clearly shows the rapid eye movements which are an essential part of paradoxical sleep.

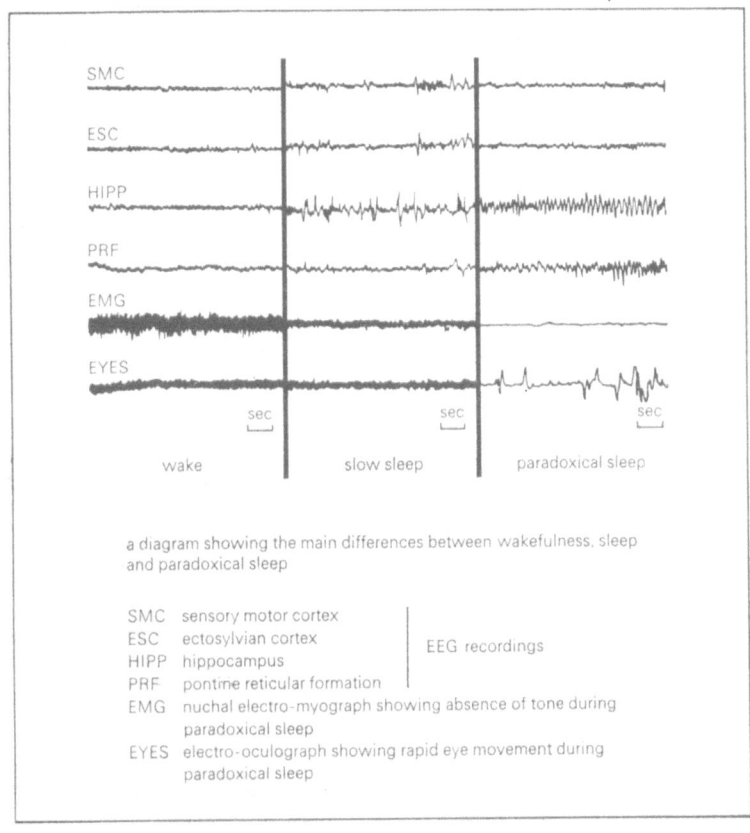

FIGURE 24 A comparison of various recordings made during different phases of wake-sleep. The similarity of the cortical recordings in wakefulness and REM sleep is striking.

ELECTROENCEPHALOGRAPHY

The electroencephalograph detects at the surface of the scalp those minute electrical changes which accompany activity by the underlying brain cells.

If a single cortical neurone discharges electrically, it is of course quite impossible to pick up the change in potential through the dura mater, skull, subcutaneous fat and scalp. However, when a group of cortical cells becomes active a change in potential is produced which can be recorded as a signal passing between two electrodes. Basically, therefore, the EEG gives us a picture of changes in electrical potential of groups of cells in relation to other cells recorded by a series of electrodes placed on the scalp. Leads from these are taken via an amplifier to a recording machine and the signal is written out by a series of pens on moving paper. The connections between the electrodes can be varied by a series of switches on the recording apparatus.

A standard arrangement of electrodes has become widely adopted. This system is known as the Ten-Twenty System (fig. 25), and con-

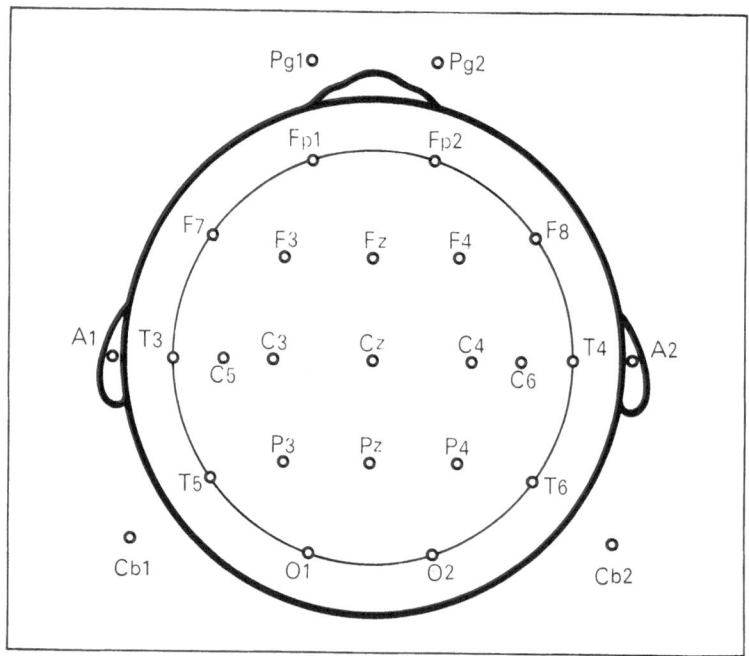

FIGURE 25 The Ten-Twenty system of electrodes.

nections can be made between one electrode and another, so that any part of the head can be monitored by using the system.

Normally about 20 electrodes are placed on the scalp and these are kept in place by a rubber cap.

A diagrammatic representation of the basis of electroencephalography is shown on fig. 26. This diagram shows the type of recording we might expect from an imagined discharge in the central region of the brain. Five electrodes are used and the tracing shows how an instantaneous discharge of this sort is recorded and how, by the direction of the wave on the tracing, the origin of the discharge can to some extent be localized.

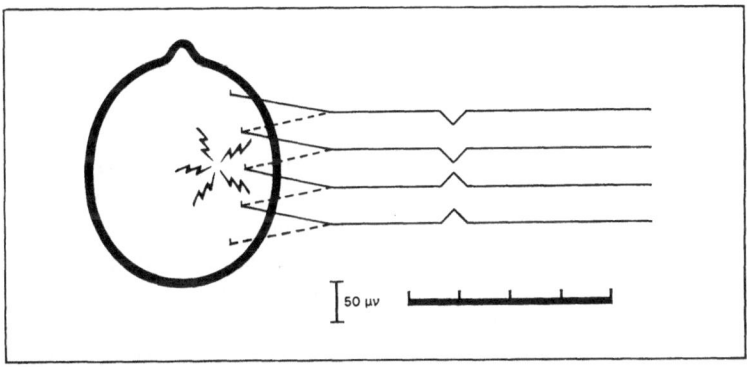

FIGURE 26 A diagrammatic representation of what happens when an electrical disturbance occurs in a group of cortical cells.

Any EEG recording will have this typical picture showing the electrodes which are in use and how they are connected. It will be seen that two lines join to form one line in the actual tracing. This diagram of the scalp, showing the placing of the electrodes, is known in EEG jargon as 'the montage'. The tracing also shows the time-scale in seconds and a scale of voltage, which is usually designated as 50 microvolts.

When the electroencephalogram is used on normal individuals they are usually lying in a quiet room and the recording is done while the patient has his eyes shut. This cuts out from the tracing any extraneous muscular activity.

The electroencephalogram has been used to study and record normal activity of the brain at rest and various standard patterns have been derived from study of the normal. Study of wave patterns has also been carried out in sleep and drowsiness and the sleeping individual shows a pattern of waves as the depth of his sleep fluctuates. Interpretation of the EEG involves considerations of frequency, amplitude, form and distribution of the waves obtained.

With the patient at rest with the eyes closed a characteristic wave pattern becomes evident on the electroencephalogram. This is a stage of drowsiness and the wave pattern is known as alpha rhythm, which can easily be recognized in an EEG tracing. Waves occur in alpha rhythm with a frequency of about 10 cycles per second and have a voltage of between 30 and 50 microvolts. Alpha rhythm is most prominent over the posterior part of the skull. Either opening the eyes or the onset of sleep will block alpha rhythm.

A rhythm of less than 4 cycles per second, delta rhythm, can be obtained during sleep, general anaesthesia, stupor or coma. Focal delta rhythm may indicate a cerebral tumour which lies superficially or an acute cerebral abscess. Theta rhythm, 4–7 cycles per second, obtained typically from the temporal region, is liable to be found in the recordings of immature personalities, aggressive psychopaths and in unstable neurotics. Theta rhythm may originate from deep cerebral tumours or from organic disease of the diencephalon.

Beta rhythm, 14–30 cycles per second, is one form of fast activity. It can be seen when the cortex is alerted and is a usual recording with normal mental activity.

Asymmetries of rhythm from the two cerebral hemispheres may arise from suppression or an increase in normal activity by one side of the brain.

Provocative techniques for the purpose of activating latent dysrhythmias include overbreathing, photopic stimulation and the use of drugs such as metrazol. Special electrodes – nasopharyngeal, sphenoidal and tympanic – may record from and reveal otherwise inaccessible foci. The technique of echoencephalography is employed to detect lateral displacement of mid-line structures in the anterior half of the cranium.

The complex condition of epilepsy embraces many dysrhythmic patterns, which vary enormously in their EEG appearance. Such dysrhythmias include high potential fast frequency discharges; high potential focal spikes (Jacksonian fit); spikes and focal slow waves

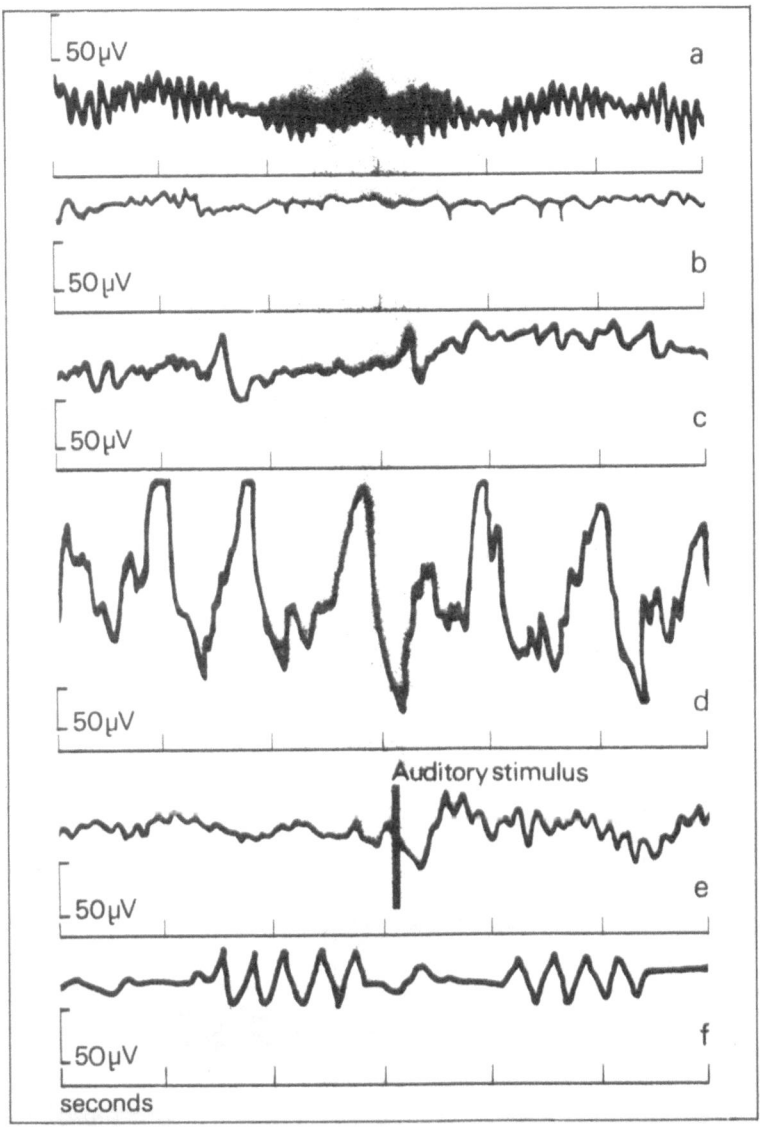

FIGURE 27 Typical electroencephalograms showing (*a*) Alpha rhythm, (*b*) Beta activity, (*c*) Theta rhythm, (*d*) Delta rhythm, (*e*) K complex, (*f*) Sleep spindles.

obtained from the temporal or frontal areas in psychomotor attacks; the classic bilateral wave and spike activity (3 cycles per second) of the centrencephalic minor attack, such as petit mal or pyknolepsy. The dramatic pattern of hypsarrhythmia, with its high potential activity, may be revealed by epileptic infants and young children.

Sleep provides many changing patterns of cortical rhythm including dysrhythmias unobtained during working hours. The changes are usually grouped into four stages of sleep (I to IV see p. 53) together with REM sleep. Stage I involves an absolute lack of spindle activity, Stage II is characterized by the appearance of sleep spindles against a low voltage background and K-complexes are seen in response to stimuli (fig. 27). Stage III has a pattern which involves high voltage slow waves, together with some spindling. In general, there are less than two wave patterns of more than 100 microvolts, having a periodicity of 1–2 cycles per second or slower occurring in every 10 seconds.

Stage IV involves an increase in delta waves, that is to say at least half or more of the record is dominated by waves greater than 100 microvolts in the 1–2 cycle per second range or slower.

REM sleep shows low voltage waves like Stage 1 but with rapid eye movements added. The main features of each stage of sleep are summarized in fig. 28.

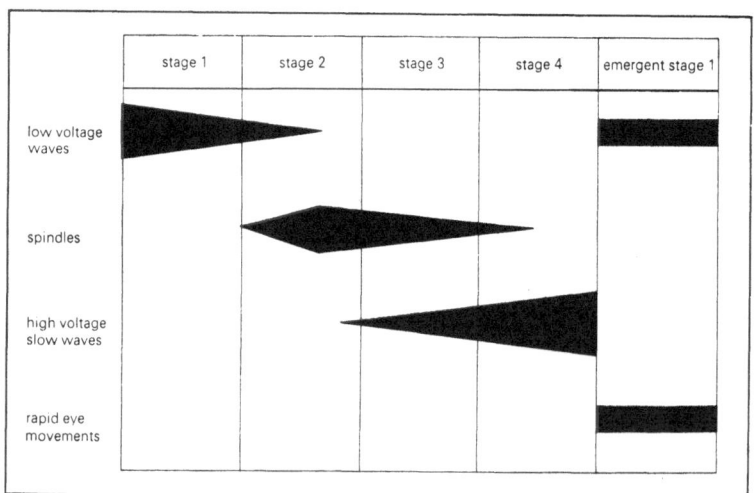

FIGURE 28 The EEG features which may be expected in each stage of sleep.

For diagnostic purposes, the greatest value of the EEG lies in the assistance it provides in problems of idiopathic epilepsy and in the detection of organic brain disease. It will be borne in mind that normal EEG recordings can still be obtained in the presence of advanced organic disease of the brain and, furthermore, that some 15 per cent of healthy persons may show abnormality in their EEG recordings. Typical tracings in grand mal, petit mal and psychomotor (temporal lobe) types of epilepsy are shown in fig. 29.

The EEG, therefore, is but an approximate generalization for areas of cerebral activity. Provided its limitations are appreciated and its recordings are interpreted with caution, intelligence and experience, it remains nonetheless a most valuable asset to the investigation of cerebral function.

DREAMS

The dream is a memory of perception experienced during sleep. As far as can be ascertained, we all dream for some 20–25 per cent of the sleeping time each night. But our realization of this, and therefore our admittance to dreaming, is of course entirely dependent on this factor of memory. Dreaming occurs with the lighter levels of sleep and is associated with the rapid eye movements (REM) of paradoxical sleep (p. 53). Dreaming is predominantly a visual phenomenon and may be in colour. The dream can result from any of many peripheral nervous stimuli – from external noise to the internal assimilation of toasted cheese – and in this manner may be considered as a particular illusion (p. 167). In the absence of such peripheral stimuli, the genesis of the dream lies in central activity of the nervous system and then has about it the more special features of an hallucination (p. 170).

Complex emotions and prevailing moods play significant parts in the formulation of the dream. Sexual emotions frequently determine and influence its contents. The depressive mood of the day is often carried into the morbid grief-ridden dreams of the night. The anxiety dream, often recurrent in nature, is a common experience and may shade imperceptibly into the nightmare – an anxiety state within the confines of sleep itself. The 'night terrors' of children (pavor nocturnus) represent acute states of fear during sleep. Marked dissociation of consciousness accompanies them, and on awakening the child has

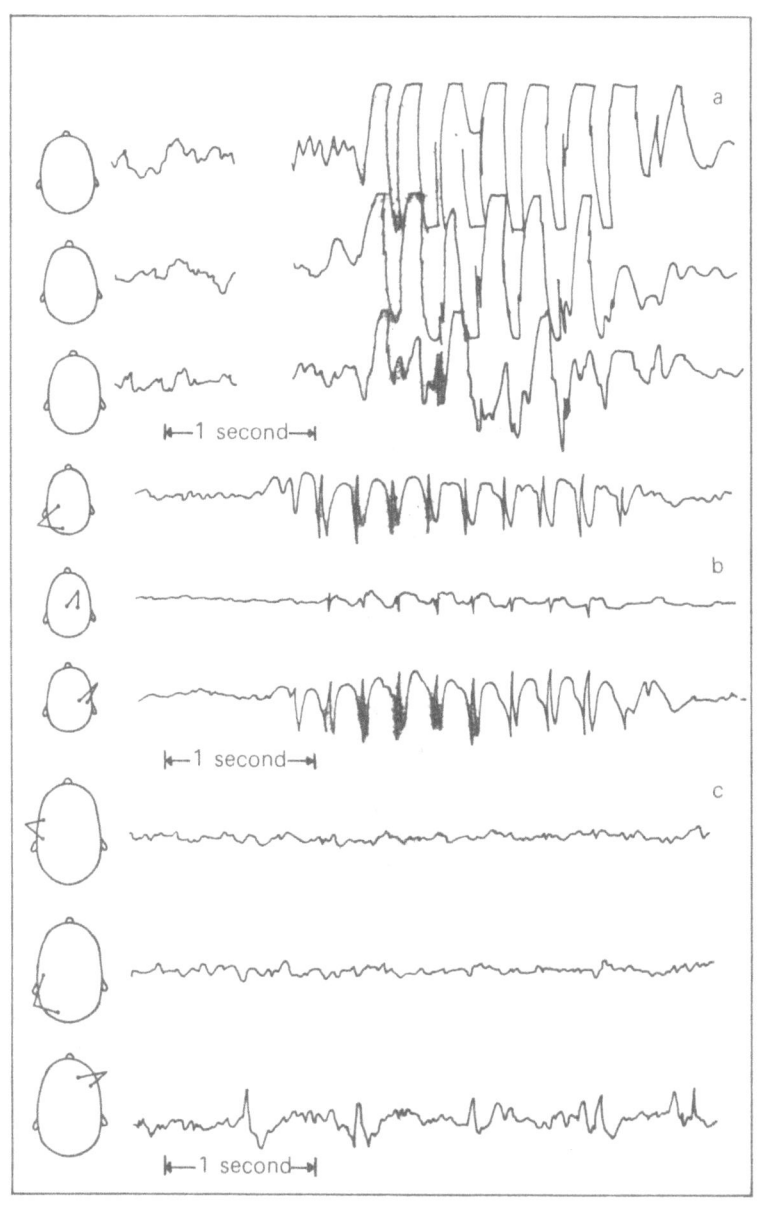

FIGURE 29 Typical EEG tracings in (*a*) Grand mal, (*b*) Petit mal, (*c*) Psycho-motor (temporal lobe) epilepsy.

no recollection of the terrifying episodes of his dream world.

These influences and their effect on dreaming are neither surprising nor altogether unexpected. In these respects, they contrast strikingly with the more esoteric tenets of psychoanalytical dream theory and dream interpretation.

The significance of the content of dreams has always been a matter of controversy. It can now be expressed as extending from those who hold that dreams are a random selection of mental processes to those who think they all stem from material which has been repressed from conscious thought.

No theory of dream interpretation is free of valid criticism. Many can be safely rejected with frank disbelief. In recent times psychiatric thought has been substantially influenced by the analytical dream theories of Freud, Jung and Adler, which have attempted to utilize the dream both as a diagnostic tool and as an agent in therapy. Freud himself visualised the dream as a grand avenue to the inscrutable workings of the unconscious mind. The prime function of the dream was to ensure continuity of sleep. Events which might disturb the sleeper and so jeopardize his slumbers – would be deftly woven into the fabric of the dream, rendering them innocuous and preserving thereby the continuity of sleep. Within the dream would be an element of conscious or unconscious wish-fulfilment.

Freud's concept of the dream – as remembered by the sleeper (manifest content) – was that of an elaborate and extravagant masquerade. It would be a collection of unconscious desires, wishes and impulses – all heavily disguised – of which the true dream material (latent content) was really composed. In any undisguised form, such unconscious material would be rejected by the conscious mind as quite unacceptable. But with appropriate disguises furnished by such dream mechanisms as Symbolization, Displacement, Condensation and Dramatization, the sleep of the dreamer would be assured. He would thus sleep on accepting, if puzzled by, the extraordinary stream of events which passed in his conscious mind.

Freudian dream interpretation proceeds therefore from an examination of the manifest content of the dream via the dream mechanisms employed, to a dénouement of the dream's latent content.

Hypnotics such as barbiturates may initially result in apparently dreamless sleep, while others such as nitrazepan may provide vivid memories of the night's dreams. It is far from clear whether the apparent increase in dreams, and particularly those with a nightmare-like quality, is real or whether recall is improved. Moreover, it has been held that the vivid dreams are therapeutically desirable.

4

THE PHYSIOLOGY OF
THE HUMAN RESPONSE

The purpose of a nervous system (p. 9) is the provision of a feedback mechanism such that an input stimulus can alter the response of the whole organism. Normal life can only exist if the response is appropriate to the input stimulus.

The input stimulus comes not only from within the body to provide internal homeostasis but also from the external environment. Indeed, the characteristic of all but the lowest members of the animal kingdom is the power of purposeful mobility in response to changes in the external environment.

Co-ordinated body responses demand knowledge of the surroundings through appropriate sensory receptors (see below), including both general receptors and those of the special senses (p. 67). Impulses from these receptors are carried in fibre tracts within the central nervous system to higher centres. These include many subcortical centres for co-ordination of muscle activity (e.g. cerebellum p. 81; reticular formation p. 84) and the cerebral cortex for interpretation of conscious sensations (p. 71).

Other cortical centres are responsible for determining an appropriate response (p. 77) and for converting this intention into actual activity via efferent impulses to the muscles. While the direct and conscious muscle activity is under cortical control, subcortical centres (extrapyramidal centres) are responsible for ensuring regulated muscle activity (p. 78).

SENSORY RECEPTORS

Numerous widely different types of sensory receptors are scattered throughout the body. All share the common function of supplying the central nervous system with information on those conditions prevailing in both the external and internal environments. Accordingly, they may be classified as exteroceptors or interoceptors.

The exteroceptors include that vast network of end-organs located in the skin, the chemoreceptors of both taste and smell and the special sense organs of sight and hearing. The interoceptors include viscero-ceptors, supplying information from the internal organs, the chemo-receptors of the carotid and aortic bodies, and the important system of proprioceptors (p. 78) – muscle spindles, tendon organs and receptors of the inner ear (otolith organs and semicircular canals).

Some of this information supplied by the sensory receptors will enter consciousness; much does not. The end-organs themselves function as transducers, converting the stimuli to which they respond into afferent nerve impulses. Stimulation of the end-organ leads to a change in the permeability of the membrane of the bare nerve ending which forms the centre of the receptor. This leads to movement across the membrane of sodium ions and hence a local potential difference (the generator poten-tial). The level of the generator potential varies with the intensity of stimulation and up to the threshold value the generator potential is localized in the end-organ and no nerve impulse is initiated. Above the threshold, intensity of sensation depends on the frequency of impulses fired off by the receptor, but with continuous stimulation of the extero-ceptors, after a period of time, fewer impulses emanate from the re-ceptor. This, in fact, accounts for the phenomenon of adaptation, although cortical inhibition may also play a part (p. 87). Adaptation is very slow or absent with interoceptors.

As the boundary of the external environment, the skin is richly supplied with sensory receptors. Doubt has been cast on the specificity of these receptors and in some instances their function remains obscure but the following are morphologically described:

Meissner's and Merkel's corpuscles and hair follicle nerve-endings (touch); Krause's end-bulbs (? cold); Ruffini end-organs (? heat); Pacinian corpuscles and Golgi-Mazzoni endings (pressure); free nerve-endings (pain).

Characteristic histological appearances also exist in many interoceptors, e.g. muscle spindles and tendon organs for proprioception.

66

Impulses from the sensory receptors travel in the sensory component of the spinal nerves, or in cranial nerve V (trigeminal) for general sensation from the face. It is important to remember that the trigeminal nerve ganglion within the skull is merely the homologue of a dorsal root ganglion of the spinal cord and is not a cranial nerve nucleus. The nerve cell for the first neurone lies outside the cord or brain (a typical arrangement is shown in fig. 30). This first neurone synapses with a second neurone which conveys the impulses of conscious sensations to the contralateral thalamic area (including the geniculate bodies) for the special senses (see below). The site of the first synapse and exact path to the thalamus varies with the sensation. Additionally the onward transmission of impulses from the first synapse depends on the interrelationship of stimulation and inhibition at that site. This is seen most markedly in the transmission of pain sensation – the so-called 'gate theory'.

There is a spatial representation of sensations in the thalamus and a limited amount of perception (particularly for pain) occurs in that region. For most of the sensations, however, a third neurone carries a sensory impulse to particular areas of the cerebral cortex for perception and interpretation.

Impulses for the unconscious sensations also enter the spinal cord through the posterior roots. They are distributed to cord and subcortical brain areas. The majority of those for proprioception reach the cerebellum (p. 81).

THE SPECIAL SENSES

The organs of general sense are concerned with stimuli applied directly to the skin. The organs of special sense, in contrast, are specialized to detect changes which occur in the more distant environment.

The eye

Light rays are concentrated on the retina by refraction at the air/corneal interface and by the lens which acts as a fine adjustment by altering its focal length under the action of the ciliary muscle. The amount of light entering the eye and the proportion of the lens that is used is controlled by the radial and circular muscles of the iris.

The retina consists of two types of receptors, the rods (for scotopic or dim light vision), and the cones (for photopic vision). The cones are responsible for colour vision and are placed centrally, in and around the fovea centralis. Light rays are concentrated in this area for high acuity

67

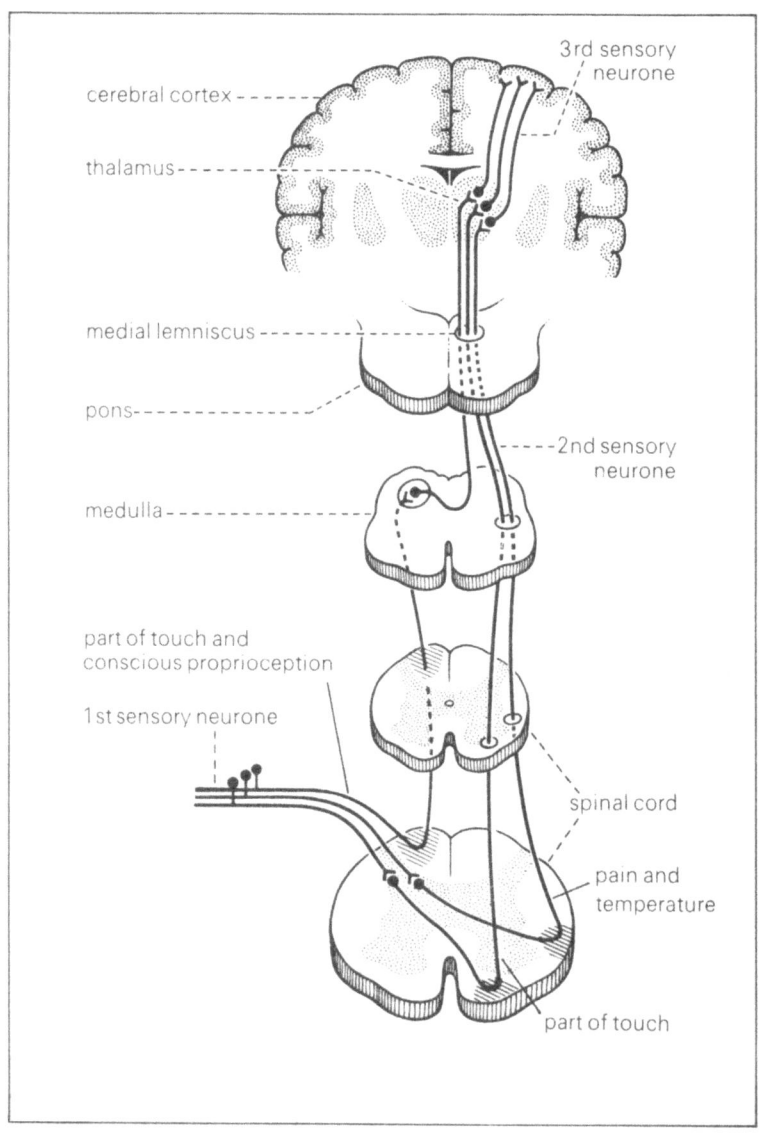

FIGURE 30 Typical arrangement of the sensory neurones.

vision. The rods, on the other hand, are distributed peripherally and are more effective than the cones where the intensity of light is limited.

Transduction of the light stimulus to the form of the nervous impulse is accomplished by chemical change in the retinal cells.

The mechanism of colour vision employed by the cones is still poorly understood. Most probably it resembles in principle that employed for vision by the rods, which is now well understood.

Rhodopsin (visual purple) is associated with the rods and consists of 11-cis retinal (Vitamin A aldehyde) bound to the protein opsin. This chemical combination occurs in the dark. When rhodopsin is exposed to light, the 11-cis retinal is changed to the all-trans form. This can no longer combine with the opsin and therefore separates from it, permitting further changes to take place which release quanta of energy. The energy so produced is utilized for the generation of nerve impulses.

The rods and cones synapse within the retina with polar cells, which in turn synapse with the ganglion cells still within the retina. Within the fovea there is a 1:1 relationship of the cones and ganglion cells, but at the periphery up to 100 receptors (primarily rods) connect with a single ganglion cell. This helps to explain the greater visual acuity at the fovea coupled with the response to a lower light intensity at the periphery (by spatial summation of synaptic transmission). Two layers of horizontally running cells within the retina are also important for the production of appropriate stimuli for cortical interpretation.

The nerve fibres which carry the impulses from the ganglion cells traverse the retina and leave the eye as the optic nerve (II). At the optic chiasma, located close to the pituitary stalk, a hemidecussation of optic nerve fibres occurs. Those from the temporal half of each retina remain on their same side. Those from each nasal half cross over. Thus each optic tract, running from the optic chiasma to the lateral geniculate body (in the course of the pathway for visual interpretation) and to the superior corpus quadrigeminum (for co-ordinating reflexes), contains the temporal retinal fibres from the eye of its own side and the nasal retinal fibres from the eye of the opposite side. The lens mechanism of the eye produces an inversion of the image on the retina. Thus impulses from the eyes, which are transmitted to one side of the cortex, convey information about what is happening to the contralateral side of the body and therefore will match the situation for other sensations.

The ear

The ear has two sensory components, that for hearing and that for position and movement in space. Sound impulses, travelling as longitudinal waves through the air, enter the external auditory meatus as pressure waves. These waves impinge upon the tympanic membrane (ear drum) and cause it to vibrate. These oscillations of the tympanic membrane are transmitted across the middle ear by movements of the ossicles – the incus, malleus and stapes. The foot of the stapes rests upon the membrane of the oval window of the cochlea (inner ear) to which the vibrations are passed.

The cochlea consists of two and a half coils of a three channel tube. The outer channels, the scala vestibuli and scala tympani are filled with perilymph, a fluid resembling extracellular fluid. These channels are confluent at the apex of the spiral (the helicotrema). The scala media, on the other hand, contains a fluid (endolymph) which resembles intracellular fluid. Vibrations in the fluid of the scala vestibuli, generated by the movement of the stapes, lead to pressure differences between the perilymph and endolymph which in turn causes vibrations of the basilar membrane. For sounds of high frequency, this membrane vibrates most at specific areas near the base of the cochlea, the exact site depending on the frequency of the sound. For sounds of low frequency, there is a more general vibration of areas of the basilar membrane which lie farther from the oval window. The frequency of oscillation of the basilar membrane will, of course, correspond with the frequency of the original air vibrations entering the external auditory meatus.

These movements in the basilar membrane cause the hair cells of the inner ear to be distorted by the tectorial membrane which in its turn leads to the generation of nerve impulses in the auditory (VIII) nerve. Synapses occur in the cochlea nuclei and medical geniculate body on the path to the auditory cortex (for conscious sensations) and to the inferior corpus quadrigeminum (for their linkage with other reflexes).

The sensation of position in space is afforded by the second component of the inner ear, the utricle and saccule. These structures also contain endolymph. On their walls, more hair cells are found and these are pressed on by small pieces of calcium 'grit' – the otoliths. Static position sense arises from the stimulation of the hair cells by the otoliths in response to the influence of gravity. Also present in the inner ear are the semicircular canals, three on each side, lying in planes mutually at right angles to each other. The differential movement of the fluid in each of these canals, signalled by the displacement of the hair cells lying within expanded portions of the canals, are responsible for our awareness of dynamic movement in space and, particularly so, for changes in that movement.

The nerve fibres from the semicircular canals, the utricle and saccule synapse in the vestibular nuclei whence there are connections with the paleo-cerebellum for integration of balance and movement, and through the thalamus to the cerebral cortex for conscious sensation.

Smell

This sense is well developed in most animals but relatively poorly developed in the human. The receptors lie in the uppermost portion of the nasal cavity above the turbinate bones. This ensures that adaptation (p. 66) from constant stimulation is reduced for, except with very concentrated odours, a deliberate 'sniff' is required to convey the air to the receptors. Stimulation of the receptors requires that the substance shall be soluble in mucus which overlies the receptor cells. Impulses from the nasal receptors are carried in the olfactory nerve (I).

Taste

While the taste receptors distinguish local environmental changes and are thus more directly allied to the normal exteroceptors, by tradition they are classed with the 'special senses'. The only taste sensations are those of bitter, sweet, salt and sour and these are perceived through special sense organs on the tongue that transmit their nerve impulses through the chorda tympani branch of the facial nerve (VII) and the glossopharyngeal nerve (IX). The finer elements of what we call 'taste' are in fact provided by the sense of smell.

THE CEREBRAL CORTEX – SENSORY AND MOTOR ACTIVITY

The major anatomical change that occurs as animals ascend the evolutionary ladder is an increase in size and complexity of the cerebral cortex (fig. 31). The cortex with certain subcortical areas is the site for cognizance of the surroundings, interpretation and for controlled movement. Cortical and subcortical activity probably depends on reverberating circuits (p. 51).

The allocation of specific functions to particular cortical areas is perhaps now hallowed more by tradition than by science. Recent

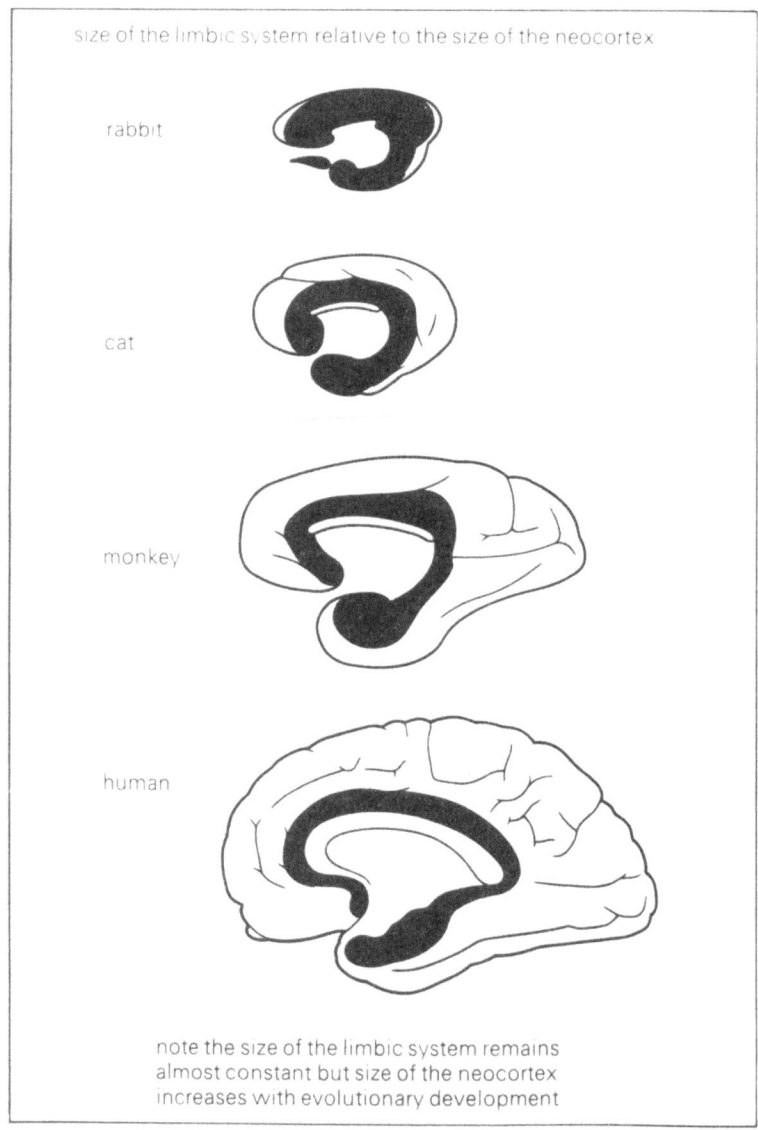

size of the limbic system relative to the size of the neocortex

rabbit

cat

monkey

human

note the size of the limbic system remains
almost constant but size of the neocortex
increases with evolutionary development

FIGURE 31 Comparison of the relative size of limbic system and cortex in different species.

72

evidence suggests that cognizance and interpretation involve close integration and simultaneous activity by several cortical and subcortical areas. Nevertheless, the concept of cortical localization of some stages in the response to the environment is a convenient one for understanding the basic principles of cortical function.

Sensory radiations flow from the thalamus to the cortex. Although there is evidence that sensory interpretation (e.g. pain) may occur at sub-cortical levels, the primary site of sensory input for interpretation lies in specific areas in the posterior part of the cortex. The impulses to these areas come from receptors on the contralateral side of the body and interpretation is based on a direct spatial arrangement linked to the receptors.

The general sensations reach the primary interpretation area in the postcentral gyrus, vision in the calcarine fissure area on the medial side of the occipital pole, hearing in the upper part of the temporal lobe and smell and taste probably in the deeper parts of the brain around the region of the uncus or upper operculum of the Sylvian fissure (fig. 32).

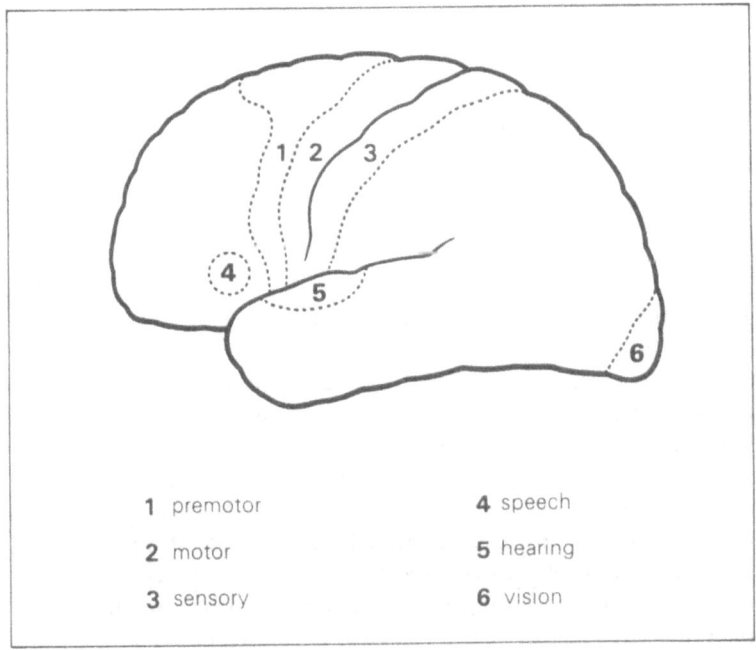

1 premotor	4 speech
2 motor	5 hearing
3 sensory	6 vision

FIGURE 32 Functional localization in the cortex of the left cerebral hemisphere.

73

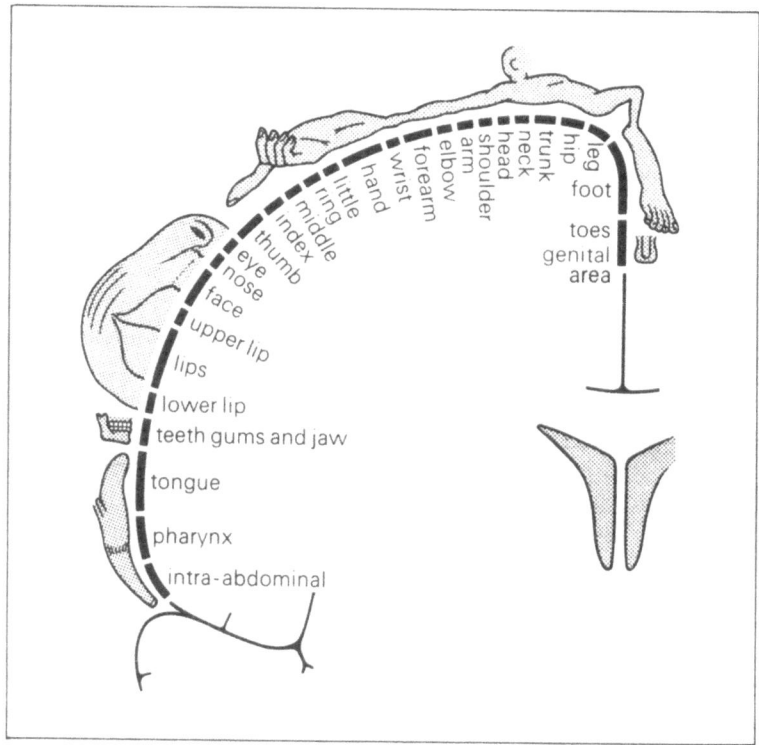

FIGURE 33 Section through the postcentral gyrus showing in diagrammatic coronal form the site and extent of sensory representation of different areas of the body.

The spatial distribution for general sensations is shown in fig. 33. For each of these sensory areas association areas have been described although there is now some doubt about the significance of these areas. One view suggested that in these areas some linking of sensation from individual receptors occurs to yield the first level of interpretation. Thus, for example, in the visual association area interpretation of shapes and colours occurs. Thus, objects can be identified and, finally, these are linked for interpretation of the overall scene. Within these association areas some form of memory (see below) of past sensory experiences must exist with which new sensations can be compared. Subdivisions of the visual and auditory association areas have been described; in particular, special areas are reputedly concerned with the interpretation of

74

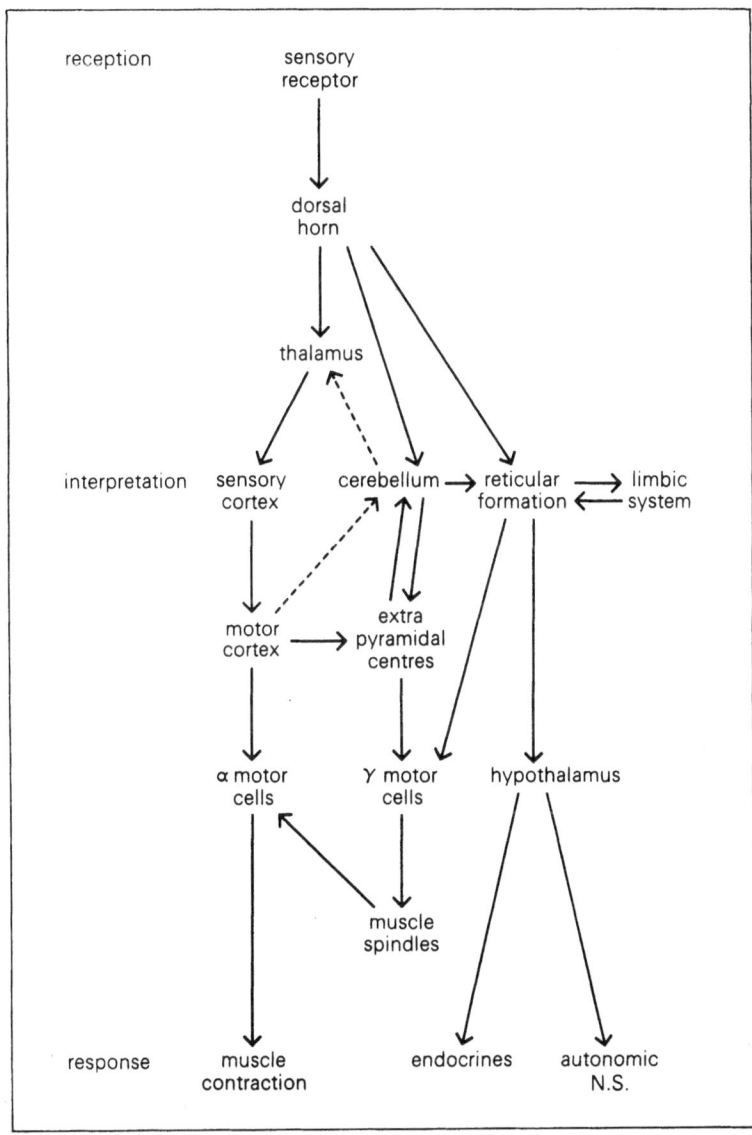

FIGURE 34 Representation of the sequence of connections from sensory receptor to muscle movement. To avoid confusion the afferent from the muscle spindles to the extrapyramidal system have been omitted.

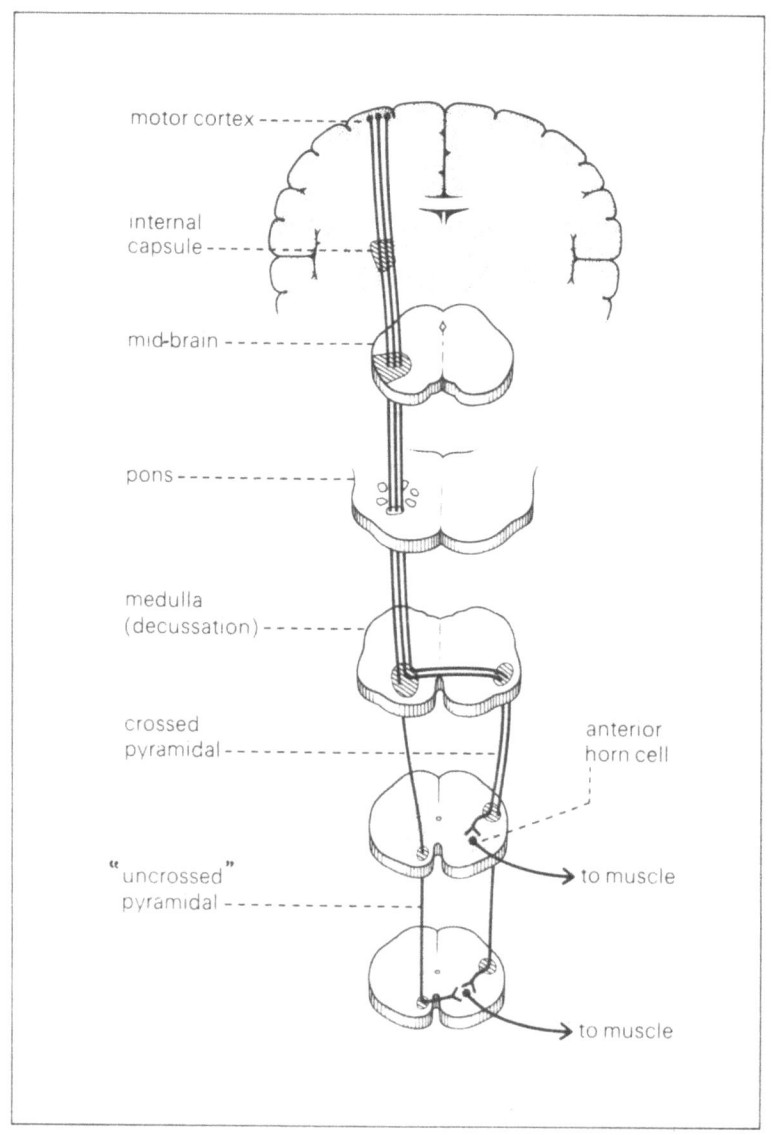

FIGURE 35 The pyramidal tract, pathway for primary motor impulses.

the written word, spoken word, etc. These are of clinical importance in the complicated neurological problems of aphasia. Full cognizance of the surroundings depends on a merging of the information from all the sensory receptors and their interpretation by reference to stored memory. According to this same theory, this takes place in a common integration area – sometimes called the 'gnostic' area which is reputed to lie in the angular gyrus. It is far more likely that full interpretation involves integrated action by several areas of the 'silent' portion of the cortex. For example the memory engram (p. 113) on which interpretation is based is represented widely and indeed bilaterally in the cortex. As with sensory interpretation, so also with overall motor control, integration of many areas of the cortex appears essential. The previous concept of a specific overall motor area is not now so widely accepted. Likewise there is currently doubt about the exact role of the frontal cortex. It was believed to be responsible for the consideration of possible overall consequences to the welfare of the individual. By suppressor and excitatory pathways, the frontal cortex either potentiated or reduced the motor responses activated by the motor integration area.

Control of the discrete movements of different muscles is present in the precentral gyrus. The representation is contralateral and portions of the body with complex movements occupy the largest area, with the feet area lying just over the medial lip of the precentral gyrus and the face and tongue being represented in the lowest portion of the gyrus. The arrangement thus parallels that seen in the sensory cortex (cf. fig. 33).

While there is representation of the individual muscles in this motor area, the area immediately rostral to the precentral gyrus controls patterns of movements. This area is usually known as the premotor cortex and is itself under some broad controlling mechanisms (including that of the cerebellum and anterior ventral nucleus of the thalamus). The whole sequence of activity from reception of an impulse through to the transmission of a response to the muscles is shown diagrammatically in fig. 34.

Representation of both sensory perception and motor activity lies in the contralateral side of the brain but the human body acts as a whole. Thus, crosswise integration must exist. Such crosslinking is seen at all levels of the nervous system via transverse interconnecting neurones.

At higher levels the interconnection occurs mainly via the corpus callosum. The corpus callosum is probably responsible for the dominance of one cerebral hemisphere. The left cerebral cortex usually shows dominance over that of the right side. The two hemispheres are however not uniform in their function and response (p. 114). Due to the contralateral distribution of representation, this left-sided dominance at cortical level probably explains the right-handedness and right-eyedness of most people. An important cause of dyslexia in which difficulties in reading persist into adulthood arises from an imbalance between dominant handedness and eyedness. Such letters as b, d, n or u are perceived as their own mirror images with consequent confusion. The reversal of these letters has been termed strephosymbolia.

MUSCLE ACTIVITY AND TONE

The voluntary muscles consist of numerous contractile cells arranged in parallel, attached either directly or through a tendon to the bone.

Controlled contraction of the muscles gives rise to voluntary movement. Such voluntary movement towards food, away from danger, is an essential component of the response of the animal kingdom to its environment.

Muscle contraction must be carefully co-ordinated if effective movement is to be achieved. The movement itself must be appropriate and antagonist, protagonist and synergist muscles must maintain the body posture. Movement is thus a carefully integrated process involving many muscle groups.

The initiation of the movement lies in the precentral area of the cortex (p. 77) and impulses are transmitted via the pyramidal tract to the contralateral anterior horn cells (fig. 35). A second neurone from the anterior horn, the α neurone, activates the muscles. The activity transmitted from the anterior horn cell depends upon the number of facilitatory and inhibitory impulses it receives. There is only one α motor neurone to any muscle fibre and the integration takes place within the nervous system. This efferent neurone is therefore spoken of as 'the final common path'.

A servo-mechanism below of stretch receptors from the muscles helps to smooth their own contraction. Two types of stretch reflex can be distinguished, the phasic stretch reflex and the tonic stretch reflex.

These servo-mechanisms depend on specialized proprioceptor cells in the muscle – the muscle spindles. Considerable variation exists but two main types of modified muscle fibres (intrafusal fibres) can be distinguished lying within and projecting from fibrous capsules, and lying parallel to the main (extrafusal) muscle fibres (fig. 36). The intrafusal

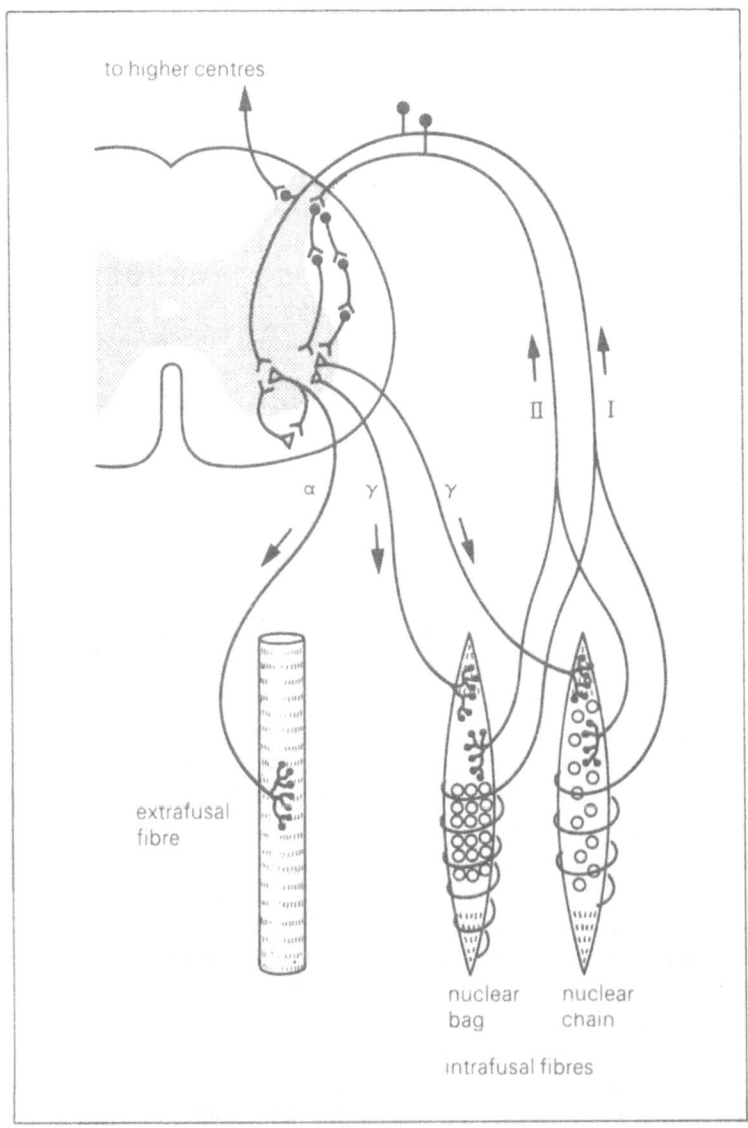

to higher centres

II   I

α   γ   γ

extrafusal
fibre

nuclear   nuclear
bag   chain

intrafusal fibres

FIGURE 36 Diagram of the main features of the anatomy and physiology of the muscle spindles.

fibres have striated polar regions with a central non-striated area very rich in nuclei. These nuclei may be clustered together (nuclei bag fibre) or form a chain (nuclear chain fibre). Both types of fibre receive a motor supply from anterior horn cells via thin conducting fibres (γ fibres). Both have an annulospiral nerve receptor which transmits impulses via a type IA fibre and a second receptor transmitting via a type II sensory fibre. The significance of the two types of spindle is uncertain.

The γ motor neurones contract the intrafusal muscle cells and the sensory fibres coming from them signal information on the degree of stretch and, in particular, compare the change of length of the intrafusal fibres relative to that of the extrafusal fibres.

Other proprioceptors occur within the tendons, 'tendon organs'. The muscle spindles lie parallel with the muscle fibres and are in consequence relaxed during muscle contraction. The tendon organs, on the other hand, are 'in sequence' and are stimulated during muscle contraction. The two proprioceptor systems are thus complementary, though the spindles are more sensitive than the tendon organs.

Impulses from the receptors enter the spinal cord in the dorsal horn. The reflexes which control tone and produce smooth activity in muscles involve both local spinal arcs and activity in higher centres. Local connection occurs with the anterior horn cell via either one synapse or several. Other connections travel to higher areas of the nervous system and particularly to the cerebellum below, and thence to the many centres in the cortex, fore-, mid- and hind-brain areas. These include not only the suppressor areas of the motor cortex, but also the corpus striatum, the subthalamic nuclei, the red nucleus and the pontine nuclei, together with portions of the reticular formation. After appropriate integration, facilitatory or inhibitory impulses pass to the anterior horn itself (fig. 37). The main efferent pathways are the facilitatory and inhibitory reticulo-spinal tract and the facilitatory vestibulo-spinal tract. The inhibitory portion of the reticulo-spinal is under cortical control via a pathway which runs through the internal capsule (fig. 37). Hence in a cerebro-vascular accident the inhibitory path is frequently damaged and the muscles show hypertonia with a spastic type of paralysis. Muscle tone thus depends on the summation of both local and higher centre controls. Disease states producing hypertonia can depend on factors influencing local reflex arcs (e.g. muscle irritation); pyramidal and extrapyramidal centres (e.g. cerebro-vascular accidents, multiple sclerosis); or diencephalic and mid-brain centres (e.g. emotions).

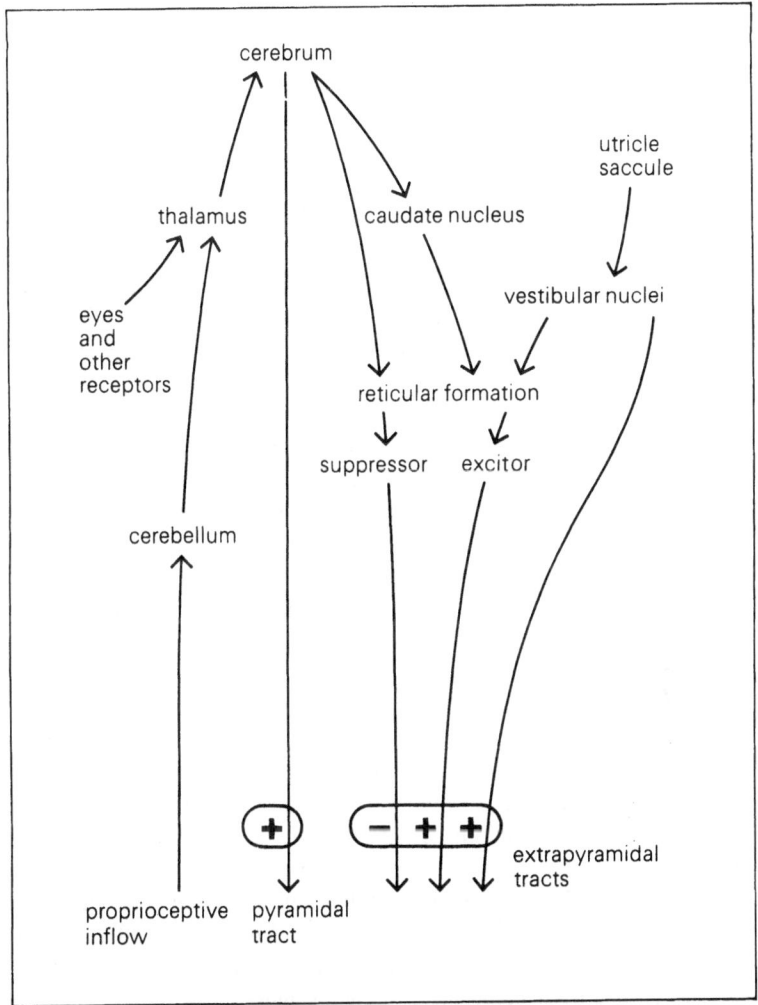

FIGURE 37 Diagram to illustrate the main interconnections that enable brain centres to influence the anterior horn cells.

THE CEREBELLUM

The cerebellum most appropriately has been termed 'the head ganglion of the proprioceptive system'. To the cerebellum, non-conscious proprioceptive information is constantly relayed – a sensory input necessary for the fulfilment of its two essential functions. These functions are firstly, the regulation and control of balance and posture and, secondly, the dynamic co-ordination of the numerous muscle groups in the production of normal harmonious patterns of muscular movement.

The cerebellum provides an excellent example of the servo-mechanism. This is a self-regulating device from which a proportion of output is returned by a feed-back mechanism for the purpose, in turn, of controlling further output. The servo-mechanisms of the cerebellum incorporate both pyramidal and extrapyramidal motor systems and the proprioceptive impulses fed back to the cerebellum from the specialized receptors in muscle (muscle spindle and tendon organs) modify further cerebellar activity whilst the co-ordination of the muscle movements is actually taking place.

Macroscopically, the cerebellum is seen as two hemispheres joined by a median vermis. Its surface grey matter is thrown into a series of fairly regular convolutions – the folia. Within its deeper white matter are found, in each hemisphere, the large crenated dentate nucleus and the accessory dentate nuclei (emboliformis, globosus and fastigius).

The microscopic anatomy of the cerebellar cortex reveals its characteristic Purkinje cells, demarcating the molecular from the granular layers of the cortex, the basket and granular cells and the mossy and climbing fibres.

Phylogenetically, the cerebellum has an older part (palaeo-cerebellum) devoted to the control of posture and balance which links with the vestibular nuclei and thence with the organs for position and movement (utricle, saccule and semicircular canals) in the inner ear, and a newer part (neo-cerebellum) controlling the intricate activity of the muscle movements.

The three peduncles of the cerebellum are composed of fibres passing to and from this organ (Table 3). These carry afferent proprioceptive impulses from the cord, additional feed-back input from

TABLE 3 Main tracts occupying cerebellar peduncles

Superior peduncle (Brachium Conjunctivum	Afferent Efferent	Anterior Spino–Cerebellar Dentato–Thalamic Dentato–Rubral
Middle peduncle (Pons)	Afferent	Ponto–Cerebellar
Inferior peduncle (Restiform Body)	Afferent	Posterior Spino–Cerebellar Olivo–Cerebellar Vestibulo–Cerebellar

both pyramidal and extrapyramidal motor systems (e.g. pontine, olivary and vestibular nuclei) and efferents to thalamus and red nucleus.

As would be expected from their functions, nuclei of the palaeo-cerebellum form their main feed-back loops with the vestibular and olivary nuclei while those of the neo-cerebellum are mainly with the cerebral cortex (fig. 38).

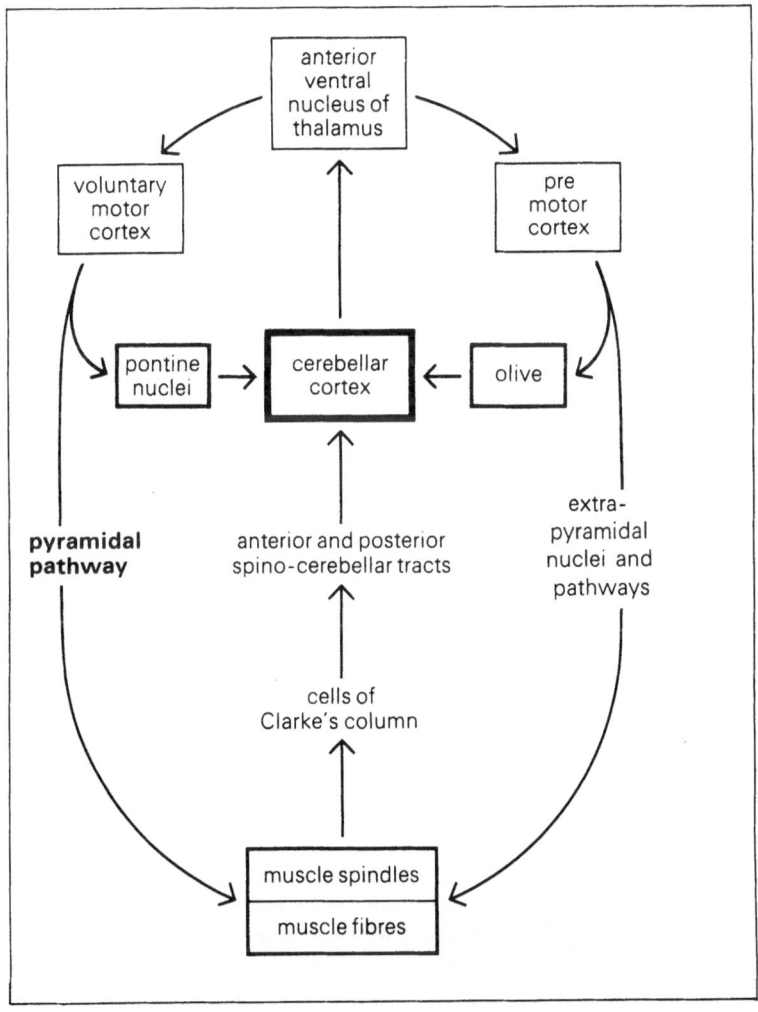

FIGURE 38 Cerebellar servo-mechanisms—for details see text.

Control of the internal environment

The appropriate response of the body to an input stimulus requires changes both in the motor activity of the body and for the control of the internal environment. For example marked muscle activity would not be possible without increased respiration and increased blood flow through the muscles.

The control of those vital body functions which maintain homeostasis – largely at unconscious levels is co-ordinated by groups of cells in the subcortical areas of the brain.

Their activity, like that of all portions of the nervous system, depends on reflex arcs involving receptors, intercalated neurones and effector organs. As might be expected, many such receptors are linked with visceral changes and their impulses are carried in the glossopharyngeal (IX) and vagus (X) nerves. Motor activity is effected via the sympathetic and parasympathetic components of the autonomic nervous system (p. 93) and the endocrine system (p. 93). The main controlling brain-stem centres for interpretation, integration and co-ordinated response are the hypothalamus and the diffuse reticular formation. Control of the body's internal environment without consideration of its corresponding response to the external environment would have little meaning. Many links therefore occur with both higher centres and voluntary motor units. Most of these links occur via the reticular formation – parts of which may be considered as a subcortical centre of conscious response, e.g. sleep-wake mechanism (p. 89) and control of muscle tone (p. 87).

BRAIN-STEM RETICULAR FORMATION

The reticular formation consists of a long chain of nerve cells located centrally throughout the medulla oblongata, pons, mid-brain and diencephalon (fig. 39). These neurones possess long and short interconnecting fibres. Surrounding the reticular formation are the fibre tracts and nuclei of the main conducting systems, many of which pass collateral fibres to the reticular neurones.

The nerve cells of the reticular formation possess many dendrites; these extend over a very wide area and show multiple synaptic connections with the neighbouring long pathways. The nerve cells vary in size from 12μ to 90μ in diameter. Their axons, which show considerable variation in both length and diameter, provide short and long linking units with slow and fast conduction velocities, relaying to ipselateral and contralateral structures. Although a number of nuclei and their connections have been defined within the reticular formation by anatomists, the physiological significance of these is not clear.

The main function of the reticular system is that of communication

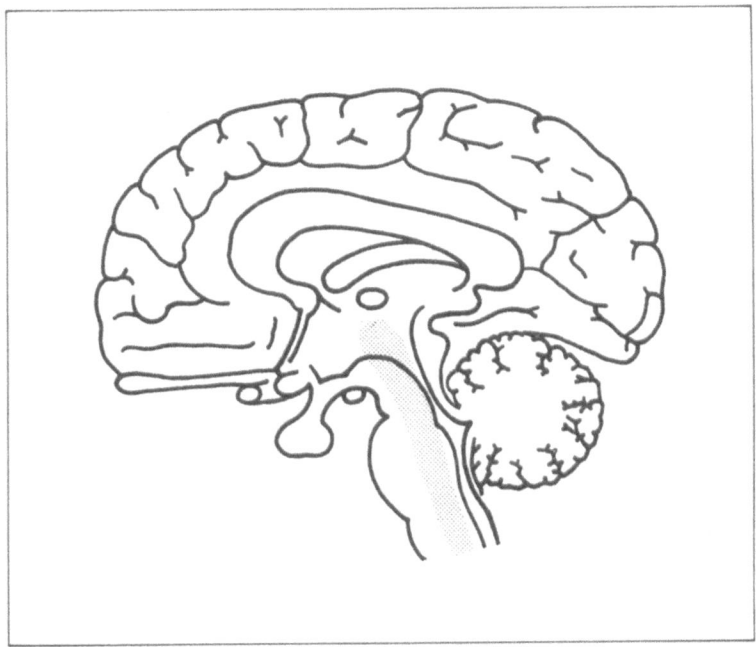

FIGURE 39 Longitudinal section of the brain-stem to show the position of the reticular formation.

between those centres of the brain concerned with the mechanisms of homeostasis and the regions of the brain concerned with thought (p. 119) and emotion (p. 122). It provides a co-ordinating system which modifies the internal environment to compensate for changes in the external environment.

A typical co-ordinating reaction of the reticular formation is the arousal reaction to danger. A man wandering dozily along a lonely, dark lane suddenly hears a movement in the hedge. He immediately becomes wide awake (cortical arousal reaction); he feels afraid (affective arousal reaction); his muscle tone increases (spinal neurone arousal reaction); his heart beats rapidly and his pupils dilate (autonomic arousal reaction);

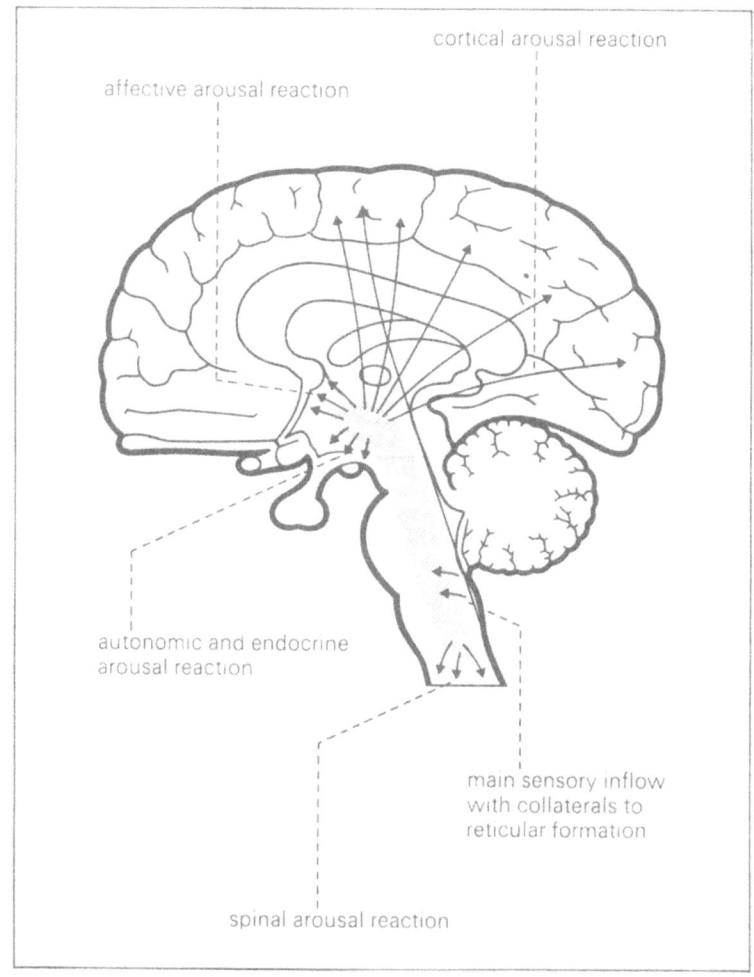

cortical arousal reaction

affective arousal reaction

autonomic and endocrine arousal reaction

main sensory inflow with collaterals to reticular formation

spinal arousal reaction

FIGURE 40 Afferent collaterals to the reticular formation and the resulting arousal reaction. Further explanation is given in the text.

and his blood sugar rises (endocrine arousal reaction) (fig. 40). There is a general increase in activity attributable to the sensory input.

Stimuli from the external environment are passed to the reticular formation in collaterals from the sensory afferent pathways and via spino-reticular pathways. By means of the long and short fibre tracts, the nuclei of the reticular formation are linked together themselves, are linked to the cortex and limbic system, and are linked to the effector-motor areas in other parts of the nervous system (see below). The animal kingdom is primarily adjusted to recognize and respond to changes in the environment. Suppressor mechanisms via fibres from the frontal cortex prevent hyperactivity of the nervous system to a sustained stimulus.

The reticular formation exerts its influence upon body activity via a series of efferent pathways.

(a) Respiratory system

Areas regulating respiration lie in the medullary portion of the reticular formation close to the floor of the IVth ventricle. Electrical stimulation has defined areas which produce inspiratory or expiratory activity. Inspiration and expiration exhibit an automatic rhythm due to reciprocal innervation of the centres. Two additional centres (apneustic and pneumotaxic centres) are postulated as lying in the reticular formation in the pons, and provide a feed-back loop modified by impulses from other parts of the body (e.g. impulses from the lung – the Hering-Breuer reflex; chemoreceptors in the carotid body) (fig. 41).

(b) Cardiovascular System

Two distinct but interconnected centres, located at the lower end of the reticular formation, regulate the cardiovascular system. One centre is concerned with cardiac activity (cardiac regulatory centre) and the other with peripheral vascular tone (vasomotor centre). Each centre is composed of reciprocally arranged stimulatory and inhibitory components.

Efferents from the vasomotor centre reach the blood vessels via the sympathetic chain and α and β receptors, and allow dilatation or constriction in different parts of the vascular system (p. 99). Efferents from the cardiac centre reach the heart via the sympathetic and parasympathetic (vagus) nerves, regulating both heart rate and force of contraction. The input to these centres originates both from within the CNS itself (e.g. from a rhythmic burst from the respiratory component of the reticular formation) and from outside receptors (baro- and chemoreceptors in the carotid sinus and carotid body area).

(c) Muscle tone

Muscle tone and muscular movements are dependent upon a balance of activity at the anterior horn cell, between impulses from local reflexes and those from higher centres, including facilitatory and inhibitory

87

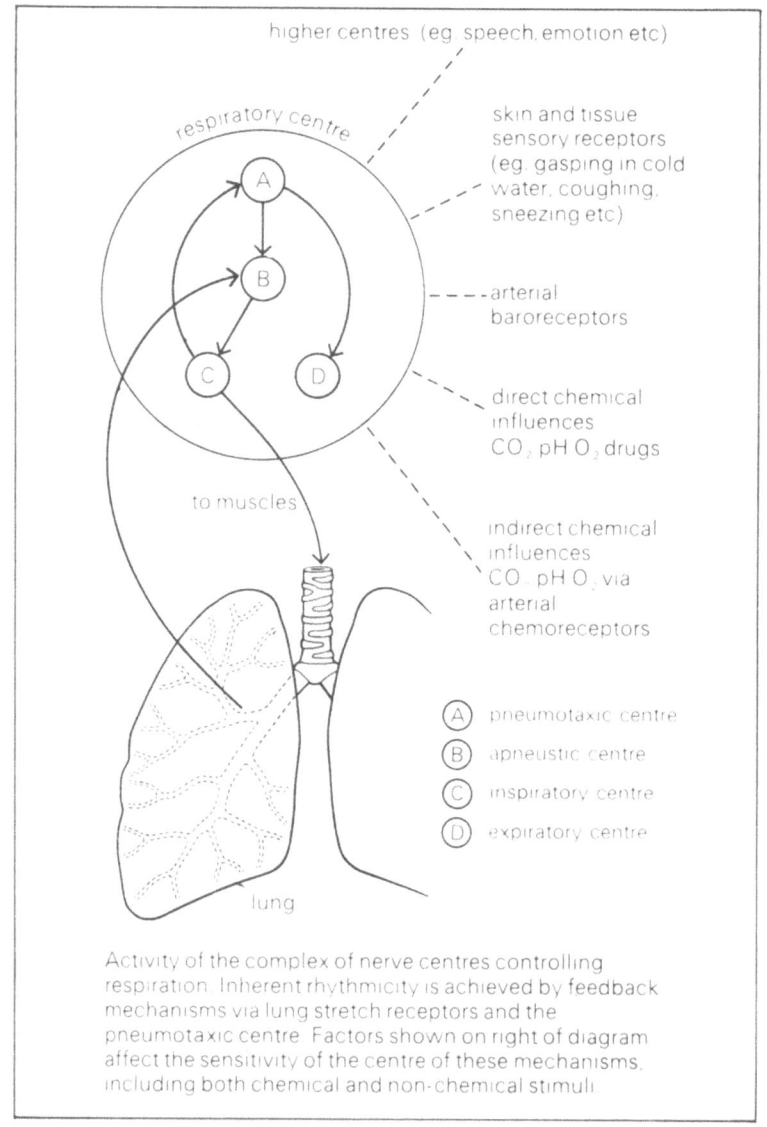

FIGURE 41 The components of the respiratory centre and the factors which affect the overall sensitivity of the centre.

impulses from centres in the reticular formation (fig. 37, p. 81). These efferent impulses run in the reticulo-spinal tracts. Afferent impulses to the reticular formation originate in suppressor areas of the frontal cortex, in the corpus striatum, the cerebellum, the tectal nuclei, other mid- and hind-brain nuclei concerned with tone and posture and from the peripheral receptors located in the muscles (p. 78).

(d) *Autonomic tone*
Although the main centre for co-ordination of the autonomic nervous system lies in the hypothalamus (p. 91), higher control may be exerted by certain portions of the reticular formation. This control may be purely adrenergic, purely cholinergic or, perhaps, a mixture of both.

(e) *Efferents to cortex*
Mid-brain section and electrical stimulation experiments have demonstrated a diffuse outflow from the reticular formation to the cortex, responsible for an arousal reaction and the sleep-wake rhythm (p. 52). Afferent impulses are derived from collaterals of the main sensory pathways (fig. 40). The cortex itself, probably through some of its suppressor areas, exerts a negative feed-back on this mechanism. This is probably the mechanism responsible for the adaptation which occurs to most sensory stimuli (p. 66).

HYPOTHALAMUS
The hypothalamus is a region within the diencephalon, lying below the third ventricle and above both the pituitary gland and optic chiasma. It is separated from the thalamus above by the hypothalamic sulcus.

The hypothalamus is composed of many nuclear masses, including those of the pre-optic area (medial and lateral pre-optic nuclei), the supra-optic area (supra-optic, superchiasmatic, paraventricular and anterior nuclei), the tuberal area (ventro-medial, dorso-medial, arcuate, lateral and posterior nuclei) and the mamillary area (medial and lateral mamillary, pre- and supramamillary nuclei) (fig. 42).

Multiple nerve connections – both afferent and efferent – relay to and from the fore-brain and mid-brain areas. The medial fore-brain bundle connects with the frontal lobe of the cerebral cortex; hypothalamo-thalamic fibres probably convey somatic and visceral sensory impulses via the thalamus to cortical sensory areas. Connections with various portions of the limbic system and reticular formation are made via the

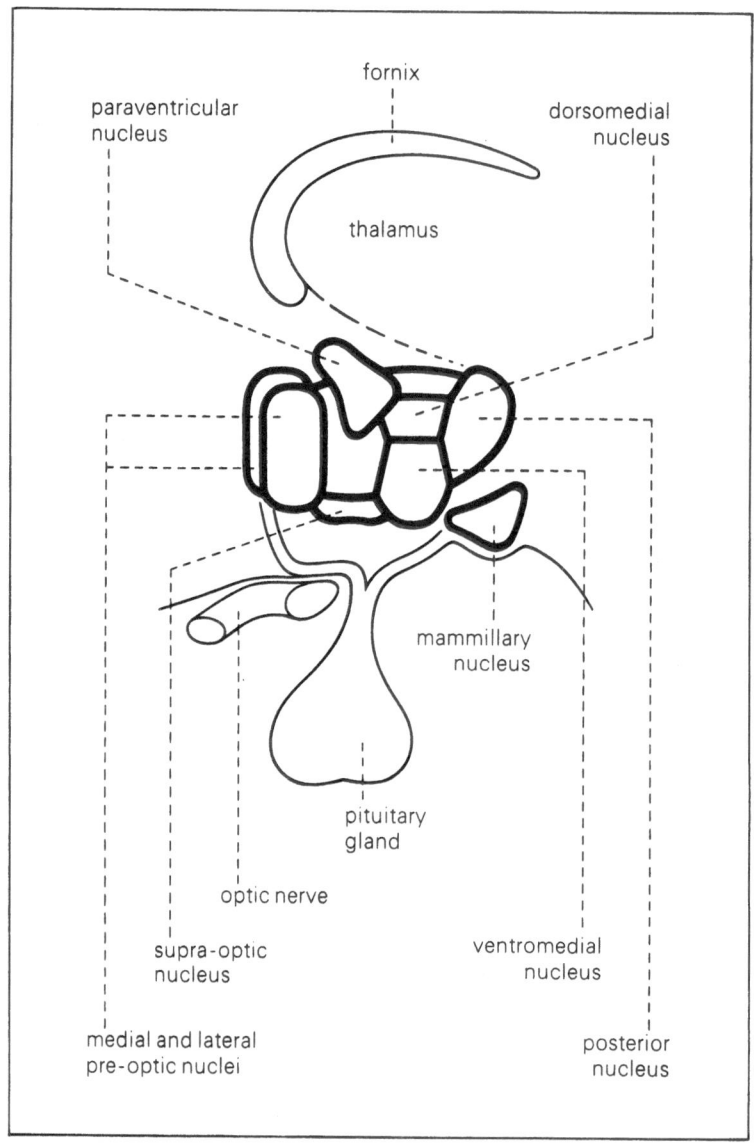

FIGURE 42 Longitudinal section of the diencephalon showing the main nuclear groups in the hypothalamus and their relationship to neighbouring parts of the brain.

fornix and stria terminalis; an efferent path travels from the supra-optic nuclei into the posterior pituitary gland and lateral hypothalamic nuclei send projection fibres via the reticular formation to bulbar and spinal motor neurones.

The functions of the hypothalamus are those of co-ordination of the autonomic nervous system and endocrine system, which control the internal environment. Since this co-ordination must be linked to the changing needs of the body, its functions are clearly related to those of the limbic system and reticular formation. Both sensory and motor areas occur in the hypothalamus for control of the autonomic system.

In experimental animals, electrical stimulation of the hypothalamus will produce increased activity by the autonomic system. Stimulation caudally evokes sympathetic activity; stimulation rostrally evokes parasympathetic activity.

In more specific fashion, the hypothalamus links the motor control of the autonomic with the endocrine system, employing sensitive receptors within its nuclei to determine changes within the internal environment and so to contribute to the feed-back mechanism.

The hypothalamus controls body temperature. Its complete destruction allows the body temperature to fluctuate with that of the external environment. The posterior hypothalamus responds to a lowered temperature and compensates by increased sympathetic activity. The anterior thalamic nuclei controls heat loss mechanisms, including panting, sweating and vasodilation.

Bilateral damage to the ventro-medial nuclei causes overeating in animals, while lateral hypothalamic nuclei ablation reduces eating to the extent of death by starvation – even in the presence of an adequate food supply. This reaction depends in part on the glucose level in the blood and experimental evidence shows that these centres have a specific ability for taking up glucose. Normal eating habits are probably the result of a balance between these two counterpoised centres. Emotion centres within the fore-brain area have direct hypothalamic connections and probably account for emotional influences on eating habits.

Other hypothalamic centres control the water balance of the body, acting both on water intake and on water loss. Stimulation of an area close to the para-ventricular nuclei increases thirst and the supra-optic nuclei contain receptors which respond to plasma osmotic pressure. The connection from the supra-optic nucleus to the posterior pituitary translates osmotic changes into variations in the release of anti-diuretic

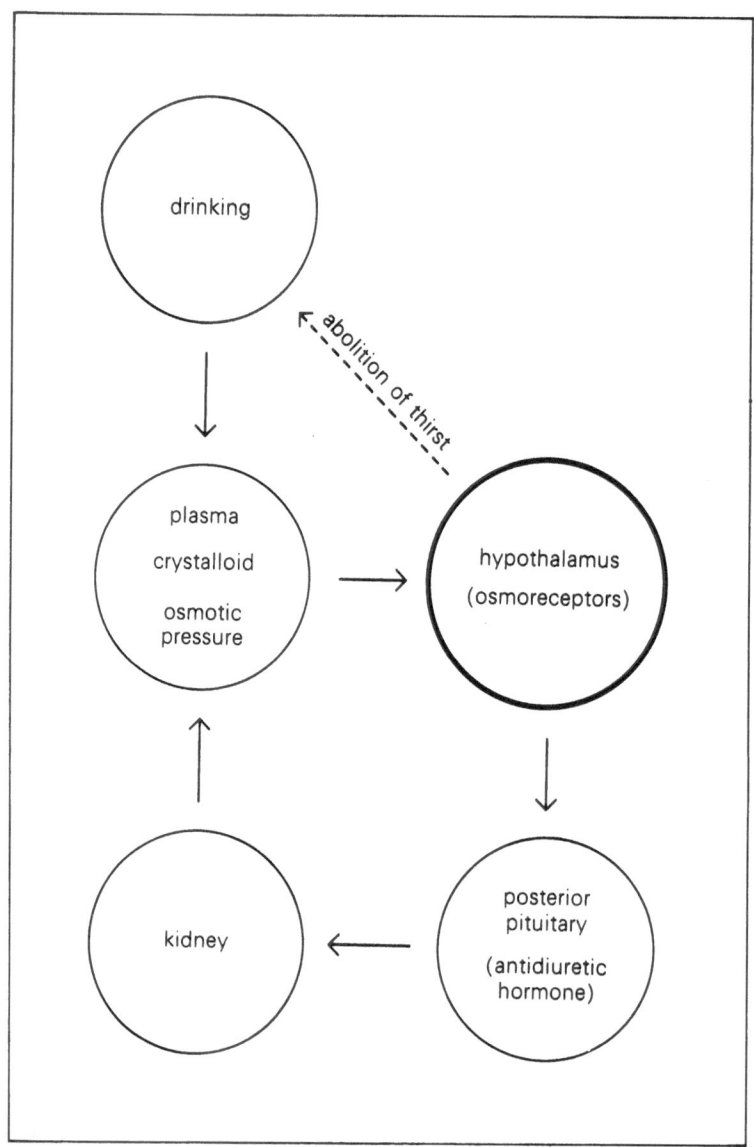

FIGURE 43 The control of body water balance by the hypothalamus and the feed-back mechanism.

hormone, and consequently controls water reabsorption by the kidney (fig. 43).

Other centres exert an overall control on endocrine activity, via the anterior pituitary. There is no direct nervous pathway from the hypo-thalamus to the anterior pituitary and chemical releasing factors travel in a portal blood system (fig. 44). The majority of endocrine activities are partly under hypothalamic control. Several of the releasing factors have now been isolated and the chemistry of many is known.

Differences in hypothalamic control exist between animals and man. In animals, for example, external influences such as light have a direct effect on the sexual cycle. Even in man, the central nervous system partly controls the endocrines via the hypothalamic-hypophyseal axis.

The relationship of the hypothalamus to other mid-brain and cortical centres is discussed elsewhere in the text. One of the most important of its links is that via the reticular formation (p. 85). By these links autonomic and endocrine systems are affected by such factors as the sleep-wake rhythm (p. 53) and the emotions (p. 123).

THE AUTONOMIC NERVOUS SYSTEM

The autonomic nervous system is composed of sympathetic and para-sympathetic divisions. Each division is recognized now to possess afferent fibres in addition to its well-substantiated efferent nerve fibres. Afferent autonomic fibres run to the brain or spinal cord in similar fashion to somatic sensory nerves but the efferent autonomic fibres reach their effector organs (smooth muscle and glands) in a manner which contrasts strikingly with their somatic motor counterparts.

The autonomic efferent pathway (both sympathetic and para-sympathetic) is made up of two neurones in sequence with a synapse between them. The axon of the first of these two neurones is termed the preganglionic fibre and that of the second is referred to as the post-ganglionic fibre.

It is characteristic of the parasympathetic division of the autonomic system that its postganglionic fibres are typically extremely short – the synapse most commonly occurring within the wall of the organ inner-vated. In consequence the preganglionic fibre is long. On the other hand within the sympathetic division, the preganglionic fibre is usually short and the postganglionic fibre is much longer. It is characteristic of the sympathetic pathway that its preganglionic fibres synapse each with many postganglionic fibres. This allows a wide spread dissemination of

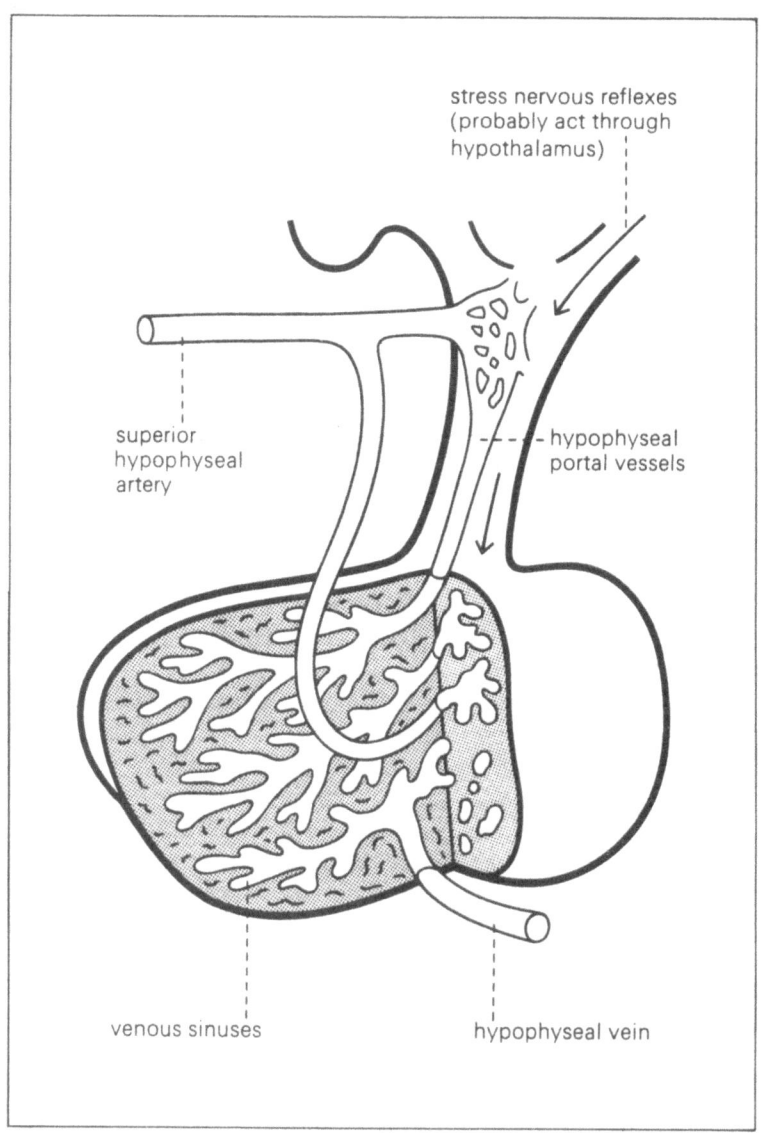

FIGURE 44 The hypothalamic-hypophyseal portal system. Releasing factors from the hypothalamus travel to the anterior pituitary (adenohypophysis) via these blood vessels to control the secretion of trophic hormones.

the original preganglionic impulse, as opposed to a rather narrow spread within the parasympathetic division.

Preganglionic fibres of the sympathetic division originate in the lateral horn of grey matter in the spinal cord of all thoracic segments and the first two lumbar. They emerge as myelinated fibres from the anterior root of the spinal nerve, forming a white ramus communicans, and run to a neighbouring ganglion of the sympathetic trunk (lateral ganglion). Here the preganglionic fibre may effect its synapse with the second neurone or it may pass through the lateral ganglion and run within the sympathetic trunk to synapse in a lateral ganglion at higher or lower level. Again it may pass uninterrupted through the sympathetic trunk to synapse ultimately in one of the ganglia grouped about the aorta or its large branches (collateral ganglia), as do the splanchnic nerves in their course to the coeliac and aortico-renal ganglia. From the lateral ganglia of the sympathetic trunk, amyelinated postganglionic fibres are returned to the corresponding spinal nerves as grey rami communicantes and are distributed to their effector organs (fig. 45).

On each side of the body, the sympathetic trunk ends superiorly at the superior cervical ganglion (representing four fused lateral ganglia). From here, therefore, intracranial structures obtain their sympathetic supply from fibres surrounding the arteries and forming periarterial plexuses (e.g. the internal carotid 'nerve').

Within the abdomen, sympathetic fibres are similarly distributed by the arteries. Massive plexuses are found on the surface of the aorta and grouped about its branches. These include the coeliac, superior and inferior mesenteric plexuses. A continuation of the aortic plexus inferiorly links with the superior and inferior hypogastric plexuses, the latter supplying the bladder, rectum and genitalia.

Among abdominal viscera, the adrenal medulla requires special mention. Preganglionic sympathetic fibres run via the greater splanchnic nerve directly to the medullary cells without any intervening synapse. These cells themselves stand, as it were, in lieu of postganglionic fibres. They also show the most interesting parallel in secreting adrenaline, compared with the secretion of noradrenaline by the postganglionic sympathetic fibres (other than those which innervate sweat glands and certain skeletal muscle vessels both of which are cholinergic).

Preganglionic fibres of the parasympathetic division originate in cells of the mid-brain (Edinger-Westphal nucleus) or of the medulla oblongata (superior and inferior salivary nuclei and dorsal nucleus of the vagus)

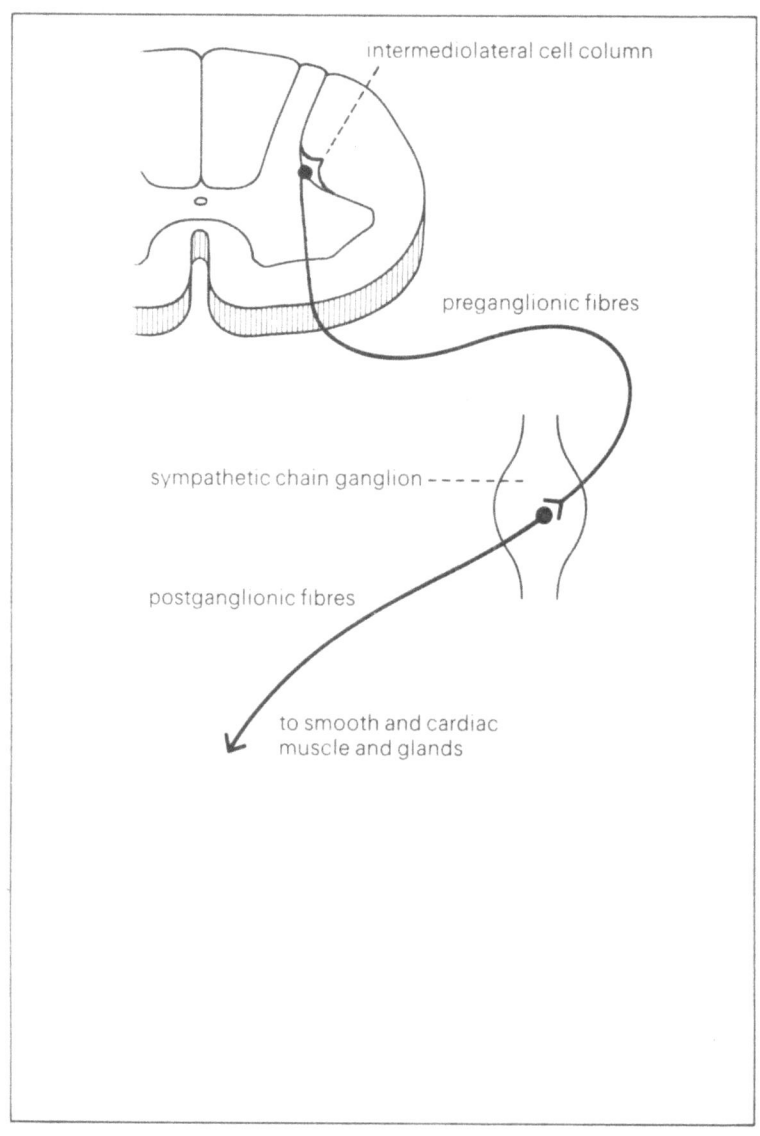

FIGURE 45 Anatomy of the sympathetic pre- and postganglionic fibres.

and in cells of the grey matter of the spinal cord in segments S.2,3,4. Parasympathetic fibres are distributed with the oculomotor (III), facial (VII), glossopharyngeal (IX) and vagus (X) cranial nerves. The ganglia in which the pre- and postganglionic fibres of these nerves synapse are:

Oculomotor (III)   *Ciliary ganglion*

Facial (VII)   *Sphenopalatine and submaxillary ganglia*

Glossopharyngeal (IX)   *Otic ganglion*

Vagus (X)   *Ganglia in thoracic and abdominal viscera supplied*

Preganglionic fibres from the sacral contribution (S.2,3,4) form the nervi erigentes – best remembered as the 'emptying nerves' from their important role in emptying the bladder in micturition and the rectum in defaecation. These fibres are also responsible for erection of the penis. The synapses between pre- and postganglionic parasympathetic fibres of these sacral segments occur – as would be expected – in the walls of the abdominal viscera supplied (terminal ganglia).

In many instances, the roles played by the sympathetic and para-sympathetic divisions of the autonomic nervous system are antagonistic (Table 4). In other instances they may be synergistic. Their balance is closely co-ordinated and controlled by the hypothalamus in the main-tenance of a remarkably constant internal environment (homeostasis) (p. 91). The hypothalamus functions not only as 'head ganglion of the autonomic' but intimately linked with this activity is its role as principal mediator for the discharge of affective impulses emergent from the limbic system in the expression of emotion (p. 122).

Cortical representation of the autonomic nervous system is found in the orbito-frontal areas of the brain.

Sympathetic arousal may be seen as a widespread and often dramatic display, classically equipping the individual for 'fight or flight'. Para-sympathetic activity, as would be expected from a consideration of the neuroanatomy involved, is more localized and more specific of effect. The general function of such activity is towards replenishing physical resources.

In both sympathetic and parasympathetic ganglia, transmission of the nerve impulse from pre- to postganglionic fibres is achieved by the release of acetylcholine. Acetylcholine again is released from the nerve endings of all postganglionic parasympathetic fibres and, furthermore, from the endings of those postganglionic sympathetic fibres which innervate sweat glands and certain skeletal muscle vessels (cholinergic fibres). Other postganglionic sympathetic fibres release noradrenaline at their endings (adrenergic fibres) as described on p. 39.

TABLE 4

	Sympathetic	*Parasympathetic*
Eye		
Iris	Pupil dilated	Pupil constricted
Ciliary muscle	Relaxed for far vision	Accommodated for near vision
Heart		
Rate	Accelerated	Slowed
Output	Increased	Decreased
Blood vessels		
Coronary	Dilated	?
Skin and abdominal viscera	Constricted	—
Skeletal muscle*	Relaxed	
Lung		
Bronchial muscle	Relaxed	Constricted
Stomach and intestine		
Motility and tone	Decreased	Increased
Sphincters	Contracted as a rule	Relaxed as a rule
Secretion	Inhibited	Increased, particularly enzymes
Urinary bladder		
Detrusor	Relaxed	Contracted
Trigone and internal sphincter	Contracted	Relaxed
Skin		
Pilomotor muscles	Contracted	—
—	Secretion†	—
Adrenal medulla	Secretion of adrenaline and noradrenaline†	—
Salivary glands		
Parotid gland	No secretion	Profuse, water secretion
Submaxillary gland	Thick, viscous secretion	Profuse, water secretion

*In skeletal muscle certain sympathetic adrenergic fibres constrict, others may relax but the main effect is relaxation by sympathetic cholinergic fibres.

†Note sweat glands and adrenal medulla fibre are cholinergic.

Two different receptors (termed α and β) exist at the periphery for catechol amines (adrenaline and noradrenaline). The α receptors are associated with contraction of smooth muscle. Conversely, the β receptors relax smooth muscle when stimulated by catechol amines. Noradrenaline shows greater activity on the α than on the β receptors.

REFLEXES WITH SPINAL AND AUTONOMIC COMPONENTS

The majority of reflexes involve only one of the two components of the nervous system – either somatic or autonomic. In certain instances, however, co-ordinated action is required from both these components; such reflexes include those for deglutition, micturition, defaecation, parturition and orgasm, and from these deglutition and micturition may be taken as typical examples.

Deglutition

The act of swallowing can be divided into three phases on the basis of the three regions through which the bolus passes from the mouth to the stomach.

In the first stage the bolus is passed from the mouth through the isthmus of the fauces into the pharynx. The food mass, either liquid or solid, is rolled towards the back of the tongue and the front of the tongue is raised against the hard palate. At the same time the mylohyoid muscles contract and force the food bolus into the pharynx. The first stage is initiated voluntarily. The cerebral cortex plays the dominant role but there must be some stimulus to the mucous membranes of the mouth to initiate the swallowing movement, cf. the difficulty in swallowing with a dry mouth.

The second stage which is a somatic reflex, is initiated when the bolus enters the pharynx. The swallowing centre lies in the medulla oblongata. During this phase the food is prevented from entering undesirable areas, and passed into the upper end of the oesophagus. The continued contraction of the mylohyoid muscles and the position of the tongue prevents the food re-entering the mouth. The posterior nares are occluded by the elevation of the soft palate. Food is prevented from entering the larynx by the approximation of the vocal cords, by the elevation of the larynx so that it lies closely under the fixed epiglottis, which acts as an auxiliary mechanism directing food away from the respiratory passages, and by the inhibition of respiratory movements. Simultaneously the pharyngeal constrictors contract sequentially and force the bolus into the upper end of the oesophagus which opens to receive it.

The bolus passes down the oesophagus and into the stomach during the third stage. The oral and middle portions of the cervical part of the oesophagus consist of striated muscle supplied by somatic motor nerves. The caudal part of the oesophagus on the other hand is composed of smooth muscle. It exhibits autonomous peristaltic activity and is under autonomic nervous system control.

Micturition

The bladder is supplied by both parasympathetic and sympathetic divisions – the action of one being antagonistic to the other. Thus parasympathetic activity brings about relaxation of the internal sphincter and contraction of the general musculature (detrusor urinae) with a consequent expulsion of urine. Sympathetic activity, on the other hand, causes contraction of the internal sphincter, relaxation of the general musculature and retention of the urine within the bladder.

As the bladder begins to fill, afferent impulses pass from its sensory receptors to the spinal cord. Efferent sympathetic impulses from cord to bladder are initiated and efferent parasympathetic impulses are inhibited. As filling continues, the pressure within the bladder stays at a low and remarkably constant level, due to a progressive reflex accommodation by the detrusor urinae musculature to the degree of filling. When nearly full, however, energetic contractions by the detrusor urinae greatly increase the intravesicle pressure and a conscious desire to micturate is experienced. Should micturition be inconvenient a voluntary restraint of the visceral reflexes is imposed by the higher centres of the brain. This results in an increased contraction of the internal sphincter and further accommodation by the detrusor urinae to the increasing volume of urine. The contraction of the internal sphincter may be assisted by impulses passing in the pudendal nerve to cause contraction of the voluntary external sphincter.

When the moment is convenient, or ultimately in spite of any attempted cortical control, micturition commences and the bladder empties. The external (voluntary) and internal (involuntary) sphincters relax and the general musculature of the bladder contracts expelling the urine. As urine enters the posterior third of the urethra more afferent impulses are initiated which induce powerful contractions of the general musculature. Contractions of the diaphragm and muscles of the abdominal wall assist the expulsion of urine by increasing the intra-abdominal pressure. At the end of the process, the final drops of urine are expelled from the urethra by contraction of the bulbo-spongiosus muscle, and the external sphincter again shuts off the bladder. These two voluntary muscles receive their innervation from the pudendal nerve (S.2,3,4).

The area of cerebral cortex responsible for the voluntary initiation and inhibition of micturition is to be found in the paracentral lobule of the brain. Other effective centres exert their influence from the hypo-thalamus and brain-stem. Emotion may greatly facilitate or inhibit the prevailing complex neural mechanisms of micturition – a fact to which both fear and embarrassment testify.

5
MAN AS AN INDIVIDUAL

In the preceding chapters we have concerned ourselves with those general responses to stimuli which occur in animals and man and the mechanisms by which these responses are made.

Nevertheless the responses of any given man, or indeed any given animal, are not stereotyped. Their individual qualities depend not only on the genetic endowment of the person or animal in question but also upon the effects of the environment, past and present. This chapter is therefore concerned with a closer examination of individual responses and moves to a large extent into the biological hinterland between psychology and central nervous system physiology.

We can examine serially the pre- and postnatal influences that lead to the mature adult (genetics p. 103, and child development p. 107) and the mechanisms that lead to an appropriate interpretation and initiate responses in the individual (sensation p. 109, perception p. 109, memory and forgetting p. 112, learning, conditioning and imprinting p. 115, language p. 119). Thence we may progress to some of the more abstract characteristics which are responsible for the individual re-sponding as an integrated person (thought, ideas and imagination p. 119, instincts and drives p. 121, the emotions and affect p. 122, the person-ality p. 126, sexuality and gender role p. 129, intelligence and intelli-gence testing p. 130, judgement p. 133).

GENETICS

The initiation of any new life occurs at the moment of fertilization of the ovum by the sperm. From this fertilized single cell all the rest of the body structure will develop. The future growth and form of the individual depends on the nuclear structure of the zygote, half derived from each parent. Thus the germ cell structure of the parent influences that of the child (heredity).

All important recent contributions from the field of genetics to our understanding of the aetiology of mental illness, render a basic knowledge of this science an essential to any study of psychological medicine.

The units of heredity are the genes and their vehicles for transmission are the chromosomes. Each gene is responsible for the building of protein (particularly enzymes) within the new cell. Genetic abnormalities thus affect the structure and function of the new cells.

Mental illness may follow the dominant or recessive influence of a single gene (monogenic) or result from the additive influence of many genes (polygenic). Thus Huntington's chorea is determined by a single dominant gene, whereas phenylketonuria is inherited as a simple recessive. The evidence for causative factors in neurotic illness or psychopathic disorders of personality favour, on the other hand, a polygenic basis of inheritance.

Human chromosomes, as present in the nuclei of all normal body cells, may be classified, numbered and arranged in a systematized order known as karyotype. Such an arrangement is the noted Denver classification (fig. 46).

These chromosomes may show extensive defects. With the larger autosomal chromosomes, defects commonly induce spontaneous abortion. With the smaller autosomes and sex chromosomes, however, such clinical conditions as mongolism (Down's syndrome), Kleinfelter's syndrome and Turner's syndrome follow upon chromosomal anomalies.

Thus an extra No. 21 chromosome (21-trisomy) accounts for the 'regular' form of mongolism, with a total chromosome count of 47. Sometimes, however, this extra chromosome is not free but becomes attached to another chromosome. This produces the 'translocation mongol' with an apparently normal chromosome total of 46. An extra one or more X sex chromosomes accounts for Kleinfelter's syndrome (testicular atrophy, sterility, eunuchoidism), often with accompanying mental defect. Combination of XXY, XXXY and even XXXXY

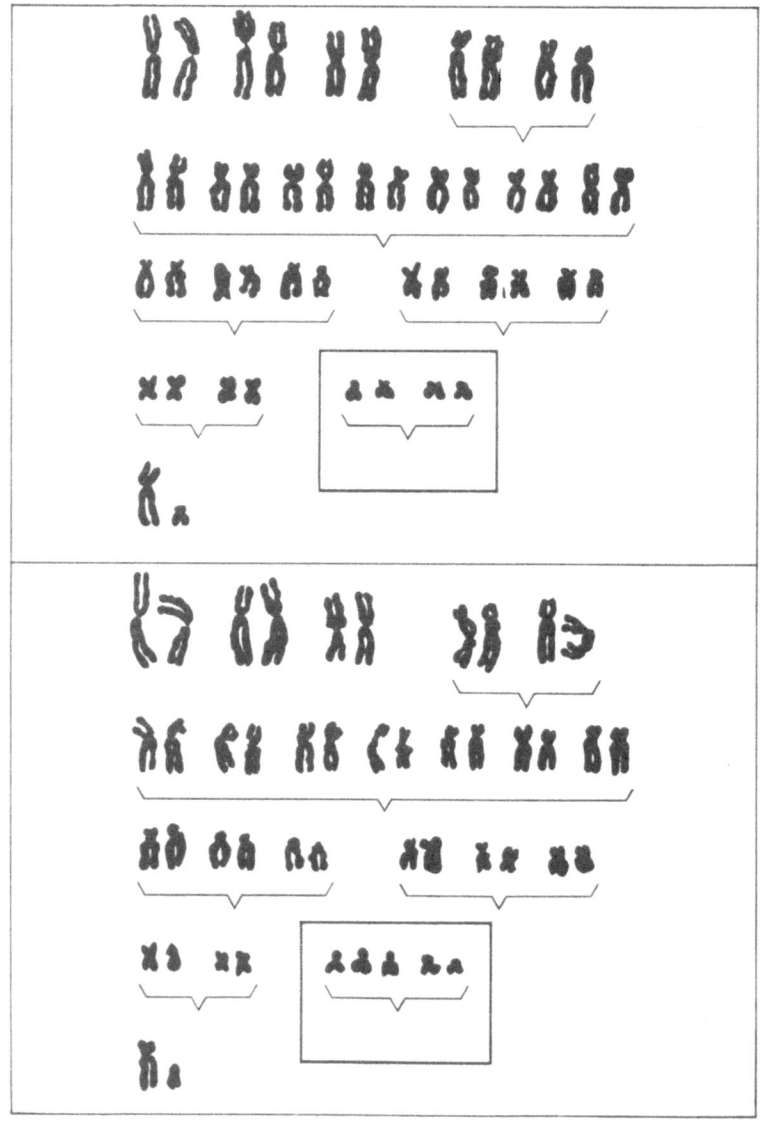

FIGURE 46 Diagram of normal chromosome pattern (left) contrasted with 21-Trisomy seen in mongolism.

occur with corresponding chromosome totals of 47, 48 and 49. An absence of the Y chromosome pattern of Turner's syndrome (dwarf woman, rudimentary ovaries, webbing of neck – only occasionally mental defect) shows a corresponding chromosome total of 45.

With many mental illnesses, including those of manic-depressive psychosis and schizophrenia, the exact genetic mechanisms of inheritance are still obscure and therefore invite conflicting hypotheses. A single dominant gene of irregular manifestation has been postulated for manic-depressive psychosis, and theories for both dominant and recessive modes of inheritance are advanced for schizophrenia.

Apart from this influence of the genes themselves, including the mutations they may undergo, their vehicles as a whole may show abnormality. These abnormalities constitute the chromosome anomalies. Each normal germ-cell, sperm or ovum, carries within it the haploid or half-number of chromosomes (23). Of these, 22 are autosomes and one is the sex chromosome. In the case of the sperm, this sex chromosome is designated either Y or X; in the ovum the sex chromosome is designated X.

At fertilization therefore the normal zygote will acquire the full complement or diploid number of chromosomes (46). Of these, 44 will be autosomes and arranged as homologous pairs, and two will be sex chromosomes. Where a sperm bearing the Y chromosome has fertilized the ovum, the resulting offspring will be male (XY); where a sperm bearing the X chromosome has succeeded, the offspring will be female (XX).

A significant proportion of mentally defective criminals have been found to carry an extra Y chromosome. This fact suggests the possibility that a gene for aggressive or criminal behaviour might be carried on the Y chromosome.

Yet another chromosome anomaly results in the 'cri du chat' syndrome. Here a substantial part of chromosome No. 4 or No. 5 is missing. The newborn infant is mentally defective and displays facial stigmata which include palpebral fissures sloping downwards from the medial to the lateral canthus. The infant's characteristic cry – like the wailing of a cat in distress – gives the syndrome its curious name.

Sometimes two or more races of cells which differ in their chromosome pattern will co-exist throughout the body. These are known as mosaics and have clearly taken origin subsequent to the initial fertilization of the ovum.

Genetic influence is further evident in the interesting correlation of physique with mental constitution. Kretschmer (1936) classified temperament according to his body-builds of pyknic, asthenic (leptosomatic), athletic and dysplastic types. More recently, Sheldon introduced his anthropometric technique of somatotyping according to the three basic components of endomorphy (predominance of gut and viscera), mesomorphy (predominance of muscle and bone) and ectomorphy (predominance of linearity). Each basic component is associated with a corresponding temperament. After appropriate measurements have been taken, an individual is rated for each basic component, according to a seven-point scale.

Kretschmer's and Sheldon's work emphasize the genetic correlation of both manic-depressive psychosis and cyclothymia with the endomorphic (pyknik) physique, and both schizophrenia and the schizoid personality with the ectomorphic (asthenic) physique (fig. 47).

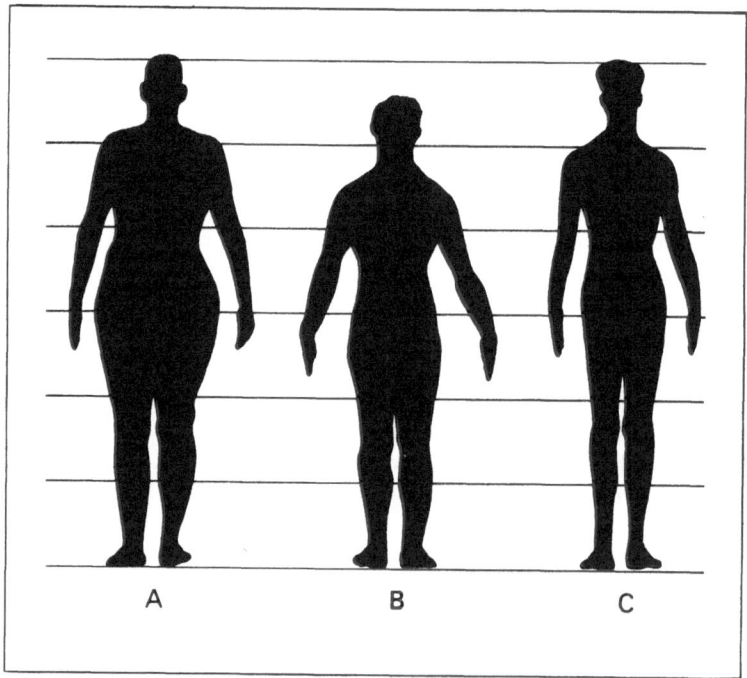

A   B   C

FIGURE 47 Sheldon's anthropometric classification (*a*) endomorph (*b*) mesomorph (*c*) ectomorph. These body builds can be correlated with temperament and predisposition to mental illness.

CHILD DEVELOPMENT

Three distinct but interacting factors determine the way that the newborn will develop through infancy, childhood and adolescence to eventually achieve adult life. These are the factors of heredity at conception, the factors of intrauterine existence, and those of the environment which exert their influence after birth. With these interacting factors it is scarcely surprising that no two children can develop exactly alike, nor that the change from infant to child or from child to adult is in any way uniform. This leads to great personal variation in interpretation of stimuli in the adult and a similar variation in the behaviour that results.

From conception, the foetus is equipped with its own highly specific genetic pattern, some of which may determine the mental behaviour of the individual throughout life. In some instances abnormal behaviour will be closely determined at conception, as exemplified by the chromosome trisomy of mongolism. In other instances the evidence suggests that the genetic endowment, though not defining exactly the developmental pattern of the child, will none the less predispose to a particular manifestation, e.g. manic depressive psychosis. The hazards of intrauterine life or of the birth process itself may result in damage to the infant's brain or interfere with normal cerebral development.

During infancy and the early years of life, the social environment is vital for the normal development of the child. Of particular importance is the parent-child relationship, since the environment of the infant is exclusively of the home. The prevailing atmosphere of parents and siblings mould the responses and behaviour of the child. Of particular importance is the demonstration to the infant of love, of happiness, of attention and of security. In childhood on the other hand the environment will include not only the home but also the school and the combination of both these influences induce further important developments in the growing child.

It appears that in the industrially underdeveloped countries the social factors of poor environment, undernourishment and lack of mental stimulation are of primary importance in adversely determining development, whereas in the industrially developed countries where social conditions are of a higher standard the genetic factors assume greater importance. It is clear that the more simple achievements are usually determined by the genetic factors, while environmental ones determine the more complex skills.

For example, the age at which children learn to speak simple phrases of two to three words is not related to social class, while the acquisition of full sentences is much more closely tied to the social class into which they have been born.

Normal development does not proceed regularly, nor are the various skills acquired at the same rate. In one child, motor skills may develop ahead of the full use of language, while in another the acquisition of the two skills may be reversed, yet neither of these patterns be considered any less normal than the other.

Early development in infancy takes place against the background of the attachment for the mother. Physical contact between the infant and its mother provides a vital means of communication. Experience is first acquired by exploration of the external world by the infant's mouth. Gradually the growing infant's need for sustained close contact with its mother is decreased and the area of potential experience for the child becomes increased enormously in space. Experience in play, particularly in play with children of the same age is an important aspect. The development of thought-processes in infancy go hand-in-hand with this growing experience and is considered in more detail on p. 226.

The use of developmental assessment tests was pioneered by the American psychologist Arnold Gesell and modern assessment tests are based upon his work. He divided developmental skills into motor adaptive, language and personal-social. He established norms for each of these skills against which any child can be assessed compared with children of the same age. The procedure is only accurate over the age of about two to three years, but below that age gross instances of deviation from normality can still be assessed. For language development, the majority of two-year-olds use single and isolated words, but by three years old two- to three-word phrases are the rule.

While it is relatively easy to assess developmental skills, it is far more difficult to find objective evidence on which to assess emotional maturity. In the newborn, emotion is limited to the response to deprivation, pain and frustration. The first expression of pleasure, often in the presence of the mother, usually occurs within the first two months. By six months the child shows different and defined reactions to anger, fear and disgust. While fear is first experienced within the first few months, by the age of two years it becomes related to more specific causes, and this phase may continue into the school age.

While the process of learning and development is one that continues throughout the life of the individual, it is the school period in which the greater amount of *formal* learning is acquired, and the development of learning skills is at a maximum during that period. This in turn is followed by the period of adolescence.

SENSATION

The term sensation refers to the elementary and primary input of information concerning the animal's internal and external environment. Sensation from the internal environment is derived from the interoceptors, numerous and widely different types of receptors scattered within the body (p. 66); while sensations of the external environment are derived via the exteroceptors distributed over the body surface. The interoceptors include chemoreceptors, baroreceptors and proprioceptors. The exteroceptors include the network of end-organs of the skin, and the special sense organs of sight, hearing, smell and taste. The majority of these special end-organs show characteristic histological appearances. The mechanism by which the receptors convert the stimuli into nerve impulses and the pathway by which these impulses produce sensation are described on page 66 et seq.

Sensation depends on the impulses from the receptors reaching the contralateral cortex and with the exception of smell are relayed to the cortex via the thalamus; general sensations are located in the post central gyrus; vision in the calcarine fissure, adjacent cortex and encroaching on the lateral side of the occipital pole; hearing in the middle third of the superior temporal gyrus and smell and taste in the deeper parts of the brain around the region of the uncus or upper operculum of the Sylvian fissure. The spatial distribution for general sensation shows a point to point representation in the post central gyrus with the impulses from the lower portions of the body represented in the upper part of the gyrus.

PERCEPTION

Perception is concerned with the meaningful interpretation of the information which reaches the sensory cortex.

Perception is one of the functions that lies within the general grouping of cognition, which embraces all modes of knowing. It thus also includes thinking, reasoning, remembering, imagining and judgement in addition to perceiving. Perception is profoundly influenced by factors

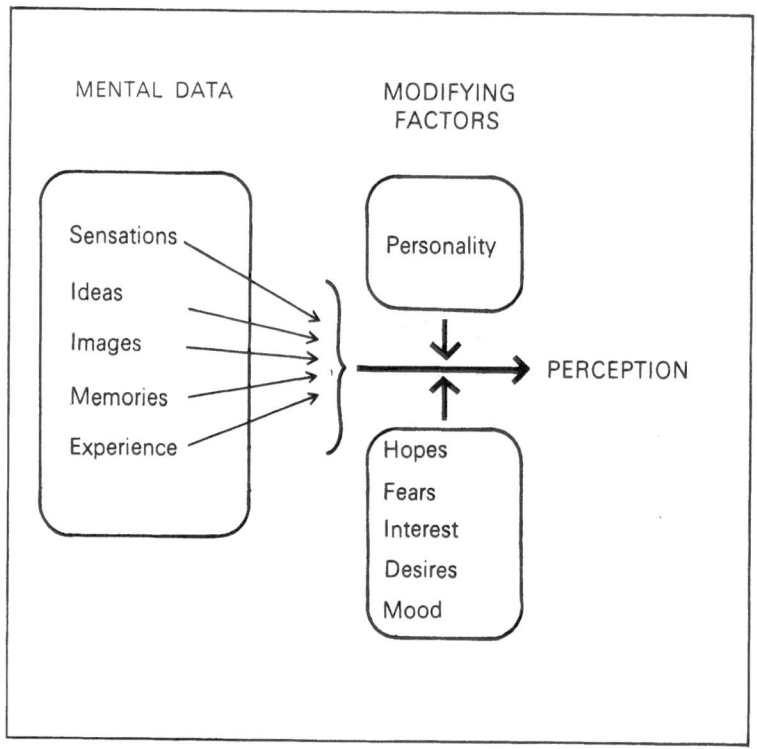

FIGURE 48 The basis of perception.

of personality. It is equally profoundly influenced by the prevailing mood (fig. 48).

Sensory information from the exteroceptors leads to interpretation of the surrounding environment, that from the interoceptors to the appreciation of the individual's own physical self – the body image. Clinically the parietal lobe of the cerebrum is overwhelmingly important in those conditions where disturbances of body image occur and where spatial disorientation exists. The reliability and completeness of the knowledge derived from sensory impressions depends not only on the accuracy of the sensory information but also on the ability of the individual to interpret this information. Perception cannot embrace all the impulses that are constantly impinging on the sense organs and thus there is a process of selection. This selection involves both the process of attention, considered below, and factors based on the emotive powers of the component portions of the whole. Among these interest plays a dominant part. Recent experimental evidence suggests that certain aspects of perception have an innate basis but that learning, that is experience derived from previous stimuli, plays a vital role. For example, in young infants the innate aspects of perception are demonstrated by different levels of interest in different patterns. Perception can be surprisingly accurate as demonstrated in perceptual constancy, i.e. the stability of external objects in respect of size, shape, form etc. despite variations in the viewing conditions. On the other hand the existence and form of classical optical illusions, i.e. distortions of perception (p. 167), imply that our interpretation of sensory input is conditioned by our past experience. Indeed our perception usually takes the form of a calculated prediction of the best fit of the input sensory information to our past related experiences. The closer the fit to previous experience, the greater the chance of perceptual accuracy leading to perceptual constancy of objects in respect of size, shape etc. On the other hand when our experience is limited or inconstant, the probability of success of prediction is reduced and wrong responses may result. This is subsequently built into the process of perception as a further aspect of learning, i.e. learning by mistakes.

Thus perception can probably be regarded as a functional activity based on input, experience and probability.

The object perceived is an inseparable part of the function of perceiving which in its turn includes all aspects of the total process that we call living.

ATTENTION AND SLEEP

The process of conscious perception cannot include the total cacophony of information impinging on the sensory receptors at any one time. Even in a single perceptual field involving only one of the exteroceptors, a limited area becomes the scene of attention – the focus for active concern. This attention may be voluntary, particularly when the person is involved in a goal directed task (p. 121) and the term concentration implies the ability to maintain voluntary attention on one focus. On the other hand, attention may be involuntary, based on the intensity, form, movement, etc., of the input stimulus.

By its very nature, attention implies a concentration upon a limited number of input stimuli and it is usually considered that the maximum number of objects which can be covered at one time (the 'attention span', i.e. that number perceived at a single glance) is of the order of six to

eight. These may be tightly grouped or widely distributed over the perceptual field. The process of attention is closely related to the process
of consciousness. In the animal kingdom a balance exists between a
state of 'arousal' and a state of 'rest' and this balance is responsible
for the sleep-wake rhythm. This constitutes a regular cycle during
which periods of wakefulness alternate with periods of sleep although
the exact pattern varies from one person to another. But sleep and wake
are really isolated portions of a more extensive continuum of sympathetic
and parasympathetic nervous system interactions. Excitation (attention) lies at one extreme of the continuum, sleep at the other, and the
state of relaxation in between. The sleep mechanism is considered in
more detail on p. 52. But, apart from this normal continuum of attention, diminished alertness occurs in various pathological states including stupor and coma (p. 171).

Since the fundamental characteristic of the animal kingdom is a
response to variations in the environment, it is scarcely surprising that
it is unusual stimuli that lead to the greatest level of attention. Conversely, monotonous repetitive stimuli reduce attention, particularly
when coupled with interoceptive impulses from a full stomach. Hence
the characteristic lack of perception which is so notable a feature of
early afternoon lectures.

Attention is an active process in which selection plays a major role
and depends not only on innate factors in the individual but also on
training and education. This selection constitutes 'interest'.

Interest is one of the essential factors in accurate perception; i.e.
the formation of appropriate memory engrams (see below) and subsequent matching of the new stimuli to these existing traces.

In spite of popular belief, attention cannot be divided. We can, in
fact, attend to but one thing at a time – though this like one's motor-car
may consist of many parts. By a very rapid switching back and forth
of attention, it is possible at a party, for example, to listen and seemingly
attend to two conversations at once. One's attention, however, is still
undivided. Each brief fragment of the conversation which has required
full attention is later mentally reconnected in its appropriate context to
produce the substance of the two conversations simultaneously overheard.

MEMORY

Since perception depends not only on the reception of sensory impulses, but also on the matching of these with past experience, it is

clear that memory – the storage of sensory information – is a vital component of perception.

It is important to distinguish between short-term and long-term memory storage processes. The short-term memory storage processes decay within a period which can be measured in seconds to hours and disrupted by mechanical, electroconvulsive and other intense stimuli (cf. the amnesia of concussion). Short-term memory is necessary for the daily routine of ordinary life, e.g. memorizing a telephone number for a period long enough to dial it. Short-term memory can be shown to be a necessary stage in the process by which long-term memory is formed. The content of long-term memory is derived from a selection from short-term memory.

The first process in memory formation is registration. This requires attention to the relevant material. Whether the attention need be active is still not resolved, though it is clear that memory formation is facilitated by conscious attempts at 'memorizing', i.e. an active process of attention.

Memory formation implies the storage of some form of trace within the central nervous system; for this trace the term 'engram' has been coined. Thus the second process in memory formation is the phase of retention. This consists of the laying down of an engram. More accurately, this process involves the formation of two consecutive and different types of engram when both short- and long-term memory are involved. There is as yet no exact knowledge of the nature of either of these engrams. Synaptic changes that facilitate the passage of subsequent nerve impulses are favoured. This phenomena of synaptic facilitation has not yet been explained. The theories include alterations of the cellular ribonucleic acid leading to the formation of new intracellular proteins; distortion of the lipid component of the cell membrane which then links with genetically determined intracellular protein; grouping together of postsynaptic receptors; facilitatory secretions from the postsynaptic membrane onto the presynaptic membrane. Such synaptic changes may lead to the development of reverberatory electrical circuits in the brain, involving the potentiation of a single nerve impulse by its rapid passage round a circuit (p. 51).

Whatever the neurochemical processes involved – and in the final analysis all central nervous system processes must result from neurochemical changes – we know something of the neuroanatomy of the memory process. Bilateral ablation of or damage to the hippocampus has a devastating effect on engram formation for short-term memory, as does destruction of the temporal lobes of the cortex for long-term memories. Although the complicated mechanisms of memory for man involve certain cortical areas, ablation experiments in lower animals have demonstrated that primitive types of memory trace can exist at subcortical levels. Even in *Homo sapiens* some of the more stereotyped memories involved, as for example in motor activities, appear to be retained at subcortical level.

While sensory impulses to the cortex are unilateral and directed to a specific zone, the work of Lashley and Sperry has suggested that different parts of the cerebral cortex are functionally interchangeable for memory storage and that the engram is stored bilaterally. Anatomical crosslinks between the two halves of the brain, particularly via the corpus callosum are vital for this bilateral memory retention. While some form of dominance of one cerebral hemisphere exists over the other – corresponding to 'eyedness' and 'handedness' – recent experiments suggest that the type of memory retained differs between the two hemispheres. The dominant hemisphere – the left one in a right-handed and right-eyed person – appears to retain a more organised type of trace. The non-dominant hemisphere concerns itself more with the random pattern of art forms.

Coupled with this difference in engram formation in the two hemispheres is a difference in function. Thus it appears that the dominant hemisphere is predominantly used for analytical thinking, such as language and mathematics, and it processes information sequentially. The non-dominant hemisphere on the other hand is probably responsible for the artistic talents, for our orientation in space, the recognition of faces and body awareness. It processes information in a simultaneous fashion and more diffusely.

In parallel with these new ideas about the site and nature of the engram have come other new ideas about its form. Previously a form equivalent to the traditional photograph had been postulated in which point to point representation existed. Recently it has been suggested that the form may be analogous to the hologram in which all parts of the original are represented at all points of the engram. This new concept accords well with the experiments of Lashley and the ability to recall a total and complicated memory on the basis of a fragment. For example, the pattern of trees on a skyline may bring back to memory the whole of the events of a holiday previously forgotten, even though the memory when evoked involves other sensations than those of sight.

There is at the moment negligible information on the factors which lead to the selection of material for transfer from the short term to the long-term memory store, or on the method by which this selection is accomplished. It does, however, appear that items which produce emotional responses are more likely to be transferred to the long-term storage process.

The final phase of memory is the process of recall, by which stored engrams are brought back for the process of perception. The stimulus to recall is frequently a sensory input similar to the one which leads to the formation of the original trace. The quantum of this stimulus may well be minute in relation to the extent of the recall it excites. It is clear that the process of remembering is not an exact one. Events as recalled are distorted according to the attitudes, interests and emotions of the individual. The psychology of testimony concerns itself greatly with such distortions of memory and the means by which quite false memories can be implanted. The results of studies under hypnosis suggest that much of the selection occurs at the recall phase and the Freudian mechanism of repression (p. 155) plays an important role in this distortion of memory. However, it appears probable that differences at the stage of engram formation also play a part. The corollary of a memory process is a forgetting process. It appears that forgetting results fundamentally from interference between the associations that are carried in the storage system. This interference may be proactive (i.e. as a result of an input occurring previously) or retroactive (i.e. as a result of a subsequent input). The greater the similarity between the two, the greater the interference and the more chance of forgetting occurring (retroactive inhibition).

LEARNING, IMPRINTING AND CONDITIONING

There is no universally acceptable definition of learning. It may be broadly defined as any change in behaviour that occurs as a result of experience, including maturational growth processes and such temporary aberrations as fatigue. The fundamental aspect of learning is the formation of an appropriate long-term memory engram and its recall.

There are three known psychological models for learning procedures. The first of these, imprinting, occurs during the first few hours in an animal's life and is seen in its most marked and relatively irreversible form in birds. By the process of imprinting young animals learn to recognize the characteristics of their parents early in life. It is now clear that imprinting shows many similarities with the properties of learning in other contexts. However, since this initial learning procedure of attachment to the parent in turn gives a stable base for subsequent development its importance should not be underrated. The second model of learning is the respondent or classical conditioning first studied by Pavlov.

Pavlovian conditioning demonstrates that if simultaneously with an unconditional stimulus (meat in a dog's mouth) a second stimulus (bell ringing) is presented, the normal response (salivation by the dog) elicited by the unconditioned stimulus can, after due repetition, be obtained by the conditioned stimulus (bell ringing) alone.

A conditioned reflex only develops if the conditioned stimulus (bell) is given with the unconditioned stimulus (food) or before it. The closer the two approximate in time and the more pleasurable the response to the unconditioned stimulus, the more rapid is the conditioning process. The build-up of a conditioned reflex is a summation of responses until a threshold is reached. If the unconditioned stimulus is sometimes omitted, then conditioning will be either delayed or even inhibited (internal inhibition). Substitution of a punishment instead of the reward produces a direct inhibition of conditioning (fig. 49). If the unconditioned stimulus is stopped, the conditioned reflex ultimately disappears (extinction). However, after an adequate period of rest the animal will again produce a weak conditioned response to the unconditioned stimulus (spontaneous recovery). The reintroduction of the unconditioned stimulus will produce increasingly stronger conditioned responses until a maximum is again reached (reinforcement). Reinforcement may be applied at any stage of conditioning to strengthen the conditioned response to its maximum.

The classical (respondent) type of conditioning is probably relevant to aspects of emotional behaviour as, for example, the conditioning by fear to a former neutral situation.

The third learning model is instrumental or operant conditioning associated with the name of Skinner.

In operant conditioning, as opposed to classical conditioning, the frequency of the response increases if it is instrumental in achieving a goal, i.e. the animal must itself make an appropriate voluntary response to the stimulus.

Operant conditioning may be effected by either a response reward system (positive reinforcement) or by some form of punishment (e.g. electric shock to the skin) when the appropriate response is not made, (negative reinforcement or avoidance conditioning). Both aspects have been used experimentally in animals and form situations for testing modification by drugs.

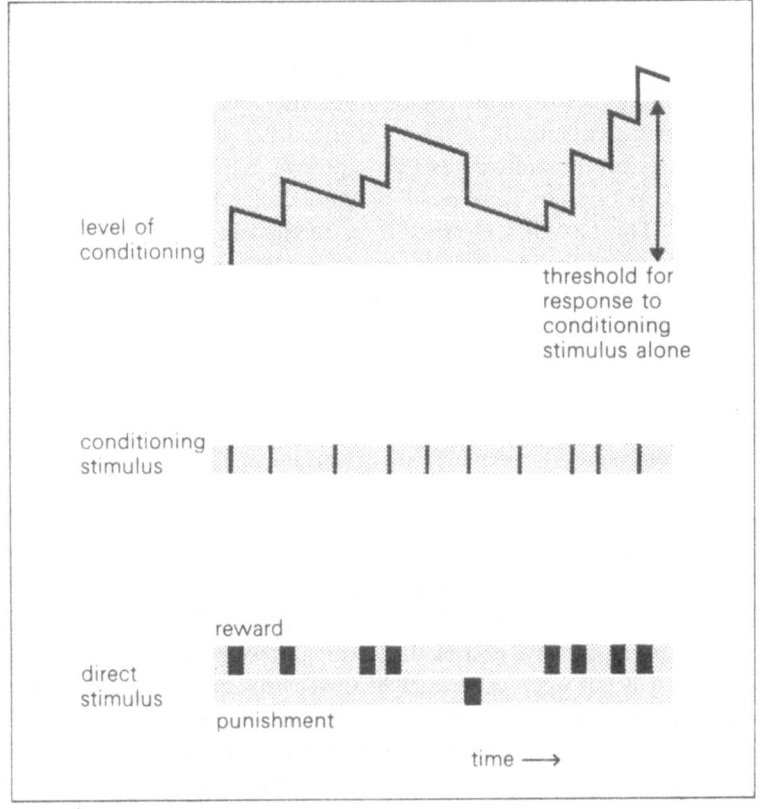

FIGURE 49 Representation of the reactions during the development of a conditioned reflex.

The mechanism of conditioning must be regarded as a stepwise process within the brain. First the beginning of the specific unconditioned stimulus must be distinguished – since conditioning is applied at the same time as the unconditioned stimulus or before it. Next, there must be reception of the unconditional stimulus and recognition of the significance between this and the specific stimulus. This mechanism must involve a time appreciation, since the more the two are separated in time, the slower is the recognition of significance. This mechanism must allow for inhibitory stimuli to negate the effect if a punishment is substituted for the reward. Once significance is recognized, a mechanism must transfer this information for long-term storage (long-term memory).

Little is known about the mechanisms involved, although it would appear likely that these are the result of alterations in the patterns of reverberating circuits. It has been suggested that the electrical changes accompanying the arousal reaction represent some form of scanning device searching out patterns of significance in the involved cortical activity. The fact that pleasurable or unpleasant sensations are desirable for conditioning suggests that the limbic system plays a part.

Operant conditioning provides an essential mechanism for teaching. Both positive and negative reinforcement techniques are used and the evidence available suggests that individuals can be distinguished who respond best either to positive or negative conditioning.

Although it is possible to analyse the learning process under experimental conditions, the natural forms of learning in life are probably more complicated. For example imitation (in children), experience, and trial and error procedures – all natural forms of learning – involve perceptual, respondent and operant conditioning processes.

Learning continues throughout life, though the most active period occurs in youth. Whilst both in animals and in man 'teaching' by peers is an important aspect of the learning process, the greater part of learning depends upon experience of the environment. In infancy and childhood play proves particularly valuable in this respect. With children in the early stage of learning, there is specificity in the learned topic (concrete learning), for example the child learns that one particular type of food is palatable but at later stages the child will derive more general and abstract knowledge from the presentation of further specific information (conceptual learning). (This is considered in more detail under Thoughts, and Ideas, p. 119.) Overall there are various constraints on the total learning ability. These include total capacity (intelligence p. 130) and the ability of different individuals to respond to different stimuli.

LANGUAGE

Language consists of a series of arbitrary symbols that are used to communicate ideas, emotions and wishes to others. In speaking, these will be symbols of thought. In writing, they will be symbols (written words) of symbols (spoken words) of thoughts. Such symbols carry meanings which are either 'denotative', i.e. that label an action or object, or 'connotative', i.e. that delineate certain qualities of the action or object. Connotative symbols by their nature involve attitudinal overtones.

The language of primitive communities is in spoken form and involves relatively few individual sounds – phonemes (not to be confused with the term 'phoneme' introduced by Wernicke for the hallucinatory voices heard in schizophrenia) that are grouped to form a large number of words (morphones). As human society develops it produces written language. For both forms of language there are rules of word order and modification, prefix and suffix use that constitute the grammar. Like all aspects of language, those of grammar are arbitrary though fixed for any specific language form. The speech centre in the brain which is responsible for the production and use of language lies in the frontal area of the non-dominant cortex and association areas have been described in relation to it. The age at which speech develops suggests that imitation of parents is an important aspect of the early learning process, while later language development shows a marked resemblance to positive operant conditioning.

The emotional tones which ramify throughout the sounds of spoken speech are of particular importance and provide a powerful, if less obvious, mechanism of communication. The German saying '*Der Ton macht die Musik*' (It is the tone that makes the music) is never more true than in the contribution of the emotional tones to speech. 'It's not what you say but the way that you say it' emphasizes this same point.

THOUGHT, IDEAS, IMAGINATION

The thought process involves a train of ideas, initiated by the existence of a concept or directed towards solution of a problem. The fundamental unit of thought is the idea. Idea is the general term used for a process not directly involved in perception but incorporating knowing, remembering, reasoning or judging. Ideas include both images which are central reconstructions of sensory experiences and those which represent a more symbolic process.

The least controlled form of thinking is fantasy which occurs in certain forms of dreaming at night and also in day dreams. Fantasy consists of a series of images which lead on from one to another. Freud considered that these were largely directed from the unconscious mind and represent wish fulfilment involving repressed material.

Problem-solving and reality-related thinking, on the other hand, normally involve a controlled but complex pattern of response. It is mediated by language (p. 119) or by symbolic codes such as those that are involved in mathematics. It therefore contrasts with fantasy, which need not necessarily include language or symbol.

Childhood thought development involves two stages: concrete thinking and conceptual thinking. In the earlier stages of concrete thought only ideas of a specific nature are involved. Those of an abstract nature are not. For example the child recognizes the particular household pet and its reactions, but cannot argue from this to the reactions of similar animals or mammals in general. It is scarcely surprising that organic brain lesions tend to impair the more abstract forms of thought and that concrete thinking is the last to be lost in arteriosclerotic brain damage.

As conceptual thought develops specific events or objects are compared and matched. Their common properties are abstracted to form a concept which will then be applied to all events or objects of similar general type. The ability of *Homo sapiens* to form concepts and to express these in symbolic terms (language) enables him to think imaginatively, solve problems, and to construct projects of a variety and complexity far beyond the limits of his normal environment, not only in terms of space but also time. The process involves assimilation, i.e. the absorption and integration of new experience into existing concepts, or accommodation – the modification of old concepts or the formation of new ones in response to the conflicting new experiences.

The Swiss psychologist Piaget has studied the time relationships of the thought process development in children and considers that there are five stages:

1. Sensorimotor stage (0–2 yrs). The infant's behaviour is determined predominantly by conditioned reflexes with negligible reasoning ability.
2. Egocentric stage (2–4 yrs). During this the thought process is entirely self-centred. Any concepts formed are very primitive.

3. Intuitive stage (4–7 yrs). The child is capable of some rudimentary form of classification without being able to describe its basis. He begins to appreciate numbers.
4. Concrete operations stage (7–11 yrs). The child handles a variety of differing logical operations but relies largely on practical situations to achieve a solution.
5. Conceptual operations stage (11–15 yrs). True abstract thinking is now achieved and this will extend into the hypothetical.

INSTINCTS AND DRIVES

The general term conation is applied to all those psychological processes which are involved in acting, willing or striving. Together with cognition and affect it formed the triad of primary psychological functions postulated by Aristotle. It covers all the determinants and mental concomitants of action whether these are purposeful or impulsive. For some aspects of human behaviour there is a clear direction towards some goal. The state which arouses and maintains the individual's activity in this specific direction is known as the motive. This motive is frequently one of the primary drives, common to all the animal kingdom and having a clearly defined physiological basis. These primary drives include hunger, thirst, sex and escape from danger. Each primary drive has a biological function of preserving the individual or the species.

The primary drives are inborn and are probably the only true instincts that exist in the animal kingdom. They should not be confused with the innate patterns that are used for their expression. The expression of these primary drives however is greatly modified by learning and particularly is this so in humans. The drives are directed towards a specific end or goal. They ideally culminate in consumatory behaviour as for example eating or copulation.

These primary drives are supplemented in humans by other motives. Some of these may be regarded as non-physiological extensions of the primary drive, e.g. greed cf. hunger. The majority of these secondary drives or motives are the products of learning. They play an important part in human motivation and many are related to the preservation of social status or self respect (e.g. keeping up with the Joneses). A heirarchical arrangement of drives has been suggested with the primary (animal) drives at the bottom and above them, in ascending order, the learned human motives. A higher level of maturation comes into being only when lower ones are already satisfied. However, the existence of starving geniuses in garrets casts doubts on the universal application of this idea.

Apart from these general motives that have a clearly defined goal – even if at times somewhat obscured – human behaviour is also governed by impulses. These are sudden decisions for action, often irrational in nature and deviating from the previous objective. An individual who makes no move on impulse, though single-minded, is often boring and an unattractive personality. One who relies solely on impulse will be so scatterbrained and unpredictable as to be almost impossible as a colleague or friend.

Both drives and impulses are analysed and equated with the conscience of the individual. The conscience contains the moral restrictions and ideals of the person. It is derived largely from the assimilation of the moral standards of his elders and with particular reference to his parents. When actions are carried out on the basis of drives and impulses which are contrary to the principles upheld by conscience, guilt is felt and may be extremely painful. The analytical schools of both Jung and Freud (p. 153) were directly concerned with drives and motives, and in particular those which had their origins in the unconscious mind.

The energy which causes the instinctual drive to lead to action is termed the libido. In Jung's original sense this covered the general energy associated with any instinctual force: it was Freud who gave it the more restricted sexual connotation.

THE AFFECT

It is difficult to offer any adequate definition of affect. Originally one of the triad of psychological functions proposed by Aristotle it signifies the subject's inner feelings at the time, as manifested by mood.

Affect is a normal concomitant of all interactions between the individual and his surroundings. When a drive, either primary or secondary, is satisfied then the feeling-tone of pleasure is experienced. Displeasure on the other hand, arises when the consumation of the drive is frustrated or obstructed. Emotions can be fundamentally divided into two classes, those with a pleasant and those with an unpleasant feeling-tone.

The pleasant feeling-tones include joy, gladness, euphoria, happiness, elation, exaltation and ecstasy. Although each of these emotions has a connotation of pleasure, there are qualitative as well as quantitative differences between them. For example the term elation implies a unified state of joy in which any aspect of disharmony is excluded; exaltation is joy with an implied grandeur attached to it; ecstasy a mystical sense. Euphoria with its general sense of well-being should not be regarded as an emotion.

Among the emotions with an unpleasant feeling-tone should be mentioned sadness, sorrow, grief, fear, dread, guilt, anger. These reactions are normally associated with the deprivation of some object held in high esteem, or of the frustration of a goal-orientated drive. Their intensity varies from one person to another under like stimuli. Variations in the emotional responses to stimuli, either pleasant or unpleasant, form important aspects of the personality (p. 126). Just as the affective response to a given stimulus can vary from one individual to another so the response in any one individual can vary. Minor fluctuations of mood occurring in normal healthy persons provide an interesting feature of everyday life. Sometimes a valid reason will account for the mood swing but many are spontaneous and inexplicable. These minor mood changes occurring from day to day cause but little inconvenience. Mild upswings are accepted pleasurably and even thankfully while mild downswings are dealt with by such harmless antidotes as an early night to bed or an agreeable evening with convivial company. It is only when the amplitude of the changes of affect, or their duration, become too great that abnormality is accepted. Within this framework of mood-swings a series of mood-reactions may be experienced, including perplexity, irritability or indifference which are related to the more common affective states.

These psychological affective reactions are associated with physiological changes. The physiological responses are dependent upon two antagonistic systems which have been termed the ergotropic (action producing) and the trophotropic (assimilation-recovery) systems. Anatomically, these correspond to the sympathetic and para-sympathetic systems respectively.

The primary site for emotional response appears to be the limbic system. Sensory afferents from the normal sensory tracts reach the limbic system via collaterals to the reticular formation (p. 86).

The limbic system (fig. 50) consists of the limbic lobe of the palaeo-cortex (cingulate gyrus, hippocampal gyrus, induseum griseum and area enterorhinalis) and related subcortical nuclei (amygdaloid nucleus,

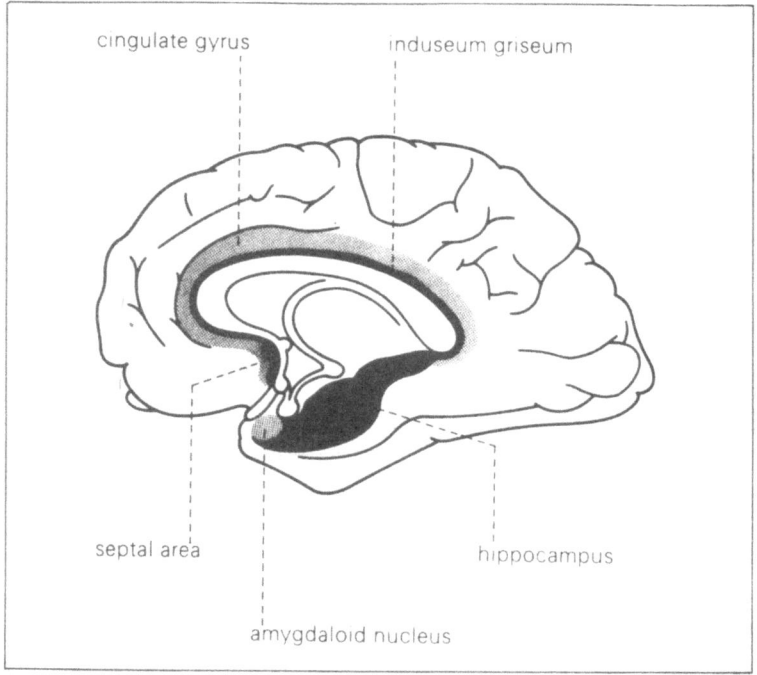

FIGURE 50 The component structures of the limbic system.

septal area and a few nuclei in the preoptic area) linked by the fornix system. The limbic system in lower animals forms a larger proportion of the fore-brain than in higher animals – due to the marked increase in the size of the neocortex in the latter (fig. 31, p. 72). Animal ablation and stimulation experiments suggest that some of the nuclei are facilitatory and some inhibitory, i.e. increase or reduce reactions of rage. The amygdaloid nuclei, anterior hippocampus, cingulate gyrus and portions of the frontal area are probably facilitatory, and the septal area and other portions of the frontal lobe are probably inhibitory. Stimulation of the hippocampus produces a general electrical discharge, and in conscious animals an interruption of spontaneous activity suggestive of a *petit mal* attack. During this reaction conditioned reflexes are absent. It would be unwise, however, to derive too much from such local ablation or stimulation experiments in view of the multiple interconnecting pathways within the system.

The nuclei of the limbic system are linked by a series of short and long fibre pathways which form reverberating circuits (Papez circuits). These link the inhibitory and excitatory components of the system with other brain areas. The main connections with neighbouring centres are:

(*a*) The hypothalamus via fornix, stria terminalis and ventral amygdaloid radiation (fig. 51).

(*b*) From hippocampus to mammillary body (via fornix), to anterior thalamic nuclei (mammillo-thalamic tract) then to cingulate cortex (via thalamo-cingulate radiation).

(*c*) A loop back to the hippocampus via the cingulum.

(*d*) With limbic nuclei of the mid-brain via the mammillary body.

(*e*) Afferent and efferent pathways between the limbic nuclei and the reticular formation both of the ipselateral and contralateral side, via the fornix and the medial fore-brain bundle.

In addition to the two controlling motor patterns of affective behaviour, the limbic system may also be responsible for the subjective

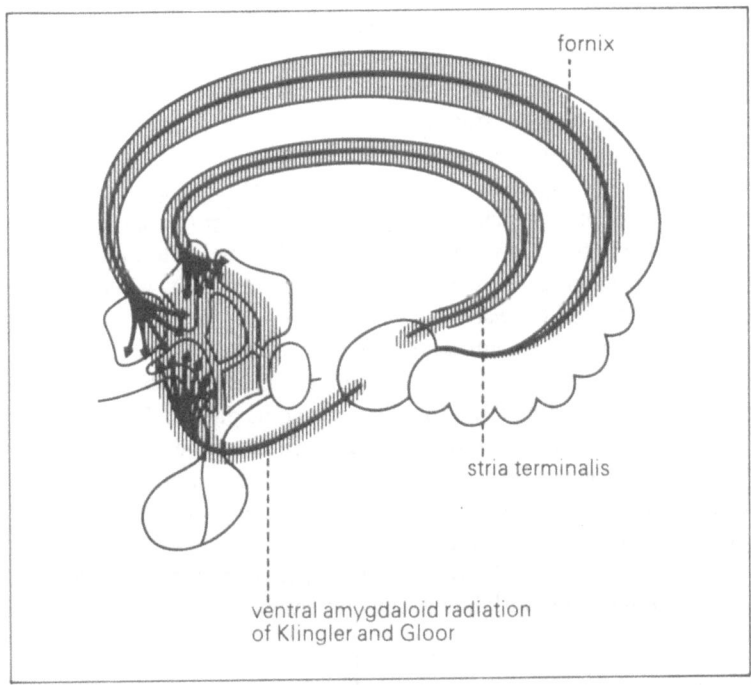

FIGURE 51 The pathways from the limbic system to the hypothalamus.

component of mood. If electrodes are implanted in various parts of the system, it is possible for an animal to give itself a mild electrical stimulus by pressing a lever. Depending upon the site of the electrodes, animals may stimulate themselves to the point of exhaustion, may avoid self-stimulation or may behave indifferently – suggesting different areas where the animal may obtain pleasurable or unpleasant affective sensations.

In lower animals, the emotional response to an external stimulus follows stereotyped pathways. In humans, conditioning plays an important role in the response – probably via fibre pathways from suppressor areas in the frontal cortex. The response is modified to correspond to learned patterns of behaviour – the 'thin veneer of civilization'.

Although little is known about the mechanism involved in the subjective component of mood, more is known of the way in which emotions alter the body activity. The linking structure is the reticular formation (p. 84), which joins together the limbic system, the hypothalamus, the cortex and the γ motor system for muscle tone. In consequence of this linking system, higher cortical activity, autonomic activity, endocrine activity and muscle tone all are directly affected by the sensory input. The body activity is modified for appropriate response to the external stimulus.

In addition to these more general body reactions to the emotions, specific motor responses occur in many individuals and again contribute to the features of personality. These include laughter (p. 144) and tears. Their exact relationship to the emotions is still far from clear for laughter may on occasion be associated with embarrassment while intense happiness can lead to 'tears of joy'.

The characteristic features of a person's emotional nature are at times referred to as the temperament, to include both the general prevailing quality of mood, its oscillations and its phases. Temperament in this sense forms an important subdivision of personality below and is in part genetically determined. Kretschmer and later Sheldon have considered temperament in relation to body build. The pyknic build (stocky build, equivalent to endomorph) is usually sociable but with mood swings (cyclothymic): the leptosomatic build (long and thin – ectomorph) is withdrawn, shy and eccentric.

PERSONALITY

No two persons can ever be exactly alike. Nor will the manner in which they think, feel, perceive or behave ever be an identical one. Each one of us will display our own special mark of personal uniqueness by which we are recognized and from which we are known. It is this very quality of personal uniqueness which constitutes what is meant when we speak of 'the personality' of an individual.

To attempt any formal definition of this intangible quality of personality can never be easy, nor will it prove to be a straightforward task. None of the definitions offered in the past can be said to be entirely satisfactory on all counts. Any attempted definition must embrace not only some unique facets and foibles which constitute the psychological make-up of the person in question, but also the interaction and response of these to the circumstances of the environment which constantly and continuously thrust themselves upon the individual throughout his existence. More simply stated, the ultimate criterion of an individual's personality will be the way that he habitually and so characteristically reacts to events and happenings in the world about him.

The structure of human personality is complex in the extreme and allows of an infinite number of variations. The personality is organized from a wealth of individual characteristics or traits, as, for example, such qualities as aggressiveness, timidity, assertiveness, frankness, shyness, secretiveness, sociability, selfishness, solitariness, persistence, irresponsibility and very many others. Thus the personality of any given individual could be visualized as an algebraic sum, in which the positives and negatives of individual traits have interacted to produce the final total. The traits themselves are relatively permanent and it is this fact that confers a constancy of quality to the personality of any person we may care to choose. With those whom we know well we have learnt to recognize the salient traits and to anticipate their interactions and we find ourselves able to predict with a remarkable degree of accuracy their behaviour and reactions. Indeed, should their reactions and conducts be found to differ in a manner totally foreign to our expectations, we might be profoundly shaken in our judgement of them and find it necessary to revise our whole concept of that person as an individual. Such incongruous behaviour, so out of character with the person we have always known, may well be a sign of organic cerebral disease as, for example, arteriosclerosis or intracranial tumour, or again may be observed with the personality changes which follow upon the organic cerebral damage of chronic alcoholism. In the natural process of ageing of the brain, a point is ultimately reached when the personality of the aged person becomes eroded and finally its structure is left but as a cartoon or caricature of its former, more youthful and robust self.

The formulation of human personality is determined by two essential factors, the contribution of heredity and the influence of the environment, each of which is complementary to the other. The genetic endowment, passed via the chromosomes of the germ cells from each parent, confers the potential mental and physical characteristics upon the new life. Thus, among many, the sex of the off-spring, its height and intelligence, its glandular composition and the highly important structure of the brain, will all, within crude limits, be determined for the new individual, to await modification by development and maturation under the subsequent influence of the environment. These inborn features play their vital role in the formulation of the new personality. Of especial interest in modern psychological medicine is their contribution to certain physical systems within the brain and spinal cord, most notably the limbic system (generation of emotion), the hypothalamus (homeostasis), the autonomic nervous system (expression of emotion) and the ascending reticular system (alerting of cerebral cortex).

The influence of the environment begins *in utero* and continues during the birth process itself. It will extend throughout the whole of the life of the individual concerned. Its greatest effects are observable in infancy and childhood, when the young personality is already emerging, but its influence is markedly evident throughout adolescence and is still active upon the mature personality of the adult when personal tragedy, sudden bereavement, material success, or chronic illness, can yet produce substantial changes in the underlying personality. In the growing child the environmental influence of home and family is of supreme importance. The moral and social settings, the presence or absence of love and security, the degrees of happiness and tolerance, the relationships with siblings or the life as an only child, all mould and modify the developing personality (p. 107). At a later stage, the situation at school, pressures from parents, relationships with teachers, acceptance or rejection by school-mates, continue to exert their important influence upon the growing personality. The experience of success or the acceptance of failure, the interactions with other personalities, stronger, weaker or just different from that of the child in question, the response to example or to indoctrination by others, particularly when strong feelings such as admiration, love, envy or hate are aroused, all provide environmental influences the effects of which may be felt for a lifetime in the mature personality of the adult.

The profound importance of personality in relation to living will at once be appreciated. Any individual who aspires to a life well-lived, in which such considerations as efficiency and success in the use of personal aptitudes, satisfaction and happiness are to prevail, must bring much critical appraisal and careful thought to factors of the environment. Though the selection of our parents remains denied to us, our choice of friends, marriage partner and daily occupation becomes of paramount significance. Employers too will devote themselves with advantage to selecting, as far as possible, the most suitable personality for the work involved, avoiding the situation of the square peg in the round hole, and to consider the interactions of this personality with other colleagues involved in any group or team activities. In vocational work, an identical approach by two individuals may attain widely differing degrees of success. Here yet again it is the nature of each individual which is at stake and emphasizes, as in so many spheres of life, that it is so frequently the personality of man – and not the method he employs – which furnishes the criterion of ultimate success.

CHARACTER

The term character implies an appraisal by others of the individual's personality on the basis of subjective criteria. In general these criteria include social, moral and ethical aspects of the motives, attitudes and behaviour that govern the response to the environment.

While the appraisal is subjective there is often close agreement between assessments made by different observers, particularly in terms of the strength or weakness of the character, i.e. the degree of organization of the response that is made by the individual.

The behaviour pattern on which others will assess the character depends not only on innate factors in the individual but also on a learning process, primarily in the social environment. This learning process involves in part imitation of parents and other respected adults, but the developing child and adolescent also develops an individual pattern often greatly influenced by his direct surroundings and friends.

GENDER IDENTITY

The gender identity of an individual is the sexual behaviour pattern, depending upon whether a male or female pattern is assumed.

that genetic factors (p. 103) are important, the effects of environmental factors, such as the mother's influence, the prevailing social conditions, and the acquisition of language play a most profound part in the development of intelligence.

Binet, who pioneered the testing of mental ability, regarded intelligence as a total combination of the qualities of reasoning, judgement and imagination, but others have regarded it in terms of the ability to undertake constructual thinking based on a clear aim. The ability to perceive relevant relationships and to educe correlates from these is an essential factor of intelligence.

From the practical point of view intelligence is often regarded as the essential quality that leads to success in academic or vocational tests. Yet by the very nature of examinations, this becomes a circular definition – 'Intelligence is what intelligence tests measure' and leading in turn to 'Intelligence tests measure intelligence'. Modern concepts of intelligence have fortunately moved far from their earlier, time-hallowed and stultified equivalents. The effects of this most necessary change are to be found no less within the field of psychological medicine than within the province of education.

For far too long the use of intelligence tests was overshadowed by the erroneous view that intelligence was an inherited characteristic of mind which could be measured with a reasonable degree of accuracy. Once determined and established by the intelligence quotient, it was considered that the best and most individual attention to schooling could do little to elevate the IQ more than a few notional points.

Too frequently, when a child's IQ was shown to be low and its lack of attainment of a corresponding order, that child would be tacitly accepted as being innately dull and little time and less effort would be spent in attempts to improve the situation for the child. The attainment of a high IQ has been said to be that which children who are good at doing intelligence tests may expect. In isolation, the IQ can be severely misleading.

Today, considerable doubt exists whether innate intelligence can ever be measured. Further doubt exists on the true nature of intelligence itself. Modern views emphasize the highly important part played by environment in the development of intelligence and in achievement, and family conditions are most likely to prove of maximum importance in individual scholastic achievement.

Studies by Stedman in the USA lay stress upon the importance of the home environment and an adequacy of nutrition in the intellectual development of the young child – in particular during the critical interval between the 12th and 30th months of life.

It is during this period of life that a child begins to develop language skills and from these emerge logical processes. It is during this period, according to Stedman, that most children develop the intellectual characteristics which they will display for life – verbal skills, memory habits and problem solving abilities – in other words, the criteria which via the IQ test society will forever judge him. The effects on the deprived child during this critical interval will manifest themselves in intellectual attainment and are of profound importance in the field of mental deficiency.

An opposing and highly controversial view of intelligence was advanced by Jensen. This postulated that some 80 per cent of intellectual capacity as established by the IQ was due to hereditary and only 20 per cent due to environment. Jensen's investigations have found

TABLE 5 A selection of intelligence tests

---

1. STANFORD-BINET (TERMAN AND MERRILL REVISION)
   Children below 7 yrs and Mentally Subnormal individuals.

2. WECHSLER-BELLEVUE (I and II)
   Adolescents and Adults
   (Largely superseded now by WAIS).

3. WECHSLER ADULT INTELLIGENCE SCALE (WAIS)
   Adults 16 yrs–75 + yrs.

4. WECHSLER INTELLIGENCE SCALE FOR CHILDREN (WISC)
   Children 5 yrs–15 yrs.

5. RAVEN'S PROGRESSIVE MATRICES
   For ages 6 yrs–65 yrs
   Often used in combination with a Vocabulary Test such as Mill Hill Vocabulary Test.

6. GOODENOUGH'S 'DRAW A MAN' TEST
   Children 4 yrs–10 yrs.

7. PORTEUS MAZE TEST
   Children 3 yrs–14 yrs
   'Adults' 15 yrs–17 yrs.

8. MERRILL-PALMER TEST
   Children 1½ yrs–6 yrs.

9. KOH'S BLOCK DESIGN TEST

---

support by Eysenck and the Jensen-Eysenck thesis has met substantial and at times bitter opposition throughout the scientific world.

Even if there is doubt about its validity, the intelligence quotient is an established and convenient index for the grading of intellectual ability. However, the limitations of the IQ must be fully appreciated and appropriate caution exercised in its determination and application. It is particularly important that the method of testing should not only involve tests for academic aptitude, but also practical tests involving the manipulation of concrete material, e.g. block designs etc. Most modern tests score these separately.

The tests consist of a series of tasks, graded in difficulty. Norms are determined for the relevant population, against which the subject's performance can be assessed. Without such standardized norms the tests are meaningless. It is important that the reliability and validity of the testing methods be determined before any new test is accepted. The tests currently available (Table 5) can be divided into those that can be given simultaneously to a group, e.g. Raven's 'progressive matrices', and those, usually more accurate but usually more time-consuming, which are given to individuals. The tests that are used most commonly now are the Stanford-Binet test in children, the Wechsler Adult Intelligence Scale (WAIS) and the Wechsler Intelligence Scale for Children (WISC).

JUDGEMENT

This is one of the factors in the character of an individual. It depends on the balance of several of the cognitive (p. 109) group of perceiving thinking, reasoning, remembering and imagining. It embraces the area of decision-making particularly when this involves the assessment and selection of alternative courses of action. Judgement can be said, with hindsight, to have been good when an appropriate selection of alternatives is made, but it is not always easy to determine the level of judgement in a person unless one is aided by hindsight. Judgement depends not only on the fundamental character of the individual but also on intellect coupled with adequate experience.

6

SOCIAL MAN

No man is an island sufficient unto himself. For better or worse, life will represent for him a complex and continuous system of interpersonal relationships with his fellow man. In the course of this endless sequence of social relationships, every individual exerts his personality upon those with whom he comes in contact – refining, coarsening, or in other ways modifying their reactions. At one and the same time, the behaviour of others reacting in turn upon the individual in question, influences, modifies and reinforces his own behaviour. It is doubtful whether the meeting of any two persons can ever leave either of them totally unchanged. Thus this two-way interchange formulates behaviour by the effect of interpersonal relationships. The study of the manner in which interpersonal relationships operate within the social structures organized by man constitutes the field of Social Psychology. From birth to death any one person finds himself operating within the setting of social groups. In number, such groups are countless and would include among them such diverse structures as the family, the team, the crowd, the committee, the social class and the nation.

Behaviour which occurs both inside and outside a social group is of special interest to the social psychologist. Why should a particular group have formed anyway? For what reason will an individual join one group yet actively avoid membership of another? How does the group influence their behaviour as individuals? How does each member behave towards the other members of the group, and also to the group itself? How do certain social groups behave towards other social groups? All these and many other questions can be posed in terms of group activities, and their answers when obtained provide us with an engaging insight into the vital interpersonal dynamics which characterise social man in his relationship with his own fellow creatures.

At this point, it would seem apposite to consider briefly certain of the allied Behavioural Sciences which relate so closely to social man. Hand in hand with Social Psychology is to be found the sister discipline of Sociology, and between these two sciences considerable overlap is evident. Since each may consider the same social manifestation from a somewhat different standpoint, it is unfortunate that discrepancies in terminology are encountered and the technical use of words in the classifications of these two sciences is by no means uniform. Sociology concerns itself with the social structures men build as they relate to each other in the pursuit of common goals. The social structures of sociology include such bodies as, for example, associations, communities, organizations and – that most fundamental of all social structures – the family. It will be seen that the social structures of sociology share much common ground with the social groups of social psychology.

The science of Ecology is that of the environment. Applied to man, it examines his interaction with his total physical and social surroundings. An important subdivision of medical ecology is the modern expanding science of Epidemiology. Epidemiology studies those factors which influence health and disease in defined populations. Findings in compared groups or communities are examined and contrasted, utilizing the sophisticated and ingenious procedures of Statistics.

The zoological science of Ethology occupies a special place in attempting to understand the social behaviour of man. This science concerns itself with species-specific behaviour in animals, most notably in insects, birds and fishes. For this reason a direct application of its principles to the behaviour of man is obviously limited, and here enthusiasm must clearly be tempered with caution, whenever attempts are made to relate behaviour occurring in the animal world to that of man. Yet if such caution is appropriately exercised, the science of Ethology offers enormous potential for our study and future knowledge of social man.

Anthropology, dealing with the life of primitive man and representing the science of culture, has very close ties with Sociology. In its social and cultural aspects it has important contributions to make to the medical field of modern Psychiatry. A branch of physical anthropology, dealing with man's division into races, is Ethnology (obviously not to be confused with Ethology above).

Political Science, Economics and History are representative of many other disciplines which fall within the wider field of the behavioural sciences.

THE SOCIAL GROUP

Since the social organization of man occurs in and through groups, it is essential that this fundamental unit of both social psychology and of sociology is clearly understood. Any motley collection of individuals does not constitute a social group but merely a human aggregate. Such a collection, for example, can be visualized as travelling upwards in a London Underground lift. Should now this lift fail, temporarily incarcerating its anxious passengers between floors, these passengers will at once interact, and will communicate with each other both by verbal and non-verbal means. This communication effectively establishes interpersonal relationships and it is this critical advent of interpersonal relationships which at once translates this collection of individuals from that of a human aggregate to that of a social group.

The number of social groups which exist in society is virtually limitless and, at one and the same time, each of us will find himself – like it or not – a member of many groups of highly diverse composition. Already during the formative years, the developing child is consigned to numerous different social groups. These are likely to include the family, the neighbourhood, village or town; the school – and within this, the school orchestra, the cricket team or dramatic society; additional groups may include the Girl Guides or Scouts, or church groups according to religion. The nationality of the child and the social class into which it is born provide wider but none the less essential groups both of which exert their profound influence upon the emerging personality of the child.

Technically expressed, a social group is one whose members observe similar norms. Such norms concern ways of thinking, feeling or behaving. To observe such norms and demonstrate compliance ensures acceptance by the group and recognition of membership. To flout such norms and dissociate oneself from their written and unwritten laws is liable to provoke withdrawal of membership by the group and the imposition of a form of social discipline or ostracism. Devices of recognition may be displayed by the group members and these can include badges, uniforms, styles of dress, forms of speech or sets of mannerisms. Social groups have been classified by Cooley into Primary and Secondary categories. The Primary group is the intimate group whose members are in regular face-to-face communication with each other. By nature, it must be relatively small. Its sentiment is on the whole one of solidarity. Its closely knit loyalties cement the identity of the group (group awareness) and it jealously demarcates itself from other groups. Such a group may be termed an 'in-group'. Typical examples of a primary group are seen in a family, a football team, or a village. The secondary group is too large in size to allow of face-to-face contact between the generality of its members. Examples would be British Rail, the BBC, Oxford University, or a large business organization such as Imperial Chemical Industries. The people of Yorkshire or of Scotland provide additional examples. The secondary group will contain within it many organized primary groups.

Membership of a group involves degrees of social differentiation. A social role is a set of obligations attached to a given position. Roles, with their concomitant obligations, are assigned to different group members by the other members of the group who will, in turn, carry expectations of a particular type of behaviour for each role-occupant. Also conferred with the role assigned will be the status attached to the role in question. Due to his simultaneous membership of many groups one individual will occupy many roles. An incompatibility of obligations assigned to different roles may produce role-strain in a given individual. Contradictory demands of different roles may lead to the more serious condition of role-conflict. Yet again certain roles of a focal nature may attract excessive demands and engender role-overload in the role-occupant concerned. The individual character and colour which a person brings to his particular role is termed his role-identity. No role can exist in isolation but relates to another member or members set in a counter position within the group. The member occupying the counter position to the role-occupant is termed his role-partner and the obligations of the role-occupant constitute the expectations of the role-partner.

LEADERSHIP

The phenomenon of leadership is a further product of the social croup. Whilst assignment of the role of leader to one group member will be substantially dependent upon his own personal qualities, his selection by the group will be equally determined by the qualities of the group members to be led. Hence an outstanding leader for one particular group may find himself little more than a nondescript member in an alternate social group. A leader, by definition, requires individuals to lead and cannot therefore exist as such in any isolated setting of his own. Within the organization of a social group the roles of members will show dependence upon the leader's role. The leader will normally excel in some aspect of the group's activities, and will influence the dynamics of the group to a considerable degree.

Leaders of primary social groups have been classified as task (or instrumental) leaders and socio-emotional (or expressive) leaders. The task (instrumental) leader is identified with the action of the group, the pursuance of its aims and the attainment of its goals. The socio-emotional (expressive) leader is concerned with the members of the group themselves, considering their needs and safeguarding their best interests. The socio-emotional (expressive) leader will usually be found to be the most liked member of the group and, as such, is able to exert a powerful influence on the action of the group. On rare occasions, one individual may combine the role of both task (instrumental) and socio-emotional (expressive) leadership for the group.

Experiments in group dynamics have studied the effects of different types of leadership upon group activity and have classified these types as authoritarian, democratic and laissez-faire.

The authoritarian leader would formulate the policies of the group. He would dictate how projects should be carried out and would criticize how they were subsequently done. Such disciplined dominance allowed minimum individual freedom on the part of the group members.

The democratic leader would suggest group policies and the manner in which these should be carried out but the action and activities required would be determined by group discussion and group decision.

The laissez-faire leader would allow each group member total freedom and would participate only when invited. Each group member would thus be free to do as he pleased, and any fulfilment of the leadership role would be negligible.

Little constructive value can be attributed to the laissez-faire type of leadership, for the leader, in practice, is a leader in name only.

Authoritarian leadership tends to be effective only whilst the leader is present. Under these circumstances group members with authoritarian leadership would apply themselves more diligently and for longer periods. In the absence of the authoritarian leader an immediate slackening or cessation of the work task would occur. Authoritarian leadership may predispose to aggressive resistance and apathy among the group members.

With democratic leadership, group members would continue working well in the absence of their leader. The work would show more originality. Hostility and aggression towards the leader and towards other group members would be markedly reduced.

These and similar group experiments, concerned with types of leadership and their interactions with the dynamics of social groups, have of course a particular and important relevance and application to such matters as teaching methods and efficiency of learning in the field of education, and to problems of management and production in the field of industry. The past half-century has witnessed a very marked change in the medical and nursing services from that of an authoritarian social climate to that of a democratic one with more humanized and happier staff relationships and a corresponding overall improvement in working efficiency.

INTERPERSONAL BEHAVIOUR

It is common knowledge that the interactions of two individuals are radically altered by the arrival of a third person upon their particular scene – two is company, three is none.

Two persons interacting together form a dyad. Their special interpersonal behaviour has a reciprocal, restricted, one-to-one quality, and each, individual in turn acknowledges and modifies his own responses in accordance with the roles and counter-positions of his role-partner.

Three persons interacting together form a triad. The dynamics of the triad differ appreciably from those of the one-to-one dyad. The triad at once provides an arena for political manœuvre. Conquest can now be achieved by division. Power can be curtailed by alliance and coalition. Ends can be adroitly played against the middle. Three persons cannot interact simultaneously, and connived interaction by two will effectively isolate the third. By such means, two members of a triad – each of whom is considerably weaker than a strong third member – can effectively isolate, immobilize and outstrip the influence of a powerful third member.

The behaviour of certain social groups towards other groups can again be most revealing. Threats from outside greatly strengthen the bonds which extend between members of the in-group and increase cohesiveness and solidarity within this group. When normal inter-group rivalry (which so often originates in a territorial cause or from competitors in a similar field of interest) exceeds sensible and healthy proportions, a number of unpleasant and even ugly consequences may follow. The attitudes of in-group members towards those of the out-group will show bias and prejudice (p. 143). Irrational suspicions press themselves greatly to the fore. Hostility emerges, which then not only reinforces the prejudiced attitudes of the in-group members – each of whom is already reinforcing the biased views of his fellow members within the group – but effectively destroys communication between the in- and out-groups concerned. This breakdown of communication, with its resulting withdrawal of group interaction with each other, serves only to inflame the suspicion, aggression and hostility felt by each towards the other group. Again, the consequent behaviour of each group now reaffirms and reinforces the sentiments held by the other. Prejudice is thus intensified and such unhappy attitudes towards the members of the out-group become in time the assimilated accepted irrational social norms, which characterize the members of the in-group.

One example of a highly organized, closely structured social group is seen in the Committee. Closely modelled on the procedure of Parliament, its members enjoy equal rights and freedom of speech under the authority of its Chairman. Its behaviour is most carefully controlled and proceeds according to a tightly written schedule of rules. Yet its gain in propriety may well prove to be its loss in originality, for in terms of initiative and action, committee procedures can too often become stultifying. Not without cause has the Committee been pithily described as 'a collection of persons who individually can do nothing, deciding collectively why nothing should be done'. If Moses had had to rely upon a committee, the children of Israel would doubtless still be in Egypt.

A less well defined and much more loosely structured grouping is the quasi-group. Quasi-groups include such elements as social classes, 'sets' of individuals (e.g. the Hunting fraternity), 'publics' (e.g. an action group of individuals determined to oppose a proposed site for a new inland airport) and crowds.

The crowd is a special example of a type of social grouping and possesses a psychology and geography of its own. It is a gathering of a considerable number of persons about some central focus of attention – 'active centre' (fig. 52). It may vary from a group of individuals gathered

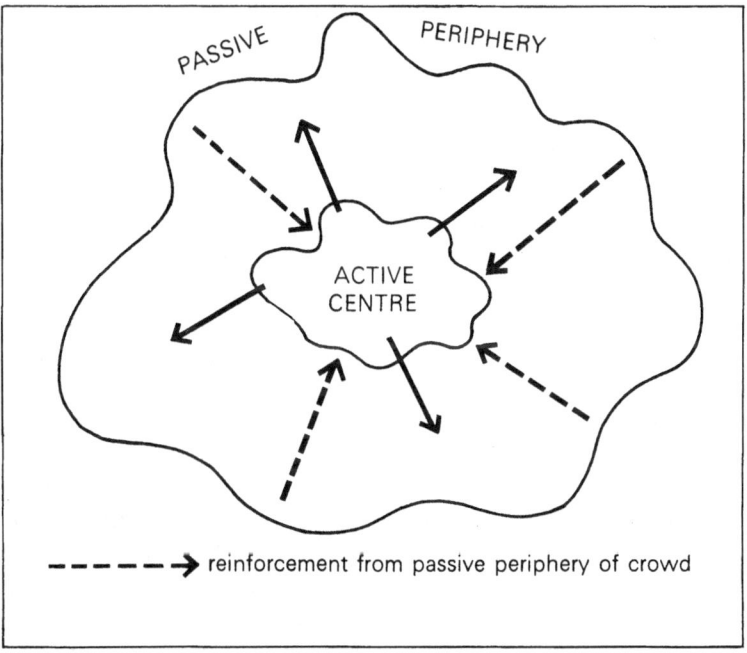

FIGURE 52 The crowd as an example of a special type of social grouping.

outside a theatre, awaiting the arrival of a film-star (passive crowd), to that of the frightening assembly of a riot (active crowd). Members of a crowd share feelings in common. They display a heightened emotionality. For them, suggestibility is increased whilst both intellectual awareness and self-criticism become decreased. Their sense of responsibility is diminished, and a disinhibition of normal social control arises. A sense of increased power is found and this runs hand in hand with the sense of anonymity experienced by the members. These members of a crowd are in very close physical contact. Normally, their grouping together is of only short duration and after the members split up and go their ways the crowd, as such, ceases to exist. From such crowds may emerge powerful leaders who will sway, control and direct the activity of the crowd. The geographical core of a crowd is formed by its central area. Here are situated its most active members and a gradient of diminishing activity spreads from the core to the periphery, where the more passive members of the crowd are to be found. The reactions and behaviour at the periphery, however, continually reinforce the activity at the core of the crowd (fig. 52). A mob is a crowd whose activity has extended beyond that of social control.

ATTITUDES AND PREJUDICES

An attitude is a persistent, learned predisposition to respond in a distinctive manner to some aspect of the environment. Accordingly, we perceive, think, feel and behave in characteristic ways towards people and things. The personality of any given individual plays a cardinal part in his or her acquisition and retention of attitudes and, *mutatis mutandis*, these characteristic attitudes provide important ingredients of personality in their intellectual, emotional and behavioural components.

In general terms, attitudes will be either positive favourable ones or negative unfavourable ones. In this respect, they contrast with interests which, apart from being more narrowly applied, restrict themselves merely to positive favourable qualities. Attitudes form an important consideration within the field of social psychology. Group attitudes are as prevalent as those of any individual. Not only will the attitudes of the prevailing social group imprint themselves upon the personalities of young individual members, moulding and influencing their development, but the continuation of membership of that social group will require in greater or lesser degree, the acceptance and sustained observance of established group attitudes. Though certain latitudes may be allowed, an initiate to the social group may expect to be taught by example, imitation and reward, or by indoctrination, coercion and punishment, the prevailing attitudes of the group – those persistent predispositions of response which are indicative of the group norms – and these will possibly remain with him for life. In instances of idiosyncratic individuals for whom particular group attitudes and their lack of tolerance are unacceptable, a schism from that group will most likely result.

Group attitudes will include those directed towards individuals, to primary groups, to institutions, to nations and to races. Since such prevailing attitudes are likely to preclude objective, unbiased appraisal of individuals or of social groups, they will promote an invalid prejudgement before the truth is established. For this reason, they are known as prejudices. Such prejudices are very commonly based on nationality, religion, the location of an individual's birth, mannerisms of speech, and the colour of the skin.

Similar untruthful and biased generalizations are called stereotypes. Stereotypes will commonly concern social, national or racial groups and falsely attribute characteristics to the members of that group, which are in fact not possessed by them. The false concepts that 'all Americans are rich' and that 'all Germans are aggressive' are typical stereotypes and are meaningless in terms of factual appraisal. The important modern medical problem of alcoholism is a further example. The vast majority of individuals who suffer from alcoholism are engaged in regular and responsible employment. Their difficulties are often concealed from all but their closest friends and families. Yet to many people the term 'alcoholic' still conjures up a stereotype depicted by the extreme music-hall caricature of a red-nosed drunken sot, who staggers through life with an uncorked bottle in each hand until, incapable of standing, collapses and passes into the deeper stages of coma. To consider the medical aspects of alcoholism on the basis of this stereotype would, of course, add nothing but further confusion to an area where clarification is urgently sought and is urgently necessary.

CULTURE AND SOCIETY

An organized social group constitutes a social institution and the sum total of social institutions constitutes society. Each social group – from that of the smallest and most intimate primary group, to the total system of social relationships of which society is composed – will possess its own distinctive culture. Culture represents a common social heritage which embodies the way in which a social group thinks, feels and behaves. With the more permanent social groups, it means that children born into their setting will be treated in certain ways, taught along specific lines, shown by particular examples, and indoctrinated by stereotyped methods. Thus those customs, beliefs, habits and rituals of that particular group will be assimilated by the young as a way of life. Later when adulthood is reached, these grown-up children will in turn impart this *modus vivendi* to their own off-spring, perpetuating their cultural heritage.

Marked cultural differences are to be found in society between existing social classes. Since society does not allow these to exist side by side on equal terms, it introduces the controversial concepts of superiority and inferiority and upper, middle and lower strata are delineated. Such stratification of society finds its counterparts in ethological studies of the animal kingdom as, for example, the pecking order in hens (Schjelderup-Ebbe) and also that of jackdaws (Lorenz). With man, the ease of movement from one social class to another – social mobility – is closely correlated with rigidity of social culture. Our present technological century has witnessed far-reaching changes which have greatly enhanced social mobility. Nevertheless, in Britain today, society remains far removed from the egalitarian concept of a classless society. By tradition its pattern of culture still fosters the structurization of a society by strata of social class, with all the political and economic problems that this engenders.

LAUGHTER

The phenomenon of laughter is but little understood in both its psychological and physiological components. Yet since laughter plays an essential part in the establishment of human interpersonal relationships, it is clearly of fundamental importance to any consideration of social psychology.

So much do we accept laughter as a shared interpersonal event that, should we observe a person vigorously laughing alone, we might well find ourselves casting doubt on his or her mental condition. Such solitary laughing or giggling provides a significant symptomatology in the field of schizophrenic illness.

The social quality of laughter can best be envisaged by the two opposing concepts of 'laughter with' and 'laughter at'. To 'laugh with' others is to recognize and accept them as belonging to the same social group as ourselves. The laughter itself will strengthen the bonds between the individual members belonging to the group. A random collection of individuals (who therefore rank merely as a human aggregate) will by 'laughter with' find themselves suddenly transformed to a human social group. This laughter has established the critical interpersonal relationships which are the *sine qua non* for any social group.

In contradistinction, to 'laugh at' is an act of social dissociation.

144

This type of laughter will produce the opposite effect to that of 'laughter with'. 'Laughter at' functions to discipline the individual (or individuals) in question for the transgression of accepted group mores. If contrition is not shown and restitution made by the offender, such continuing derisory laughter from the social group will effectively expel him from their membership. Such 'laugher at', with its built-in corrective qualities by ridicule, is effective in preserving the observance of those norms which characterize a particular social group. It thus ensures the continuing observance and conformity in such matters as opinions, manners, dress and behaviour.

The alienating effect of unsuitable and inappropriate laughter is by no means confined to psychotic patients. A forceful example can be found in that misguided technique much now in vogue among radio and television broadcasting. It has become a practice among such broadcasters, when the standard and performance of comedy is low, to relay simultaneously with the unfortunate and would-be comic act, a recording of an audience laughing vigorously. The gales of hearty laughter are synchronized to coincide with the apologies for jokes and humour delivered by the performer.

The trickery of this 'canned laughter' deceives no-one. No doubt it is the dream of the broadcasters to unite the performer, the viewers or listeners, and his team of sychophantic laughing ghosts in one hilarious in-group. Alas! The absence of 'laughter with' is all too painfully obvious. Its effect is to alienate an audience from the very silly charade and to produce the response of 'laughter at'. Since, in this instance, this measure of social discipline can only prove totally ineffective, irritation and annoyance will occur in the audience, and the ultimate sanction is invoked by an abrupt switching-off the set.

The most recent research in this interesting subject now subdivides laughter into seven main categories:

(1) *Humorous laughter* – as occurs in response to an amusing and witty joke.
(2) *Social laughter* – that which integrates the individual into a social group.
(3) *Ignorance laughter* – that which is used to conceal a lack of genuine knowledge, employing a joke as an immediate smoke screen.
(4) *Derision laughter* – as seen among children who will laugh at physical disability in other children.

(5) *Anxiety laughter* – as may occur immediately after an anxious crisis is safely passed, or for example in the response of Londoners during World War II when the Blitz was at its worst.

(6) *Apologetic laughter* – as occurs when a joke is made to divert attention from a blunder or social gaffe.

(7) *Ticklishness laughter* – the laughter which occurs in response to being tickled. This is still unexplainable though theories are advanced, including the biological theory of self-defence. By this, it is postulated that in a non-violent way the tickled person gives warning to the tickler to stop, whilst simultaneously submitting and defending the sensitive parts of the body.

MENTAL IMAGERY

Mental images are produced by activity in the association areas of the brain. For each sensation we experience (relayed to the projection areas of the cerebral cortex, when stimulation of the peripheral sensory receptor occurs), a corresponding mental image may be evoked at will. Thus we can visualize the face of a friend or run through a familiar tune in our head, and in the majority of persons such visual and auditory images will be those most easily evoked and most clearly appreciated. But with even more effort and perhaps less clarity, we may be able to conjure up, for example, the smell of petrol, the feel of wool, the warmth of a fire, the chill of ice, or the muscular sensations which arise when a heavy suitcase is carried. In many respects, mental images fall between the normal sensory experience itself and the hallucination of central nervous origin (p. 170), yet the mental image lacks the essential clarity of either of these two phenomena and, furthermore, demands considerable effort and concentration to prevent its fading. Mental images can be sub-divided into memory images, which result from past experience, and constructed images, which may be objects of fantasy. Mental imagery plays a most important part in the process of remembering. Mental images of a form so vivid as to approximate to the sensory experience itself are termed eidetic images. Whilst occurring quite commonly during the years of childhood, it is unfortunate that the capacity to produce eidetic imagery is but rarely sustained in adulthood.

7

SCHOOLS OF PSYCHOLOGY

The principles of psychology are as old as mankind itself yet as an independent science psychology is one of the youngest. This paradoxical state of affairs can be readily understood by a brief review of its interesting history – from psychology as a division of philosophy to the scientific psychological knowledge gained almost exclusively during the past 100 years which has established psychology in its current position pre-eminent among the Behavioural Sciences.

Throughout the ages – from the Graeco-Roman era until the latter part of the nineteenth century, psychology existed as an integral and essential division of philosophy. In ancient times, Plato, the father of philosophy, emphasized the importance and superiority of mental processes. His views inspired much psychological inquiry and no little psychological speculation. His teachings on the immortality and special qualities of the psyche or soul (in marked contradistinction to the soma or body) have been severely misrepresented in medical thought which leaned so heavily and for so long upon the false concept of a dichotomy of mind and body. Today we are only just emerging from these prejudices.

Aristotle, Plato's pupil, produced among many impressive works, his important treatise on the mind *De Anima* and also his classical psychological essay on 'Memory'. The Pythagorean School had accurately postulated that the seat of the mind could be found in the brain – as opposed to the many fanciful and ingenious loci throughout the

147

body which had been advanced. Hippocrates, in addition to his important studies in inherited factors and predispositions to mental illness, taught on the disorders of cerebral function and their role in mental illness and in sanity.

With its traditional approach to the exploration of new frontiers of knowledge and with its formidable prestige in learning, it is easy to visualize how philosophy influenced, overshadowed, and even retarded, all psychological thought to the seventeenth-century philosophers and beyond. Change was, however, coming. The views of the British seventeenth-century philosophers Hobbes and Locke, which favoured the concept of association in explaining learning and remembering, initiated a gradual emergence of the first and senior, if poorly defined, school of psychology, the Associationist School.

The Associationist School (p. 151) gained and maintained its ascendancy in psychological thought throughout the eighteenth and greater part of the nineteenth centuries. But by the latter part of the nineteenth century, many of those who pursued the new and engaging lines of psychological inquiry had grown grossly dissatisfied with the traditional methods of philosophic thought and exploration (so characteristically employed by the associationists) and which relied on subjective introspection. They found such methods outdated and unsympathetic to the new climate of scientific discovery from which were emerging so many of the sister disciplines of research. The revolutionary advances in the fields of physiology, biology, physics, and chemistry impinged inexorably upon the nature and methods of psychological study.

It was Wilhelm Wundt in 1879 who set up the first psychological laboratory at Leipzig. In so doing he dramatically marked the dawn of a new era in psychological research by founding the new science of experimental psychology. The far reaching effects of the atomic theory of chemistry, whereby seemingly incomprehensible matter could be explained in terms of elements, atoms and molecules, had already inspired great hopes that mental processes might likewise be reduced to basic units and then subsequently synthesized to more complex forms. In marked contrast to the philosophic approach which relied upon imaginative, subjective and questionable introspection, Wundt now required in his laboratory factual, objective data measured by experiment. Wundt's theories, which stressed the synthesis of conscious experience from sensations and feelings, were further developed by the Structural School of Psychology born in Germany and in the

United States of America most notably by E. B. Titchener (1867–1927). With the passage of time, however, much of the basic doctrine of this school was superseded by the newer theories of the schools of psychology that were emerging.

The beginning of the twentieth century witnessed the origin of a new school of psychology which, for better or worse, was to blaze its remarkable trail throughout all corners of the world. This was the School of Psychoanalysis (p. 153) originating in Vienna in 1900 and founded by Sigmund Freud. This School rejected the avenues of approach of the existing schools of psychology and with a refreshing audacity advanced the revolutionary and highly controversial theories of unconscious motivation. Central to these new theories was the role of the dynamic unconscious mind in both healthy mental activity and in the occurrence of mental illness. Freud's distinguished associates in this school, Carl Jung and Alfred Adler later disengaged themselves from the School of Psychoanalysis, each to form his own particular school. Jung founded the School of Analytical Psychology and Adler the School of Individual Psychology.

The Gestalt School (p. 157) introduced another new approach to psychological theory. Founded in Germany in 1912 by Max Wertheimer, Wolfgang Köhler and Kurt Koffka, it stressed the importance of '*gestalten*' or 'wholes'. Such 'wholes' would posses qualities of their own and would not merely represent the total sum of their integral parts. In isolation, such integral parts may differ widely from their very selves when these form part of a *gestalt*. Therefore little would be gained in knowledge of the *gestalt* by attempting to analyse its component parts. The prime interest of the Gestalt School lay in problems of perception. Much of their attention was devoted to the perception of patterns, the mechanics for which were to be found in the innate organization of the sensory field. Gestalt theory found a wide application. Learning, memory, behaviour and social psychology, among other special interests, were studied extensively according to gestalt principles.

The Behaviourist School (p. 160) introduced a new and highly controversial approach to psychology. Founded by J. B. Watson in America in 1912, it sought to explain all psychological phenomena in terms of simple physiological functions. It denied the existence of any conscious experience and sought to explain behaviour by stimulus-response units – the reflexes. From aggregations of these essentially simple units, more complex patterns of behaviour could be built. The conditioning of reflexes was of vital interest. In place of mentalism, the behaviourists substituted neural mechanisms. To the Behaviourists, the prevailing method of introspection as a means of psychological inquiry was particularly abhorrent. The attempts of this school to provide a mechanistic theory of mental processes has provoked much valid criticism of their beliefs and methods from present-day psychologists. The behaviour therapy (p. 246) of modern psychiatry is based on the clinical application of selected principles of the Behaviourist School.

Over and above the major schools of psychology, of which mention has been made, a number of less circumscribed schools, of groups of psychologists, and also individual psychologists themselves, exerted considerable influence on the growing mass of psychological knowledge which was emerging in the twilight era which spanned the later part of the nineteenth century and the earlier part of the twentieth century. Among these we may include the Functional School with John Dewey (1859–1952) and J. R. Angell (1869–1949) working together at Chicago, America; William McDougall (1871–1938) both in England and America, with his Hormic School of purposive activity – such purposive, goal-seeking theories providing the basis for McDougall's doctrine of instincts; Adolf Meyer (1866–1950), who advanced in America his psychobiological theories and applied these with great effect in the field of clinical psychiatry.

In a nascent field of scientific learning, where so much awaited discovery and where so little could be claimed to be known, it is not surprising that groups of persons with common interests working in relatively restricted areas of study, should find themselves congregated into particular schools. Yet the advent of greater knowledge has brought about a reformation and natural evolution, in the course of which the transition of rigid boundaries has led to a merging of artificially segregated schools and a consequent loss of stereotyped identity. Today, much of our interest in these isolated schools of psychology is historical. Yet this appreciation of the past promotes our comprehension of the present. To understand our present position in both psychology and clinical psychiatry, an academic knowledge of the historical background promotes a greater awareness and a greater clarity in our appreciation of the modern problems that confront us.

Schools of Psychology

THE ASSOCIATIONIST SCHOOL

The Associationist School of Psychology, whilst not rigidly demarcated, represents historically the senior of the individual schools of psychology. Its influence spanned that transitional period of time during which psychology was emerging from its role as a subordinate to philosophy to establish itself as a science in its own right. Accordingly, the chief interests of this school – learning and remembering – were dominated by the methods and ways of thinking of the philosophers. Indications of its concepts can be found in philosophical writing from the time of the early Greeks to the seventeenth-century philosophers, Thomas Hobbes (1588–1679) and John Locke (1632–1704). Subsequently, the names of David Hartley (1705–1757), David Hume (1711–1766), Thomas Brown (1778–1820), James Mill (1733–1836) and his son J. S. Mill (1806–1873) became prominent in Britain among the followers of this school and in Germany those of J. F. Herbart (1776–1841), H. Ebbinghaus (1850–1909) and G. E. Müller (1850–1934) were most noted. An American psychologist, E. L. Thorndike (1874–1949), contributed greatly to the theories of animal learning and extended the boundaries of Associationism.

The essential period of some two centuries of psychological thought during which the Associationist School held sway falls conveniently into an earlier period preceding the final decade of the nineteenth century and a later period subsequent to this. The early Associationists devoted themselves to 'mental philosophy'. By means of detailed introspective observations, they addressed themselves to the phenomena of sensations and attempted to reduce mental processes to a basic mechanism of association.

Aristotle, in his classical treatise on 'Memory', had demonstrated that when memories are stimulated by other ideas, the relationship is an associative one determined by three factors – similarity, contrast and contiguity. These three factors furnished 'the laws of Association'. The Associationist School attempted to simplify matters still further, reducing them to one factor of contiguity in experience, and on this basis they sought to explain mental activity. Thus, ideas occurring in groups or sequences would be determined by past experience and would link together sensations which had occurred together, or in succession. The Associationists sought to explain remembering and learning in terms of associations of past sensory experience and

151

considered all mental activity to be attributable to the association of ideas. Hermann Ebbinghaus (1850–1909) devoted much of his attention to the problems of remembering and forgetting. For his experiments on rote-learning (learning by heart) he employed 'nonsense syllables'. These were meaningless syllables such as kel, seb, gar, devoid of built-in associations. He established the 'memory span' – for the number of syllables which could be retained and repeated after a single reading. The techniques of learning series of these syllables, including the effects in economy by 'over learning' and the rate at which the nonsense syllables were forgotten enabled him to produce graphically his famous 'curves of forgetting'.

The views of E. L. Thorndike (1874–1949) were closely allied to those of the Associationists, though he preferred to be known as a 'connexionist'. His classical animal experiments were made with cats in puzzle-boxes. The puzzle-box was designed to open if a latch were lifted or a loop of wire pulled, or some similar simple escape mechanism were activated. A hungry cat was placed in the box and was then observed to determine which method it employed, and how long it took, to effect its escape from the box. At first the cat would claw at random until eventually, by chance, the latch would be lifted or the loop be pulled and the cat would gain its freedom. On being returned to the puzzle-box, a repeat of the previous activities would take place but generally the number of random movements would prove less before the cat escaped. This decreasing trend would continue on subsequent occasions until ultimately, when placed in the box, the cat would at once go to the catch or loop and release itself from the box. At this stage, learning is complete. By noting the time required for each trial and the number of trials undertaken, the results can be plotted graphically as a 'learning curve'. This familiar curve is produced by most animals when under test for experimental learning.

From his experiments, Thorndike deduced that animal learning occurred simply by trial and error, without any capacity for understanding the problem. This process of motor learning, moreover, obeyed three laws:

(1) *The Law of Frequency.* The movements most frequently performed tend to be repeated.
(2) *The Law of Recency.* The movements most recently performed tend to be repeated.

(3) *The Law of Effect.* Right movements are stamped-in by the satisfaction of success. Wrong movements are stamped out by the dissatisfaction of failure.

Thorndike's concept of animal learning as a series of blind motor responses has encountered much criticism and many exceptions can be taken to his postulates. In escaping from the puzzle-box, for example, the cat will employ a totally different sequence of motor movements to attain the same end results. In changed circumstances, the cat will show adaptive behaviour – as also will quite humble laboratory animals. A major antagonist to Thorndike's theories was Wolfgang Köhler (p. 159) who applied Gestalt principles to animal learning and who believed that understanding and 'insight' could be found in problem-solving by animals, even of a relatively simple kind, providing that the problem set was within the limited capacity of the experimental animal.

THE SCHOOL OF PSYCHOANALYSIS

The School of Psychoanalysis was founded by Sigmund Freud (1856–1939) at Vienna. 1900 is a convenient date to accept for its foundation and the term 'psychoanalysis' should always be properly reserved for the strict doctrines of Freud, although modifications of Freudian theory have been utilized as a basis for subsequent schools of psychology. The School of Psychoanalysis is a school which, of all prevailing schools of psychology in the early part of the twentieth century, was to exert the greatest impact upon the field of mental exploration and was to influence medical, scientific and even artistic thought in a most profound and far reaching manner. Freud's two distinguished associates, Carl Gustav Jung (1870–1962) and Alfred Adler (1870–1937), unable to accept many aspects of Freudian theory, most notably the role of sexual factors emphasized by Freud in mental motivation, ultimately dissociated themselves from the School of Psychoanalysis, each to form his own psychological school (of Analytical Psychology (Jung) and Individual Psychology (Adler)). More recently other followers of Freud – the Neo-Freudians – have sought to modify the tenets of the School of Psychoanalysis, adapting and replacing much of the biological theory with those drawn from the sociological sources. Such Neo-Freudians include Eric Fromm, Karen Horney and Abram Kardiner.

Freud's theories of psychoanalysis were essentially born of medical practice. Having qualified as a doctor at Vienna University, he worked for some years as an academic scientist in physiology. However, lacking the financial means to support himself or a family whilst pursuing such academic research, he resolved to set up in private neurological consulting practice in Vienna. Before so doing he travelled to Paris to study the treatment of hysteria by medical hypnosis under J. M. Charcot (1825–1895). Later he continued his studies in hypnosis at the rival school in France at Nancy under the direction of H. Bernheim (1837–1919).

Freud's treatment of his neurotic Viennese patients by means of hypnosis met with indifferent success and he sought a more satisfactory and more reliable method. He was aware of the non-conscious material that could emerge from patients in the course of their hypnotic trances and sought to explore this important and uncharted area by alternative methods. In this respect, he found the practice of 'free association' effective and utilized this together with examination of his patients' dreams and such phenomena as slips of the tongue and pen, certain forms of wit and art, as a means of discovering those motivations which lay behind the patient's conscious thought. In the course of such exploration, he found that a patient might display considerable unconscious opposition to prevent such motivations from becoming consciously appreciated. This was 'resistance' and the progress of psychoanalysis lay in recognizing and overcoming such resistances.

It was central to Freudian hypothesis that each human act or emotion resulted from an earlier determining cause – the principle of 'psychic determination'. Free will was thus inadmissible. Motivation arose from the influence of the dynamic unconscious mind and in such motivation sexual factors played a pre-eminent role. Freud visualized the mind as stratified in three layers – the conscious, the pre-conscious and the overwhelmingly important unconscious. The contents of the unconscious were closely guarded by the censor which prevented unconscious material from gaining access to the conscious mind. The conscious mind would include those thoughts and feelings of which one is aware at any given moment. Closely linked with it, and allowing free interchange, is the pre-conscious mind containing those thoughts, memories and feelings which, at will, can be readily recalled into consciousness. But exerting by far the greatest influence on human thought and activity is the unconscious mind, the content of which can never emerge directly into consciousness. Thus, unconscious mental activity remains unconscious and any knowledge we have of its workings is obtained by skilled oblique interpretation on the part of the psychoanalyst. By nature the unconscious mind, according to Freudian theory, is infantile and egocentric; its dynamic primordial energies are amoral and obey the pleasure–pain principle; these energies easily transfer from one unconscious process to another. Impulses, memories and emotions which are too painful or too embarrassing for acceptance by the conscious mind would be banished from consciousness to the unconscious mind by the mechanism of 'repression' and would be effectively prevented from re-emergence by the efficient action of the censor. Thus, the dynamic influence from within the unconscious may greatly disturb and stress the conscious mind, inducing guilt, tension, anxiety and other features of neurosis until a controlled ventilation by psychoanalytical procedures could allow a corresponding emotional release. At times, the conscious mind may employ certain devices to reduce the effectiveness of the unconscious influence. These are the ego-defence mechanisms and include such devices as rationalization, identification, projection, displacement, reaction formation, repression and dissociation.

Freud later supplemented these theories by his concepts of the id, ego and super-ego. The id he considered was almost wholly unconscious and consisted of unorganized, instinctive impulses which sought immediate gratification. The ego was equated in greatest measure with the conscious self in contact with the external environment. At a somewhat later stage in mental development, the super-ego was fashioned. This, corresponding very approximately to what is usually known as conscience, functions as a strict and punitive arbiter of moral values and issues.

It was essential to Freud's theory of psychoanalysis that the libido or main source of mental energy stemmed from the sexual instinct – a dogma which invoked disagreement with both Jung and Adler. Jung's concept of libido was not a restrictive one and embraced widely that abundance of mental factors which produce a will to live. Adler's concept of the libido was essentially a social one, an urge based on a striving for superiority over other members of a social group and producing a will for dominance and power. Again, it was central to Freud's theory of the neuroses that the cause of the neurosis lay in the past. The greatest operative factor here was the period of infantile sexuality. Freud considered sexual development in the infant and young child to proceed via three principal stages. The first of these is the oral stage, at a time when pleasure and satisfaction are chiefly obtained by sucking and mouth contact; the second is the anal stage when pleasurable sensations and satisfactions are obtained from bowel movements; and the third is the genital stage when ageeable sensations and satisfaction may be obtained from manipulation of the genitalia. Conflict between the taboos of society and the developing young individual's interests may occur at any stage and the effectiveness in resolution of the conflict by the young child, or lack of effectiveness of such resolution, is liable to determine the emergence of neurosis at a subsequent time of life.

A further testing ground for the developing young child was postulated in the Oedipal situation. According to Greek mythology Oedipus unwittingly killed his father and, having solved the riddle of the Sphinx, equally unwittingly married his mother. Freud utilized this story to depict the attachment for the mother, which occurs with a young developing boy's libido, and the resulting rivalry experienced for the father. The converse situation in the case of a young developing girl is known as the Electra situation – again from a somewhat similar Greek story of the daughter of Agamemnon and Clytemnestra. Failure of resolution of the Oedipal or Electra situations by the developing child would again, according to psychoanalytical theory, give rise to neurosis in later life.

In contradistinction to these theories of Freud, both Jung and Adler believed that the causative factors in neurosis lay in the present. It was Jung's view that neurosis arose when situational demands made upon an individual exceeded the quantity of mental energy he was capable of summoning, and an inability to resolve the presenting problem or crisis would be followed by regression to earlier and less sophisticated childish activities. Adler believed that frustration of the drive for superiority could precipitate a retreat into illness as an alternative means of exerting power. He was concerned with 'organ inferiority', and how an individual's attempts to compensate for feelings of inferiority may be translated into the exaggerated state of 'over compensation'. His concept of 'masculine protest' must be understood in terms of the times in which he lived (when males were regarded as the superior breed), and the fact that striving was essentially towards superiority.

THE GESTALT SCHOOL

The Gestalt School of Psychology, as its name suggests, is German in origin. Literally translated, the German word '*Gestalt*' would approximate to the English words 'form' or 'configuration'. But with greater advantage the term '*Gestalt*' should be remembered as signifying 'whole' since the Gestalt school, whose prime interest was perception, addressed itself to the study of *Gestalten* or 'wholes'.

This school was founded at Frankfurt in 1912 by Max Wertheimer (1880–1943), Wolfgang Köhler (1887–1967) and Kurt Koffka (1886–1941). To these names must be added that of Kurt Lewin (1890–1947) who extended Gestalt concepts by way of his dynamic Field Theory.

The Gestalt school most vigorously challenged and refuted the fashionable pre-occupation of the Associationists and other contemporary schools of its time for attempting to break everything down to elements or basic units when studying mental function. Such an approach, they claimed, was erroneous and mental phenomena could only be studied as 'wholes' and not as an aggregation of individual parts. Indeed, they demonstrated how such a 'whole' will possess properties of its own which could never be ascertained from an examination of its component parts studied in isolation; and furthermore, the nature of the 'whole' will prove to be very much more than the sum of its individual parts. Whilst originating in the study of perception, Gestalt principles have been extended to far wider fields throughout psychology and physiology. These include thinking, learning and the important field of social psychology.

A fundamental of Gestalt theory is that the organization of the sensory field is innate. That is to say, the manner in which, for example, particular shapes (such as squares, circles, triangles, systems of dots, etc.) are perceived, and the important tendency to organize numbers of these into particular groupings, are born within us. For this reason, Gestalt theory is sometimes described as nativistic. The mechanism of grouping relies on certain factors of organization, notably:

(1) Proximity – those units which are close together will tend to be grouped together.

(2) Similarity – those units which are similar will tend to be grouped together.

(3) Continuity – those units which form part of a continuum (e.g. a straight line) will tend to be grouped together.

(4) Closure – those units which take part in forming a recognizable shape or figure – even when gaps exist between the individual components, will tend to be grouped as that 'closed' figure and the gaps conveniently ignored.

In addition, the nature of the groupings will depend also upon the past experience and higher mental activity of the observer via the factors of familiarity (if one grouping approximates to some figure already known) and set (an intentional search for a particular configuration).

A perfect example of the operation of these factors in the organization of the sensory field can be observed by anyone who cares to look at the sky on a frosty night. The stars have been grouped by the ancients into the constellations of astronomy, and their groupings accord with Gestalt principles – even though made some thousands of years before Gestalt theory was formally proposed. The constellations are determined by apparent closeness (e.g. the Pleiades); by similarity of size and brightness (e.g. the Plough); by continuity (e.g. the face of Taurus); or by closure (e.g. the Dolphin).

Wertheimer's original studies in perception had produced some highly significant observations of apparent motion. If two electric light bulbs A and B are set apart and are then switched on and off alternately, a most interesting phenomenon may be observed. If the intervening time interval between illuminating each bulb is a relatively long one (e.g. one second), we would see, reasonably enough, the bulbs flashing alternately. If the intervening interval is very short (e.g. one-thirtieth of a second), the eye cannot discern this rapidity and the two bulbs would be seen as if each were burning continuously. However, and here is the remarkable phenomenon of apparent motion, if the time interval is adjusted to a critical value of one-fifteenth of a second, then bulb A appears to move across to the position of bulb B and then back again to its original site, repeating this sequence of events so long as the critical frequency is maintained.

This phenomena, of course, is that of the motion picture at the cinema. As the film is viewed, actors can be seen moving energetically yet smoothly in many different directions. Movements by different persons in different directions can be observed simultaneously. Yet the cinematograph projector merely throws onto the screen a series of still pictures – albeit in sequence and at a critical frequency. All movement is thus supplied by the mind of the observer and in accordance

with Gestalt principles. The mental phenomenon of vision provides a dynamic whole and does not represent an aggregate of individual disjointed parts.

Wolfgang Köhler applied Gestalt psychology to problems of animal learning. Dissatisfied with the automatic trial and error theories advanced by Thorndike, he demonstrated that problem-solving by intelligence is evident in animal learning, providing that the problem set is one which falls within the grasp of the animal in question. Köhler concerned himself with the occurrence of 'insight' in the animal under observation. Insight, from the Gestalt view, implies a reorganization of the perceptual field. Elements previously appearing unconnected would, with this reorganization, now be perceived as contributing to a Gestalt. The reorganization may occur slowly with a correspondingly gradual dawning of the solution. But more typically, the reorganization would occur quite abruptly with the answer perceived in a sudden flash.

The classical experiments of Köhler were made with apes during the First World War when Köhler was interned at Tenerife. Köhler stressed that for problem-solving in animals the problem must fall within the capacity of the animal under experiment, and furthermore, this animal must be able to inspect the total situation. With these conditions fulfilled, degrees of 'insight' may be observed in animals of quite lowly levels.

Köhler's experiments with apes involved such devices as placing a banana out of reach from within the cage but leaving a bamboo stick nearby. The apes would rapidly solve this problem, employing the stick to pull the banana into the cage. The next stage was to place two sticks within the cage (neither of which was long enough on its own to reach the banana) which could be joined together to form one longer stick. Köhler's most intelligent ape solved this problem and used the combined single stick to obtain the banana, and furthermore retained this knowledge when re-tested the following day. Modifications of this experiment were made by placing boxes within the ape's cage, which when piled upon each other would allow access to a banana suspended above the animal's head. Köhler's studies appeared in his famous book *The Mentality of Apes*, published in 1917. Serious doubt was cast on the 'insight' nature of the learning process when it was subsequently demonstrated that the sudden solution of the problem was only found in apes who had reached maturity in the jungle and hence acquired experience there.

The Fundamentals of Psychological Medicine

Kurt Koffka applied Gestalt theory to many special fields of mental activity – cognitive, affective and conative – including his impressive work on memory and his interesting studies in behaviour.

Kurt Lewin, with a special interest in Child Psychology, extended the principles of Gestalt Psychology to the sphere of Social Psychology. His dynamic 'Field Theory' sought to explain motivation in human behaviour. The field of Lewin comprised a life-space containing both an individual and psychological environment. The structure of this field at any moment could influence not only the behaviour of the individual, but also the behaviour of others within their setting of social groups.

THE BEHAVIOURIST SCHOOL

The Behaviourist School of Psychology was founded in America by J. B. Watson (1878–1958) in the year 1912. This school claims many distinguished followers among whom may be mentioned Karl S. Lashley (1890–1958), E. C. Tolman (1886–1959), Clark L. Hull (1884–1952) and B. F. Skinner (born 1904).

It was Watson who appropriately stressed that psychology was not the science of consciousness, as hitherto thought, but was in fact the science of behaviour. In Watson's view all behaviour was sensorimotor and was built up from simple stimulus–response units – the reflexes. From these simple units, habits could be formed and the conditioned reflex would provide the basis of learning. Even thinking and emotion were explained along these lines. Watson believed thinking to be sensorimotor activity which originated in underlying muscular responses. Emotion represented patterns of visceral and glandular motor activity without any need to postulate conscious involvement.

Most central to Watson's behaviourist theories was his denial of conscious experience. 'Consciousness' to him was anathema; and since, as he pointed out, it could be neither assessed objectively nor investigated scientifically, he relegated it contemptuously to the realm of metaphysics.

Watson's views, which may be conveniently summarized in the one word 'reflexology', were dramatic, extreme, and – with the wisdom which comes from hindsight – untenable in many instances. They reflected a bitter discontent with the prevailing nineteenth-century theories of psychology, still very much entrammelled with their philosophical handicaps. Watson sought inspiration and guidance

from the important new scientific advances in physiology and by the application of these to the theories of psychology shook his complacent contemporaries to the core of their speculative and introspective hypotheses. Yet with considerable modification, Watson's forthright and outspoken views provided the basis for the work of the later Behaviourists and have ultimately, of course, heralded the development of the important Behaviourist theory as understood and practised today.

The contribution of Karl Lashley (1890–1958) was a predominantly neurophysiological one. His classical experiments involved the mechanics of learning in rats whose brains had been experimentally damaged. Lashley removed whole areas of the rats' brains and observed the effects of these on the rats' capacity for learning. From his experiments Lashley formulated two principles:

(1) *The principle of equipotentiality.* This states that, with certain exceptions (e.g. the visual cortex), one part of the cortex is potentially the same as another in its capacity for learning.

(2) *The principle of mass action.* This states that the more cortex remaining, the better the learning.

The results of Lashley's experimental work now rendered impossible his earlier acceptance of Watsonian theory. He required, by his observations, a substantial alteration of early behaviourist concepts to account for human behaviour.

The views of E. C. Tolman (1886–1959) again differed in very marked fashion from Watson's original concepts. From his own experiments with animals, Tolman concluded a number of 'intervening variables' must be introduced between the incoming stimulus and outgoing response. Any consideration of 'purpose' had been dismissed by Watson in the spate of his wholesale rejection of introspective consideration. Tolman, in contradistinction, emphasized strongly the role of purpose in the determination of individual behaviour and his own brand of Behaviourism has been termed 'purposive behaviourism'. The effects of Tolman's hypothesis produced considerable division between subsequent adherents to the Behaviourist School.

Clark L. Hull (1884–1952) was closely drawn to the concept of Pavlovian conditioning. Whilst still utilizing the basis of Watsonian theory, Hull accepted Tolman's concept of 'intervening variables' introduced between stimulus and response. He favoured the concept of drives or needs and classified these among the intervening variables. His

work on conditioning led him to observe that reduction in need or drive plays an all important role in the reinforcement of the learning process.

The work of B. F. Skinner (born 1904) has exerted its profound effect on modern psychological thought and has contributed greatly to the enhanced reputation which modern behaviourist theory and practice enjoy today, not only in the academic field of psychology but also in the clinical field of psychiatry. Skinner emphasized the important technique of 'operant conditioning' in learning (p. 115). For Skinner, conforming to traditional behaviourist theory, behaviour was built from reflexes – the stimulus-response units (S-R). 'Operant conditioning' derives its name from the environmental nature of the process since the animal concerned must operate on its environment for the reinforcement of its activity to occur. With the technique of operant conditioning, highly complex patterns of behaviour can be achieved, all based on conditioning of the basic and simple stimulus-response units. By reinforcing only those desired responses, animals can be taught to play simple musical instruments and to engage in other ingenious activities. In the course of experimentation, Skinner introduced his famous 'Skinner Box', a somewhat sophisticated puzzle-box into which the animal to be conditioned would be placed. The Skinner Box, for example, could be arranged with a bar inside, and set up so that pressures upon this bar would release a pellet of food from an overhead hopper. If a hungry rat is placed in the box his movements at first will be random. Sooner or later, it will by chance press the bar and will be immediately rewarded with a pellet of food. Thus the arrival of food *reinforces* the bar-pressing activity and the more frequently the bar is pressed the greater the amount of food available to the rat. Should the overhead food hopper be emptied and not re-filled, the rat will continue to press the bar but no pellets of food will be forthcoming. Quite soon the frequency of the bar-pressing by the rat will fall – showing the phenomenon of *extinction* of the operant response when reinforcement no longer occurs. The sophistication of the Skinner box can be increased by, for example, the introduction of a small electric light. The mechanics of pellet release can then be adjusted to occur only if the light is on. In this way the factor of *discrimination* can be introduced since reinforcement of the rat's bar-pressing activity, by the arrival of food, only occurs when the light is on. Thus, the rat quickly learns to press the bar when the light is illuminated but not if the light is switched off.

Operant conditioning, of course, is relevant to human activities no less than in experimental animals. But caution must be exercised when attempting to translate findings from the experimental setting to the experiences of daily life. A world which functioned purely in Skinner's terms would indeed be an alarming habitat.

Behaviourist theory may rightly explain many of the important means by which both animals and human beings learn and adapt their activities. But fortunately, as it stands today, it can never adequately account for so much that is manifestly inherent in the highly complex, intelligent and creative qualities which epitomize the activities of the human psyche.

Part II
Abnormal psychological reactions and their management

8

IMPORTANT DISORDERED PSYCHOLOGICAL REACTIONS

DISORDERS OF PERCEPTION

Perception (p. 109) is concerned with the meaningful interpretation of the sensory information either in terms of the external environment or of the individual's physical self. It has an innate basis but will, in addition, involve the learning process, for interpretation must depend on previous experience.

Perception may be disturbed by misinterpretation of the pattern of peripheral stimulation and result in *illusions*. Or perceptual interpretation may be based on false beliefs and result in *delusions*. Again, central perception may occur in the absence of appropriate peripheral stimuli and produce the rather dramatic perceptual experiences of *hallucinations*.

Illusions. An illusion is the misinterpretation of peripheral stimuli. It is in fact a perceptual mistake. In its simplest form it results from inadequate input stimuli (e.g. mistaking the shadowy outline of a tree in the dark for a man). Some illusions have a simple physical basis as, for example, the reflection of light in a mirror or the reflection of sound producing an echo. More complicated illusions can be deliberately generated by the presentation of stimuli in a form or pattern designed to mislead perception (e.g. optical illusions, perspective in paintings – fig. 53 and fig. 54). Illusions are repeatedly experienced by all normal people. They may be increased in certain emotional states (e.g. fear) and can be associated with delusions in mental illness.

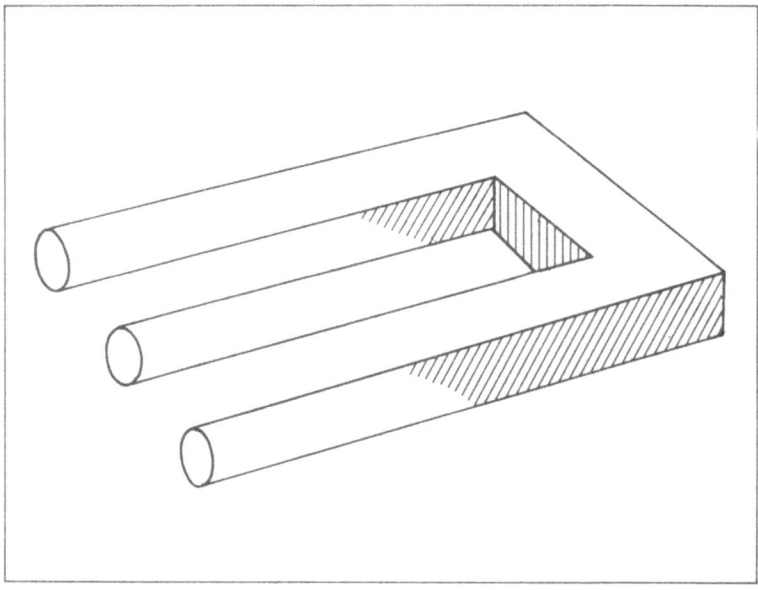

FIGURE 53 An illusion – the impossible figure.

Delusions are perceptual misinterpretations which are based on false beliefs. In assessing whether the beliefs are unreasonable it is essential to take into account the racial, social and cultural background of the individual. Delusions may be classified as normal or pathological. Delusions show great variation in intensity, content and duration not only between one person and another, but also in the same person at different times. They often closely reflect the mood of the individual. Thus depression can give rise to delusions of guilt or nihilism; mania to grandiose delusions; fear or jealousy to persecution ideas. The content of the delusion may be correlated with the mood of the individual but in psychotically disturbed persons there may be complete disparity between the delusion content and the emotional response to it, e.g. hilarity about the imminent end of the world.

While delusions by definition must be held with conviction at some stage, the degree of conviction can vary and the patient can gain some 'insight' into the falseness of the belief. Delusions may be varied and unsystematized but are frequently systematized, such that if one of them is accepted as a reasonable precept, the others flow from it by a logical

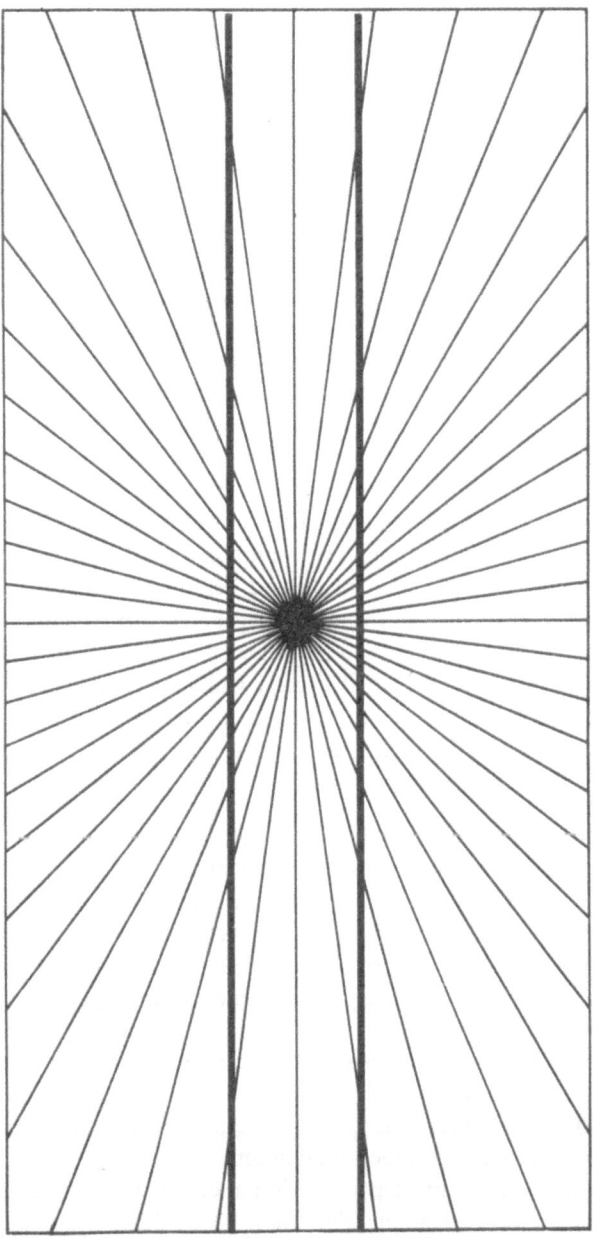

FIGURE 54 The Hering illusion. The vertical lines appear to be curved.

thought process. In the paranoid disorders, delusions are typically systematized and persistent but those of mania are fleeting and often related directly and immediately to the input stimulus.

Hallucinations have a certain similarity to illusions. Whereas illusions are false interpretations of existing stimuli, hallucinations occur in the absence of appropriate peripheral stimuli. They may be associated with any of the sensations, but those with an auditory basis (e.g. voices) are most common; for some there is a more abstract modality (e.g. the feeling of strength being drawn away).

Hallucinations are quite commonly experienced by normal people (e.g. hearing a telephone bell ring) and may be encountered especially when falling asleep – hypnapompic hallucinations; or when waking – hypnagogic hallucinations. The dream provides a special example of a normal hallucination. Pathological hallucinations can occur throughout a wide range of mental illnesses, from schizophrenia to hysteria, and should not be regarded as pathonomonic of a psychosis. Some of the most extensive hallucinations are found in toxic delirium. Pseudo-hallucinations (described for vision and hearing) occupy a somewhat contraversial position between mental imagery and formal hallucinations.

Although it has been stressed that illusions and hallucinations occur regularly in the life of normal beings, and that all these perceptual abnormalities are found in a broad range of mental disorders, they are encountered most frequently and most typically in schizophrenia (p. 188); and in the symptomatic psychoses (p. 201).

DISORDERS OF ATTENTION AND MEMORY

Levels of attention show considerable fluctuations. At one end of the spectrum can be found total attention where concentration is most acute, and at the other end complete absence of attention as may occur in sleep. Between these extremes are found the varying degrees of attention encountered in everyday life and which depend upon that equilibrium established by the ergotrophic and trophotrophic portions of the nervous system. One aspect of the degree of attention prevailing is the formation of an immediate memory imprint, and this leads to a more permanent subsequent memory engram. Factors of memory are thus closely related to degrees of attention.

A frequent complaint of psychiatric patients is that of difficulty in attention and concentration. This may be marked in patients with organic brain diseases and with accompanying dementia. Localized brain damage may also produce 'selective inattention' which occurs when stimuli projected onto an area of local damage in one hemisphere fail to be perceived in competition with stimuli in an unaffected area. Disorders of attention may be divided into those in which a reduced level of awareness of the surroundings is present and those in which an increased awareness exists as, for example, in states of hyper-excitability.

A mild reduction in awareness of the surroundings is termed 'diminished awareness'. Greater degrees involve narrowing of consciousness (e.g. hysterical fugue) or clouding of consciousness, and the states of torpor, stupor and coma. Clouding of consciousness may have a physiological basis in the state between wakefulness and sleep, but it is more commonly pathological and determined by conditions which affect the normal functioning of the brain. These may be toxic states, metabolic disturbances or due to structural damage to the reticular activating system disturbing cortical activity. It presents as a state of apathy or indifference with some excessive drowsiness and failure of registration of memory. Slowed performance in simple arithmetical tests may be found and there will be slowing in the EEG. The common causes include the toxemias, uremia, diabetes and hypoglycemia, barbiturates and alcohol as well as space-occupying lesions in the skull and conditions of epilepsy.

In delirium there is disorientation for place, time and person, and friends are misidentified. Behaviour is often restless, disorganized and purposeless and there may be hallucinations. Delirium, which is often worse at night, may occur from a more severe degree of any of the metabolic disturbances which can produce clouding of consciousness. It is also found in the patient with senile dementia who is suddenly removed from his normal surroundings and presented with unusual visual cues to the environment. Delirium as a response to infection occurs more commonly in children than adults.

Dissociation between consciousness and behaviour may occur in 'automatism'. This may occur from psychological conflict, drug intoxication or a trance state but is frequently seen in the postictal phase of epilepsy. Hysterical fugue can be regarded as an example of automatic behaviour.

A pathological loss of consciousness in greater degree is seen in the conditions of narcolepsy and catatonic schizophrenia where the patient may lapse into sleep or stupor. Unlike the normal sleep process narcoleptics may lapse into a state of unconsciousness while walking, eating or sitting and talking.

At the other end of the consciousness scale but still leading to a patchy inattention are the states of hyperexcitability including mania and the reactions to the amphetamine groups of drugs. Here the attention may temporarily appear to be heightened but this is only of a fleeting character and distractibility is a cardinal feature.

'Insomnia' is the inability to sleep for that normal length of time which is associated with a particular individual. The need for sleep varies from one person to another and any complaints of insomnia should be examined in the light of that person's normal sleeping habits. The complaint of insomnia must be regarded as a symptom and as far as possible treatment should be directed to the underlying cause. There may be physical reasons for the difficulty in sleeping or remaining asleep, e.g. thyrotoxicosis, nocturia etc., but the physician should be alerted to the possibility of emotional disturbance as the basis for the insomnia.

In the anxious patient the usual complaint is of difficulty in getting to sleep because problems crowd in as the patient tries to relax. On the other hand, depressed patients generally find that sleep comes reasonably rapidly but that they wake early in the morning and cannot then get to sleep again.

Disorders of memory rarely involve too acute a memory retention (hypermnesia) but the more common phenomen is a failure to retain memories – amnesia. Hypermnesia is found rarely as a normal pheno-menon. It is seen in a certain percentage of children. It may also be associated with pathological states including hypomania and paranoid psychosis.

In contradistinction to hypermnesia, which is rare, amnesia is an all too common complaint. Loss of memory may be seen in patients with most organic or functional mental reactions, retrograde amnesia relating to events before the onset of the illness or trauma, anterograde amnesia to events after it. From the pathophysiological point of view loss of memory may result from failure of registration, failure of reten-tion or failure of recall. In psychosis, e.g. agitated depression, the ab-normality lies in the altered registration. The retention of short-term memory traces, rather than long-term memory traces, is more affected in organic brain diseases, e.g. infections, neoplasms or arteriosclerotic degenerations. This suggests that the essential pathological process involved is a failure to lay down short-term memory traces with minimal loss to the permanent memory trace. On the other hand in hysterical amnesia, the psychological mechanism involved is probably that of repression and it is probably the recall mechanism which is involved. This can be confirmed by the improvement in memory which can take place in such patients under hypnosis.

9

PSYCHIATRIC DISORDERS
AND THEIR
CLASSIFICATION

The past two decades have seen major advances in our understanding
of the physical changes which underlie many psychiatric disorders. In
consequence, these advances have found a radical and effective application in the field of psychopharmacology. This successful application
has in turn promoted a decline in the importance of earlier psycho-
dynamic hypotheses which have attempted to explain and offer a
rational therapy for the mental illnesses.

It might have been hoped that this could also imply that the classification of mental disorders would be made more meaningful, particularly if a single descriptive classification could be achieved, capable
of modification as aetiology becomes better understood. Unfortunately,
a multiplicity of systems of classifying mental illness still exists which
has led to serious difficulties, not least those of comparing psychiatric
observations from different centres.

In broad terms, psychological illness may be divided into the neuroses
and the psychoses, with the additional important groupings of mental
deficiency and personality disorders, including their special sub-
grouping of psychopathy. Such boundary as exists between neurotic
and psychotic illness cannot be clearly demarcated nor can the psychoses
themselves be rigidly defined. In consequence, many of the current
systems of classification will exhibit variance according to the opinion of
the classifying authority – a situation which calls for the greatest caution

if designated illnesses from two or more classifications are compared. A suggested simplified classification is shown in Table 6. A psychosis is perhaps best considered an illness of the mind in which disruption of the personality is manifest within a setting of substantial morbid mental symptomatology. A neurosis, on the other hand, displays less florid mental symptomatology and minimal disruption of personality.

TABLE 6 Working classification of the most common psychiatric diseases.

NEUROSES
   Anxiety states
   Obsessive—compulsive disorders
   Hysteria
   Neurotic depression

PSYCHOSES
   Schizophrenia
   Paranoid disorders
   Organic psychoses
   Affective psychoses
      Psychotic depression
      Manic-depressive psychosis
      Manic states

PSYCHOSOMATIC DISORDERS

HYPOCHONDRIASIS, NEURASTHENIA

MENTAL SUBNORMALITY

PERSONALITY DISORDERS

Variation in those features which characterise the human psyche are not necessarily pathological. Undulations of mood are common to us all – to the medical practitioner no less than to his patient. Anxiety is a purposeful reaction to the environment and provides an essential driving force of life. Most of us at times have shown the paranoid tendency of 'blaming our tools'.

The medical practitioner has therefore two problems to face when dealing with any patient with a suspected mental illness. Firstly, is the change a pathological one or does it fall within the range of normal response to the varying environment? Secondly, what is the nature of the illness, the management of the patient and the treatment required?

The neuroses

ANXIETY STATES

Of all the psychological phenomena encountered in medical practice, none is seen more frequently than anxiety. Such anxiety however will not necessarily be of psychiatric importance.

Anxiety *per se* is not pathological and provides an essential driving force of life. Its alerting influence heightens awareness and anticipation and increases perception. Efficiency and performance are each enhanced by it and at times these advantages may be sought deliberately, e.g. by athletes.

The anxious personality – though not of itself suffering from mental illness – is the born worrier of life. Such individuals function against a background of apprehension and fear which fluctuates in its intensity. Habitually bent on crossing the bridges of life far in advance of ever reaching them, much mental energy is dissipated in anticipating hypothetical future crises, whilst being in a position to do nothing for their resolution. Such crises as may in the course of time confront the anxious personality are infinitely more simple in reality than ever postulated in anxious anticipation.

For this type of personality, a world without worry would be incomprehensible – even when day to day events are set quite fair. By no means infrequently, the anxious personality will with very good insight confess that should the day ever dawn when he found himself quite free of anxiety, he would at once realize that something was very substantially wrong. Such personalities, of course, effectively employ their anxiety as a considerable source of drive.

The mental stresses of the anxious personality are readily converted to somatic symptoms and concern for the physical state of health is common. Hypochondrical fears are readily in evidence – particularly with the more dramatic forms of illness, such as coronary thrombosis, cerebral apoplexy and the well-known forms of cancer. Preoccupation for medical dictionaries, text-books and television programmes dealing with disease, is a further familiar finding among anxious personalities.

Since illness and worry go hand in hand, a distinction must be made between anxiety which contributes in a causative fashion to the disease and that which occurs in a secondary capacity from the illness itself.

Such secondary symptoms are extremely common and furnish the greater part of all anxiety observed by the medical practitioner. These symptoms moreover are not confined to the patient, but are found as frequently and severely among the close relatives. Theirs is the anxiety which often initiates the attendance of the patient at the doctor's surgery.

No clear-cut line demarcates these minor and purposive quantities of anxiety from those major amounts which represent the morbid anxiety of mental illness. Nor will approximate equivalent amounts of anxiety affect different individuals in any similar way. In terms of medical practice, it is more helpful to envisage a 'quantitative anxiety-continuum' against which must be set the personal tolerance of the individual. Qualitatively too, the type of stress evoking an anxiety response will be highly selective and will vary enormously from individual to individual. Severe anxiety disrupts normal psychological function; cerebration may decline to a level of near mental paralysis and in a setting of abject fear. Such degrees of anxiety constitute an obvious mental illness; pathological degrees of anxiety are designated 'morbid anxiety'.

Morbid anxiety

The features of morbid anxiety are characteristically those of apprehension and dread. Its focus may switch in mercurial fashion from one concept of menace to another – the phenomenon of 'free-floating anxiety'. Alternatively, the morbid anxiety may attach itself with limpet-like tenacity to any one of a variety of incongruous concepts, manifesting itself as intense fears – the so-called phobias (fig. 55). From agoraphobia (fear of open spaces) to xenophobia (fear of strangers) impressive lists of these phobias may be found in the earlier psychiatric text-books. These are not separate illnesses but specific attachments that morbid anxiety may select.

In many instances the genesis of morbid anxiety will be simple. It results pre-eminently from the stress of conflict between the specific needs of the individual and those realities thrust upon him by life. The circumstances of employment, finance and domestic life are fertile fields of conflict in which such individual factors as shattered pride, thwarted ambition and disappointment are powerful operants. Responsibility with insufficient support will generate major degrees of morbid anxiety in those psychologically vulnerable to stress of this kind.

The role of sexual difficulties in the genesis of anxiety, no less than the role of anxiety in the genesis of sexual problems, is complex and far

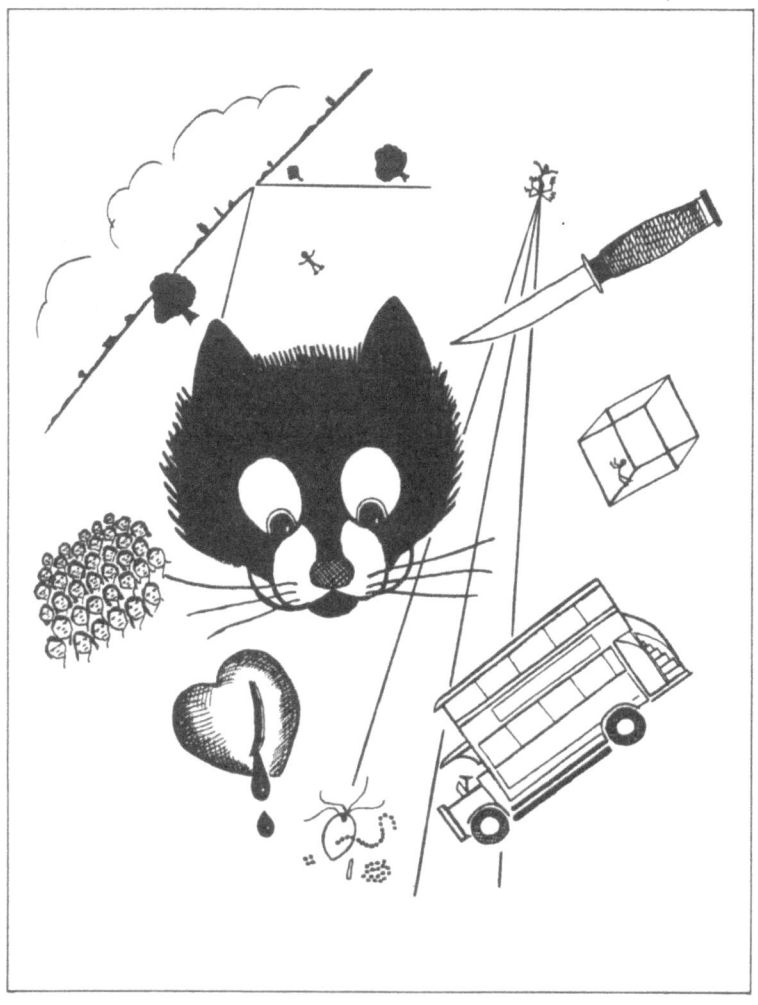

FIGURE 55 Common attachments of Morbid Anxiety illustrating fear of cats, crowds, heights, open spaces, sharp objects, enclosed spaces, blood, germs and travel.

reaching. The potential of the sexual field for the production of morbid anxiety is increased enormously by prevailing ignorance and superstitious taboo. However, the Freudian view (p. 153) which sought to explain morbid anxiety solely on the basis of unsatisfied sexual arousal cannot be accepted.

Morbid anxiety relays its effects via the hypothalamic region of the brain to both sympathetic and parasympathetic components of the autonomic nervous system and via the anterior pituitary to the endocrine glands (p. 93). Thus anxiety will present not only by mental symptoms, but by somatic manifestations resulting from an imbalance of the two components of the autonomic nervous system and of the endocrine glands.

The mental symptoms of morbid anxiety are set against a background of increased irritability, apprehension and an awareness of tension. An ill-defined sense of impending catastrophe may co-exist with a host of isolated fears, among which the fear of insanity occurs with overwhelming frequency. Morbid introspection, often coloured by accompanying depression, breeds hypochondriacal fears of physical illness. Concentration becomes impossible and memory is thereby faulty. Sleep, an early casualty of anxiety, is disrupted. Considerable difficulty in getting off to sleep precedes a night of anxious dreaming or nightmares: fitful waking may occur during the night with the patient in a state of panic and bathed in perspiration.

The somatic symptoms of anxiety are legion. They include pallor, dilated pupils, dry mouth, sweating and tachycardia with hypertension. There is a heightened muscle tone and frank trembling or fine tremors may be seen. Nausea, vomiting and diarrhoea are indicative of the general hypermotility of the alimentary tract. Parasympathetic overactivity is further evidenced by frequency of micturition. Spontaneous orgasms may add to the patient's distress.

The psychosomatic implications of morbid anxiety are extensive and necessitate careful evaluation in physical disease (p. 211). Asthma, angioneurotic oedema, peptic ulceration, ulcerative colitis, migraine, hypertension, hyperthyroidism and neurodermatoses require special mention, as also do menstrual irregularities and many pelvic disorders of women. Anxiety represents a common cause of obesity, for eating supplies a simple means of allaying tension.

In childhood years, when the cerebrum has yet to triumph over primitive visceral response, morbid anxiety is responsible for many common behaviour disorders. It causes problems of feeding, elimination and sleeping no less than undesirable habits and emotional outbursts.

Diagnosis

Morbid anxiety is seen most commonly in association with a background anxiety state where genetic factors lower the threshold for worry or stress. Such persons tend to be 'born worriers', commonly show obsessional traits and quite frequently a tendency to depressive reactions. A history of recurrent nervous stress or earlier 'breakdown' is usual, and often the family history reveals similar anxious traits among close relatives.

Just as anxiety may manifest itself in the form of apparent somatic illness, so physical illnesses are usually accompanied by a variable amount of anxiety. One of the most difficult problems is the separation of the primary anxiety state from a normal degree of anxiety occurring in other illnesses.

Morbid anxiety may be a prominent symptom of any mental illness known to us. Its extreme limitation as a diagnostic agent will therefore be at once appreciated. A large proportion of morbid anxiety observed in medical practice is released by minor depressive illness, though depressive symptoms may not at once be obvious in its presentation. Intense morbid anxiety can emerge in close conjunction with obsessive-compulsive illness.

Management

The treatment of morbid anxiety by the medical practitioner effectively commences at his initial interview with the patient. Both the manner and conduct of this consultation will prove of paramount importance in subsequent therapy. The patient's narrative must be heard in full, uncritically and – an important feature if the practitioner's time will permit – unhurriedly. Reassurance should be given on individual issues as each arises, together with any practical counsel which may be indicated for their solution. It is important to reassure the patient by an explanation of the symptoms and by enlightenment on their mode of origin. Emphasis should be placed on the very favourable outcome of illness of this kind.

Where there are somatic complaints, a full physical examination should be made to dispel authoritatively the patient's concern for his somatic symptomatology. An effort should be made to restore as speedily as possible a satisfactory cycle of sleep. A good diet and adequate exercise are helpful in assisting the patient's general state of health and therefore increasing his resistance to the stress.

Such elementary psychotherapy is an important feature in the practitioner's management of morbid anxiety. More ambitious psychotherapeutic measures may bring their own complications and are best left in the hands of a qualified psychiatrist. A description of the techniques is given in Chapter 11.

The psychotherapy, whether of an elementary or ambitious type, and reassurance should be supplemented by appropriate medication, preferably a tranquillizer or, failing this, a simple mild sedative. Among the tranquillizers which are very effective in the control of morbid anxiety are the benzodiazepines of which one of the most effective is diazepam. These drugs will reduce the anxiety whether this presents as a mental disturbance or causes somatic symptoms. They are effective in anxiety ranging in intensity from a minor condition covering a transient crisis to a chronic state capable of causing gross disturbances in the functioning of the individual. They may also be given with benefit as adjuvant therapy in the anxiety states which are secondary to other illnesses. A more extensive description of the anxiolytic drugs is given in Chapter 12.

OBSESSIVE-COMPULSIVE DISORDERS

Attempts to manipulate the forces of destiny by pagan and supernatural practice are made by us all at some time or another. Perhaps the rabbit scut or four-leafed clover carried to the examination room, perhaps the magic word before the croupier's wheel has come to rest. When mental stress runs high the human mind seeks solace for itself in devious avenues of thought and in curious patterns of behaviour. We realize, of course, the absurdity of our actions – yet, why be sorry when we can at least be safe? In other words, like all obsessive-compulsive symptomatology, it is much easier and less painful to accede to the illogical than to resist and to cope with the ensuing emotional distress.

Obsessive-compulsive phenomena are very common among children, and are a natural aspect of their normal behaviour. Avoiding cracks in the pavement, often visualized as chasms descending to an infernal world, intricate ceremonials before mounting stairs or knocking rituals before entering doorways, all, for the imaginative child, serve to ward off evil influence. During development to adult life many of these features recede, some, however, persist, a situation to which the countless superstitions testify. While some of these features will be found in most of us, certain adults will show them to a substantial degree in the course of their individual behaviour. For this type of person, the term 'obsessional personality' is used. Typically they show an overdeveloped degree of conscientiousness combined with an aspiration to high standards – 'perfectionists'. They often dangle these standards ahead of themselves so that as one standard is reached the level itself is tantalizingly raised. In such a personality there is rarely satisfaction with a job well done .They become at the same time their own slave and exacting taskmasters. An exaggerated sense of orderliness is found in some aspect of the individual's life, although this orderliness may not be present throughout the remainder. This may be in manner of dress, in handwriting (fig. 56), or for example in the obsessional housewife, the exaggeration of house-proud characteristics. There is an inclination to parsimony, rigidity of habit and an inflexibility of thought, and since doubt and indecision are common the obsessional personality has a tendency to check and re-check repeatedly. Such personalities form of course but one of the many different types which collectively compose that wide range we term 'normality'. Under favourable circumstances and in appropriate occupation, the drive of the obsessional, his precision and high sense of duty often render him among the most valued members of our society.

Morbid obsessive-compulsive disorder

No certain boundary exists between those upper limits of exaggerated though normal obsessional traits of the personality and the lower limits of their corresponding neurotic illnesses. The essential feature by which we may regard the characteristics as reaching a level of an illness is the obtrusion into consciousness of undesired ideas and thoughts, the contents of which may be unpleasant, senseless and acutely distressing. Feelings of compulsion to perform certain acts may accompany the obsessional thinking. An important characteristic of obsessive-compulsive illness is the unavailing struggle of the patient to rid himself of the demands of these unwanted thoughts with its ensuing conflict, tension and mounting degree of anxiety. In advanced form this will produce the obsessional type of phobia.

The normal individual can gain some little insight into the tension produced by these obsessional problems by remembering the difficulties, not passing from one to another as was the opinion of Pythagoras, who held that a transmigration of the soul ; but that the soul is given to every infant by infusion is the most received and orthodox opinion. And the learned do likewise agree that this is done when the infant is perfected in the womb, which happens about the twenty-fourth day after conception.

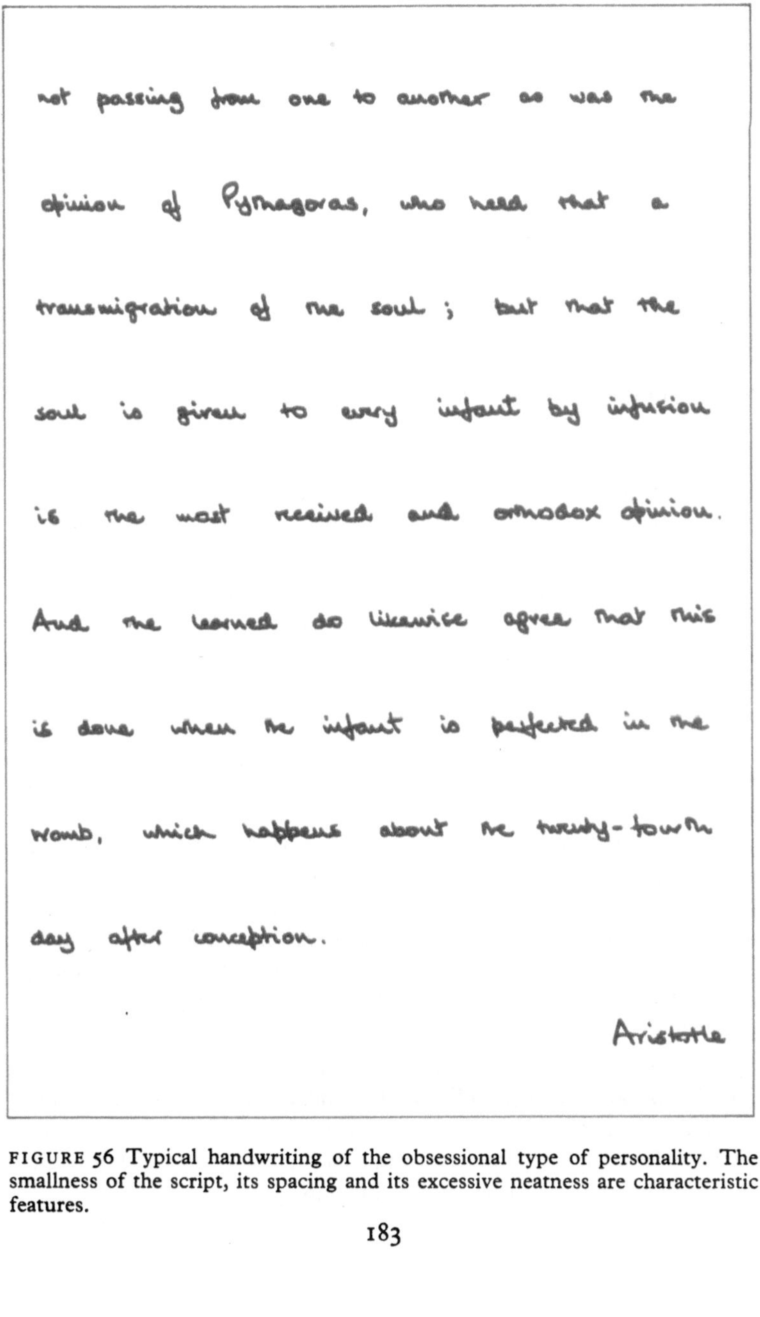

Aristotle

FIGURE 56 Typical handwriting of the obsessional type of personality. The smallness of the script, its spacing and its excessive neatness are characteristic features.

frustration and ineffective mental manœuvres to which he may resort in an attempt to rid himself of a persistent fragment of tune which inexplicably keeps running through his head.

Diagnosis

Not only does obsessive-compulsive illness occur *per se* but its symptomatology may be indicative of other mental illness. Any psychological stress with accompanying anxiety can induce a transient phase of obsessional symptoms in those so predisposed. Depression with its affinity for the obsessional personality will produce a similar symptomatology, and organic disease of the brain can precipitate obsessive-compulsive features.

Although minor obsessive-compulsive symptomatology may prove of little more than annoyance to the individual, advanced forms of obsessive-compulsive illness can be utterly incapacitating. The conflict between the compulsive nature of the obsession and the fear of yielding to it is the main reason for this gross incapacity. This is accentuated by the doubt and indecisiveness of such personalities which leads to a greater and greater number of checks being made.

Typical and traumatic examples are the tracing of recurring motifs of patterned wallpaper, dressing rituals, washing rituals, number patterns in those who have to utilize numbers frequently, e.g. accountants, and fear of compulsive obscene phrases in upright pillars of the community, e.g. clergymen.

Management

During his assessment of both the nature and extent of an obsessive-compulsive symptomatology, the medical practitioner will be wise to seek an opinion from a psychiatric colleague. When such symptoms arise, as they commonly do, within the structure of a second, underlying mental illness, their treatment will clearly be that of the underlying illness in question. Hence the effective treatment of morbid anxiety, depression or schizophrenic disorder will secondarily relieve obsessive-compulsive features which may be present in the course of these illnesses. With obsessive-compulsive illness itself, treatment can pose a number of very difficult problems. Frequently this illness is found to be one of long-standing and, as such, may prove disappointingly resistant to therapy – including specialized psychiatric procedures. Nevertheless, such resistant cases may still show phases of fluctuation when improvement will be observed for no apparent reason.

In general terms, psychotherapy of a supportive kind, with explanation of symptoms and enlightenment of those special features of personality which enter into the illness, will afford valuable help to the obsessionally ill patient. Furthermore, some reorganization of the daily life, if possible directed to the avoidance of circumstances found by experience to aggravate the disorder, will prove helpful.

Medication plays an important part in the relief of obsessive-compulsive symptoms, particularly when these are accompanied by depression or mounting degrees of anxiety and tension. Such medication may with advantage take the form of an antidepressant, simple sedation, or the use of appropriate tranquillizers, e.g. diazepam which has been shown to be an extremely valuable drug in the relief of obsessive-compulsive disorders, when marked degrees of anxiety and tension are present.

HYSTERIA

The feature common to all cases of hysteria is a breakdown in central nervous system integration. This breakdown usually occurs as a reaction to stress. In individuals with normal stability such a breakdown will occur only as a result of an exceptionally severe degree of stress, but in an unusually susceptible person a minor degree of distress may precipitate hysteria. There is evidence to suggest that this susceptibility to hysteria is associated with the extroverted type of behaviour pattern and some familiar pattern seems to exist. Central to hysterical symptomatology is the phenomenon of 'dissociation'.

The hysterical personality

Among the different types of personality which are recognized in life, the hysterical personality is a more obvious one.

Its essential features can be found in the dual traits of immaturity and inadequacy. From these arise that need for marked emotional dependence upon others, as also do the exaggerated demands for attention and affection. The traits foster furthermore the craving by this personality to be accepted by others as being something far greater than it really is. Lacking an adequate central stability, the hysterical personality is liable to display a chameleon-like versatility. Role after role may be switched or rejected to capitalize on the advantages of the moment. Affective response is typically forced, artificial and shallow. In the sexual field, an outward display of enticement and encouragement contrasts markedly with a limited or absent capacity for performance.

In so many aspects, the hysterical personality inhabits a world of childish make-believe and utilizes the unreal values appropriate to childhood. Like the thwarted child, resenting its lack of independence, it seeks to impress others with its own importance; like the over-indulged child, frustrated at not gaining its own way, it revels in dramatic scenes of histrionic behaviour so reminiscent of a childish tantrum.

The hysterical personality employs many and devious means to attain its ends. Threats of suicide are extremely common. Though frequently empty, they can never be taken lightly for the hysteric is notoriously liable to overplay his or her hand and what was intended as a suicide gesture may well end as the consummated act.

The involved manipulations of the hysterical personality are characteristically bids for dominance from a position of natural weakness.

Diagnosis

Hysterical symptoms may take innumerable forms. There may be disturbances of sensation such as anaesthesia or paraesthesia or other neurological symptoms such as ataxia; spastic or flaccid paralysis; choreiform or athetoid movements and tremor. Other manifestations include loss of vision, gynaecological complaints, difficulty in breathing or in swallowing, abdominal pains and peculiar dermatoses. Mental disturbances include double or multiple personality. In some cases, a hysterical fugue or trance (fig. 57) follows a traumatic experience but in others it is an escape from a disagreeable situation.

The differential diagnosis of hysteria is full of difficulty, not least the necessity to make certain that no organic lesion is present. It should be possible to show that the symptom is a response to some conscious experience which has a strong personal significance to the patient. Even so, it may sometimes be very difficult to decide between symptoms due to organic disease and those of hysterical states, particularly in later life when there may be a hysterical overlay on pre-existing organic lesion.

Management

No simple formula can be advanced for the treatment of hysteria. Each case will obviously be assessed on its highly individual merits and therapy devised accordingly. A detailed case history will be taken and a careful physical examination must be made to exclude an underlying and contributing organic illness. The personality of the doctor for better or worse will play a vital part in the attainment of any degree

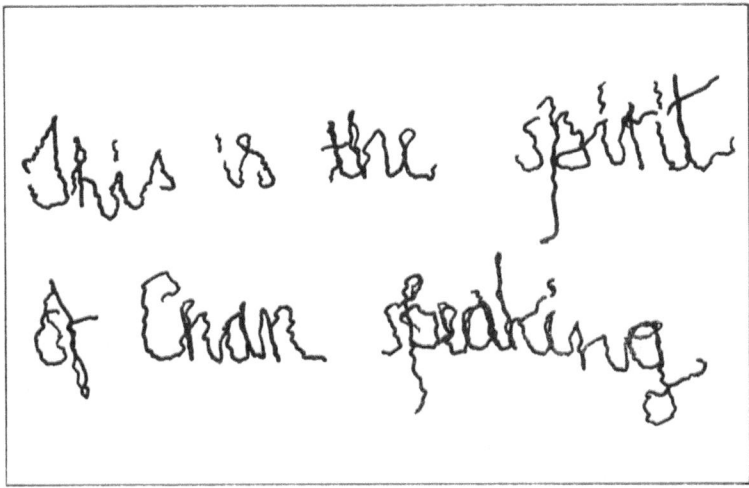

FIGURE 57 Automatic writing from a state of hysterical trance. Female hysteric aged 42 years. Persuaded to dabble in spiritualism by friends, she was hailed as a 'medium' and became possessed of an evil spirit named Chan.

of success. It is for this reason that unskilled and unqualified persons may achieve outstanding success in the treatment of this neurosis where eminently qualified persons may fail. There is a possibility of curing an acute hysterical reaction by simple suggestion and a heavy dose of a sedative. A chronic hysterical condition is, however, one which may demand all the resources of psychiatric therapy to effect any permanent improvement. The basis of successful treatment is suggestion and this may be done either over a long period or in single intensive association under hypnosis or under light anaesthesia. Abreactive methods may also be used. It is thus clear that the management of hysteria requires the attention of a physician skilled in the use of these particular techniques and referral is therefore advised.

Apart from the use of mild sedatives to secure reasonable sleep and tranquillizers to allay anxiety, drugs are of little benefit in the hysterical states.

NEUROTIC DEPRESSION

Neurotic depression is by usage considered to include the 'reactive' form of depression rather than the less comprehensible 'endogenous' type of the illness. These two sub-groupings are, however, by no means mutually exclusive and in some instances an illness may assume certain

187

features of each and considerable overlap may be present at times.

For this reason depression falls into the fields of both neuroses and psychoses and is considered as a whole in the group of Affective Disorders under the term Affective Psychoses (p. 202).

The Psychoses

SCHIZOPHRENIA

The incidence of schizophrenia in civilized nations shows a remarkable level of consistency at approximately one per 100 of the population.

Schizophrenia should be visualized as a 'splintered mind' – a psyche fragmented by the impact and progression of an illness, within the course of which the normal capacities for behaviour – perceiving, thinking, feeling, and physical movements – exhibit disorganization and disintegration in varying degree (fig. 58).

Schizophrenia should not be thought a single entity. Its name embraces a whole constellation or cluster of psychological illnesses of similar form. In many cases, where clear-cut and typical symptoms can be observed, the diagnosis will be a very obvious one. Yet in other instances, drawn more from the periphery of this composite group of diseases, the problem of diagnosis may prove one of extreme difficulty to be disputed at length and with considerable disagreement by highly competent psychiatric authorities.

Schizophrenia, most characteristically, reveals itself during the years of young adulthood. So much of its tragedy – until the arrival of modern drugs and methods of treatment – lay in the prospect of a life-sentence of hospitalization conferred by this psychosis. Too frequently such patients degenerated slowly in the chronic wards of mental hospitals, forgotten by the world and incapacitated more and more by their deterioration, until death – sometimes as much as half a century or more later – mercifully relieved them of the final stages of their illness.

The origins of schizophrenia

Still today, the aetiology of schizophrenia remains a subject for anyone's inspired guess. Though much has been postulated and counter-postulated in the pursuit of elusive, possible causes, our wealth of findings to date is quite inconclusive and the inferences drawn from these are highly speculative.

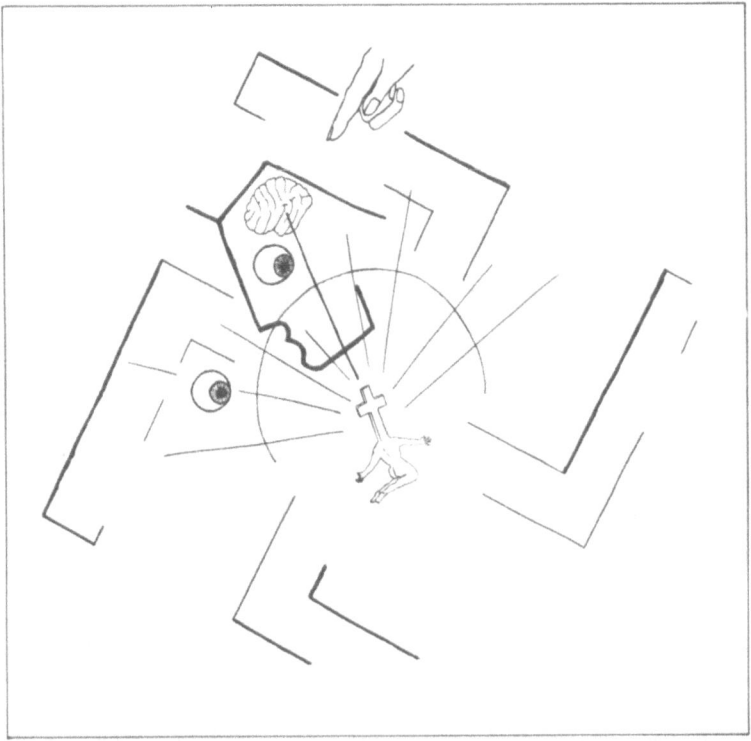

FIGURE 58 Drawing by male paranoid schizophrenic patient aged 37 years illustrating his dream. Many significant features of the symptomatology of this illness are shown. A two-dimensional face contrasts with the three-dimensional eyes – one of which is dissociated entirely from the face. Both eyes are turned to the supplicating figure of religious mystique, from which deliverance and salvation from the mental illness is sought. A finger of accusation, directed at the brain and coercing its activities, indicates the intense ideas of reference experienced by the patient.

The reversed swastika (with its persecutory associations) suggests arms and legs in headlong flight from the evil agents of external influence.

Genetic studies rightly stress the important and decisive role played by the mechanisms of heredity in the transmission of schizophrenia. Geneticists, however, are by no means agreed on the manner in which this transmission occurs. Conflicting hypotheses therefore exist with preferences for single genes of dominant, recessive, or intermediate type, or again for polygenic inheritance from the additive influence of multiple genes. Linked with these theories of inheritance is the interesting affinity which schizophrenia displays for the ectomorphic type of physical habitus.

The conflicting 'breed' and 'drift' hypotheses, which attempt to explain the greater incidence of schizophrenia among the lowest social classes, exemplify the major differences in outlook which have existed between genetic and environmental standpoints.

Pharmacological and biochemical studies contribute greatly to current aetiological theories of schizophrenic illness. Gjessing earlier showed how the periodic phases of stupor and excitement in catatonic schizophrenia could be equated with a retention of nitrogen within the body, and how compensatory excretion of nitrogen occurred during the intervals which followed such phases.

The hallucinogenic compounds – mescaline, LSD[25], psilocybin and psilocyn – have been found to induce psychotic states reminiscent of schizophrenia and therefore promoted much speculation for a pharmacological basis of schizophrenia in terms of these 'model psychoses'. Some biochemists look to the faulty metabolism of nor-adrenaline and adrenaline – each chemically closely related to mescaline – as significantly responsible; others favour quantitative disorders of cerebral serotonin and similar neuro-transmitters within the brain. Deficiencies of cerebral enzymes no less than defective carbohydrate metabolism have been advanced with enthusiasm as possible causative agents.

Attention was focused on the 'pink spot', produced on chromatographic paper allegedly by a substance excreted in the urine of non-paranoid schizophrenics, and dubiously hailed as DMPE (dimethoxyphenylethylamine) – a further mescaline-like compound. This 'pink spot' theory however was later shown to be invalid.

A toxin, taraxein, has been claimed to exist in schizophrenic blood. The possibilities that schizophrenia may be an allergic response or an auto-immune disease caused by a circulating antibody have also been put forward.

Psychoanalytical theory has traditionally sought to attribute schizophrenia to the sequelae of infantile experience and has viewed its symptomatology as regression to early narcissistic levels. Attempts have been made to explain schizophrenia in terms of adverse familial and social factors (see below). Other theories seek to resolve the mysteries of schizophrenia on the basis of a psychosomatic response to emotional stress.

From this net-work of conjecture, the possibility that schizophrenia may originate in an inherited dysfunction of metabolism is a tempting one. This theory – from the many postulated – may one day be proven as lying closest to the truth.

The interpersonal relationship between the family and the child in its early years has been closely studied. Attention has been drawn to the phenomenon of the 'double bind' as causative in schizophrenia. The 'double bind' indicates the conflict which may occur in communication between the mother and her child by a simultaneous process of attraction and repulsion. Thus the mother may state verbally to the child 'I love you' and yet the emotional tones may indicate with an equal clarity 'I hate you'.

An alternative concept in considerations of maternal influence in the production of schizophrenia is that of the 'schizophrenogenic mother'.

Clinical varieties of schizophrenia

Schizophrenia, most conveniently, may be sub-divided into four broad clinical varieties – simple schizophrenia, hebephrenia, catatonic schizophrenia and paranoid schizophrenia.

Simple schizophrenia declares itself in late adolescence or early adulthood and characteristically displays a gradual mental decline with marked blunting of affect. Delusions and hallucinations are conspicuously absent. Such simple schizophrenics gravitate more and more to the lowest strata of life and contribute regularly to the unemployable and to the ranks of vagrants and of prostitutes.

Hebephrenia, occurring in the early twenties, again exhibits a very prominent blunting and incongruity of affect. Fantastic delusions and hallucinations are experienced by the patient (fig. 59). Curious mannerisms and antics are displayed together with other aspects of childish inconsequential behaviour. Inane giggling and inapposite grimacing are very common. A progressive deterioration of the personality ensues, establishing the prognosis in hebephrenia as least favourable among the clinical varieties.

In catatonic schizophrenia, symptoms of motor disorder predominate. Characteristic changes in muscle tone are found in the waxy flexibility, the extraordinary statuesque posturing, and the facial contortions encountered in this disease. Phases of stupor may alternate with outbursts of excitement, and automatic obedience, echolalia and echopraxia are frequently in evidence.

191

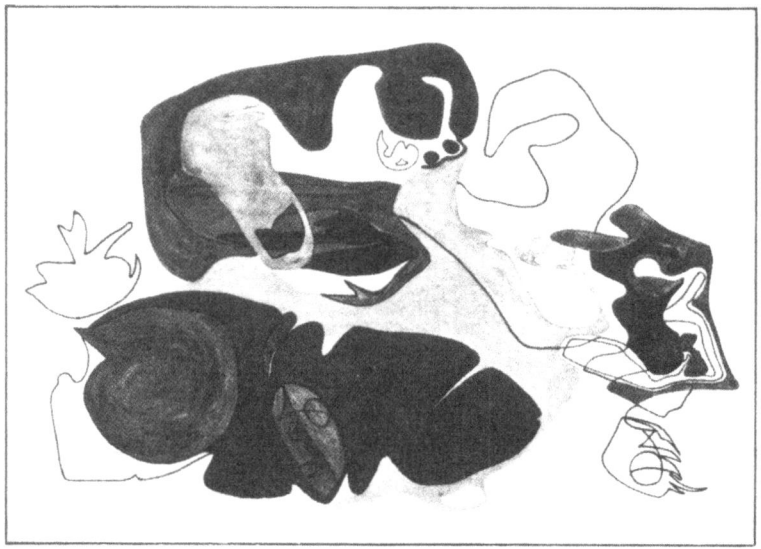

FIGURE 59 Painting by male hebephrenic patient aged 25 years. Such painting may represent to the withdrawn schizophrenic patient the only remaining means of communicating to those about him the intense inner turmoil of his mind.

Paranoid schizophrenia, in contrast with the other clinical varieties, occurs at a much later age – usually about the middle thirties. The dominant feature of this type of schizophrenia is to be found in the remarkable delusions of persecution expressed by the patient, often incorporating ideas of grandeur. The turmoil of the patient's mind is projected upon the world about him, and the most involved suspicions – intricately systematized and unbelievably complex – then emerge from his distorted appraisal of events and circumstances around him. Hallucinations of bodily interference by external agents are very common. The tendency for deterioration is less in paranoid schizophrenia and the prognosis, correspondingly, is much more favourable.

Diagnosis

In 1896, Kraepelin's unification of a large number of hitherto seemingly heterogeneous illnesses under the one concept 'dementia praecox' has constituted one of the greatest milestones of psychiatric history. Later, in 1911, dementia praecox was re-designated 'schizophrenia' by Bleuler – a change which has found universal acceptance.

The symptomatology of schizophrenia embraces disorders of thought, emotion, perception and motor function, with degrees of aberration which show no relationship one with the other. When possible it is important to differentiate between the primary symptoms of schizophrenia, i.e. those arising directly from the disease process, and secondary symptoms, i.e. those resulting from the patient's mental reactions to the havoc of his own psychosis. The primary symptoms are diagnostically vital; the secondary ones may serve, in a number of cases, to confuse the picture.

The thoughts of the schizophrenic frequently exhibit 'tangential' qualities and progress in a manner reminiscent of the knight's move in chess. He senses that his private thoughts are no longer his own but overheard and manipulated by other persons. Subsidiary ideas may intrude to the point of 'overinclusion'.

The primary delusion which emerges without apparent cause completely 'out of the blue' is a fundamental feature of the schizophrenic thought disorder. The patient, for example, suddenly becomes aware with an unshakeable conviction that he is the reincarnation of Napoleon.

Further evidence of thought disorder may be found in the patient's spoken and written word. Normal words and phrases acquire different meanings to the schizophrenic and stilted patterns of phraseology are employed. Curious neologisms reminiscent of Lewis Carroll's 'Jabberwocky' are liable to be coined, and idiosyncrasies, mannerisms and stereotypes may be strikingly evident in the patient's handwriting.

Emotional disorder of the schizophrenic shows incongruity of affect, compared with the thought process. The typical reaction is a blunting, with finer feelings lost and replaced by an apparent coldness and callousness. Giggling or laughing under the most inappropriate of circumstances readily occurs.

Disorders of perception show themselves as illusions and hallucinations. Auditory hallucinations occur with the greatest frequency. Voices may echo the patient's thoughts as if these were spoken aloud; they may command or direct him, they may criticize his actions or at other times may comfort or encourage him. Haptic hallucinations of physical interference, frequently with sexual connotations, are common.

Kurt Schneider has grouped the symptoms of schizophrenia into those of first rank and second rank. His symptoms of the first rank are principally those of the ego-disorder – the cardinal feature of schizophrenia – and as such are of high diagnostic value.

Management

The important feature of the initial management of the schizophrenic patient is an accurate diagnosis coupled with an assessment of response to drug therapy. It is important to assess whether the patient can return to useful or semi-useful life, within the surroundings of the family community.

In many cases of schizophrenia hospitalization is desirable once the disorder is suspected and in all cases a psychiatric opinion is essential.

Though hospital care, with its specialized techniques and nursing, is still indicated in acute exacerbations, the duration of such temporary periods of hospitalization is becoming progressively shorter. This is due to the rapid control of symptoms which is now possible by the use of neuroleptic drugs, emphasis on active rehabilitation and the policy of social care of the schizophrenic patient within the community.

When the management of a schizophrenic patient is undertaken within the family circle, advice to, support for and not infrequently treatment of other members of the family become highly important considerations of therapy. The responsibility of such a patient may at times be demanding in the extreme, even for the most robust. The relatives are likely to be subjected to social, economic and emotional strains, which at times may seem scarcely tolerable. Moreover, among these relatives may be some who are suffering from an attenuated form of the same psychosis.

It is therefore important to interview directly the relatives concerned with the management of the schizophrenic patient at regular intervals. During such interviews, symptoms and signs of emotional disorders should be sought. Specifically, it is important to look for the early stages of both anxiety states and depression, and give appropriate advice and if necessary treatment.

It would be foolish to suggest that, at our present stage of psychiatric knowledge, schizophrenia can be cured. Nevertheless the effective control of the symptoms by adequate medication under medical supervision enables many schizophrenic patients to lead useful and near normal lives. This provides the further inestimable therapeutic advantage which comes from a restored ability to earn a living and to maintain a rightful place within the community.

An important feature of the management of the schizophrenic, once their total disorientation has been controlled, is to stress the ultimate aim of their return to a useful life within the community.

A number of psychiatric drugs developed within the past fifteen years have enabled the more florid symptoms of schizophrenia to be effectively controlled. In doing so, they have brought the treatment and management of the schizophrenic patient more and more within the sphere of the patient's own doctor under a psychiatrist's guidance.

The standard drugs for the treatment of schizophrenia are the phenothiazines and butyrophenones. A more detailed description of the use of the neuroleptics is given in Chapter 12. At times, the addition of an anti-depressant, such as amitriptyline, to the classical neuroleptic compound may prove of very great help as depression is often an accompanying factor in these cases. Tranquillizers such as the benzodiazepines allay anxiety and facilitate a more direct and easier approach to the anxious schizophrenic patient but have no direct effect on the primary disorder. These drugs are also a great help for the patient's family. A safe, mild sedative compound, e.g. nitrazepam, may be given to improve sleep in the disturbed schizophrenic.

PARANOID DISORDERS

The bad workman blames his tools. Most of us at some time are bad workmen. The conscientious, law-abiding motorist successively charged with a series of petty offences for inappropriate parking, may feel an element of personal discrimination against him and develop irrational ideas of victimization.

The ne'er-do-well in life is rarely at any loss to explain that, but for the jealousies encountered from less endowed individuals or the inescapable adversities of circumstance, life would have carried him to the top on the crest of its successful wave.

Such tendencies to seek both cause and explanation for our shortcomings in external agents rather than from within ourselves are characteristically human. So too is the tendency to exteriorize our emotional disturbance, defect of personality and inner conflict onto our surroundings and then to perceive these defects as originating from the environment. This unconscious practice of self-deception represents the psychological mechanism of projection – an essential mental phenomenon in the pathology of paranoid disorder.

The origins of paranoid disorders

Genetic endowment may greatly predispose to paranoid disorder – an influence which can be seen in the paranoid personality no less than in those paranoid reactions which accompany such inherited mental illnesses as schizophrenia and manic-depressive psychosis.

Transient paranoid reactions, however, may be found with surprising frequency in normal, healthy individuals and occur in response to the stress of environmental circumstance. Acute personal disappointment, dismissal from employment, the shock of bereavement or the impact of divorce – all are common enough causative factors. Such reactions are normally short-lived and may last only a matter of days or even hours. Feelings of a deprivation of rightful entitlement are usually much in evidence and to these may be added subsidiary notions that others, by concerted and organized activities, have been working to this end.

Factors of isolation play a vital role in the genesis of many paranoid disorders, and these can act as powerful operants where prejudices due to class, colour, creed, race and religion already exist. The political refugee, alone in a foreign country whose language he can hardly speak, may evolve striking trends of paranoid thought as may the prisoner condemned to solitary confinement in gaol.

The psychoanalytical theory of paranoid disorder is based on the concept of repressed homosexuality. Freud's explanation of the psychopathology involved states that the homosexual idea 'I love the man' undergoes unconscious change to the contradiction 'I hate the man'. This, in turn, by the mechanism of projection is yet again re-arranged and appears in consciousness as 'The man hates me'. In this manner, psychoanalytical theory seeks to explain delusions of persecution and related paranoid phenomena.

Paranoid disorders may arise secondarily from obvious physical deformity, or from underlying physical illness – of which chronic deafness is a classical example. Infection, exhaustion, organic disease and degeneration of the brain, pernicious anaemia and post-operative conditions may all be cited as further examples. In this respect, it will be readily realized how frequently paranoid features accompany many illnesses of the aged. Arteriosclerotic and senile disorders and the dementias of various origin, all show a high incidence of paranoid symptomatology.

Chronic alcoholism or the taking of drugs may prove a potent source of intense paranoid delusions and these may or may not be linked with an accompanying sexual impotence. Mental defectives, within their wide range of both mental and physical handicaps, are very prone to exhibit paranoid disorders. Paranoid delusions may be acquired by contagion, as when one healthy individual assumes the delusions of a paranoid person who lives in close contact – the phenomenon of *folie à deux*.

Affective disorder – most notably depression – is an important and frequent cause of paranoid manifestations. Such change in mood in conjunction with the cardinal features of guilt (often of a sexual kind), feelings of inferiority and insecurity, will be found to account for a very high proportion of all paranoid disorders encountered in practice.

The paranoid personality

Within the broad spectrum of human normality many examples of paranoid personality abound. In their eccentric fashion they bring a degree of colour, confusion, exasperation and quandary to the more prosaic measure of everyday life. The paranoid personality is typified by features of secretiveness, unwarranted suspicion, resentment and hostility. Such individuals, sensitive, shy and solitary by nature, maintain an attitude of mistrustful alertness to anticipated attack from others. They readily take offence; they sense threats in the most neutral surroundings; they misinterpret remarks and actions; they spend hours and days in petulant fault-finding while they elaborately nurse grievances and pursue them in senseless litigation.

The prevailing sense of personal inadequacy may be transformed by overcompensation into feelings of superiority with characteristic grandiose behaviour. The paranoid personality provides the cranks and fanatics of life with bees in their bonnets or chips on their shoulders. The pavement orator, the barrack-room lawyer, the inexhaustible writer to Crown, to Parliament and to the Press all exemplify the paranoid personality in action. The classical triad of the paranoid personality is provided by features of insecurity, inferiority and guilt.

Paranoid illness

The range of paranoid symptomatology is understandably wide. It extends from the border line of normality with the heightened sense of self-awareness and accompanying minor ideas of reference (e.g. belief that others are passing derogatory remarks) through intense delusions of jealousy (e.g. the conviction that adultery is being committed by an innocent spouse) to florid persecutory delusions of grotesque content, sometimes accompanied by hallucinations. These florid delusions are

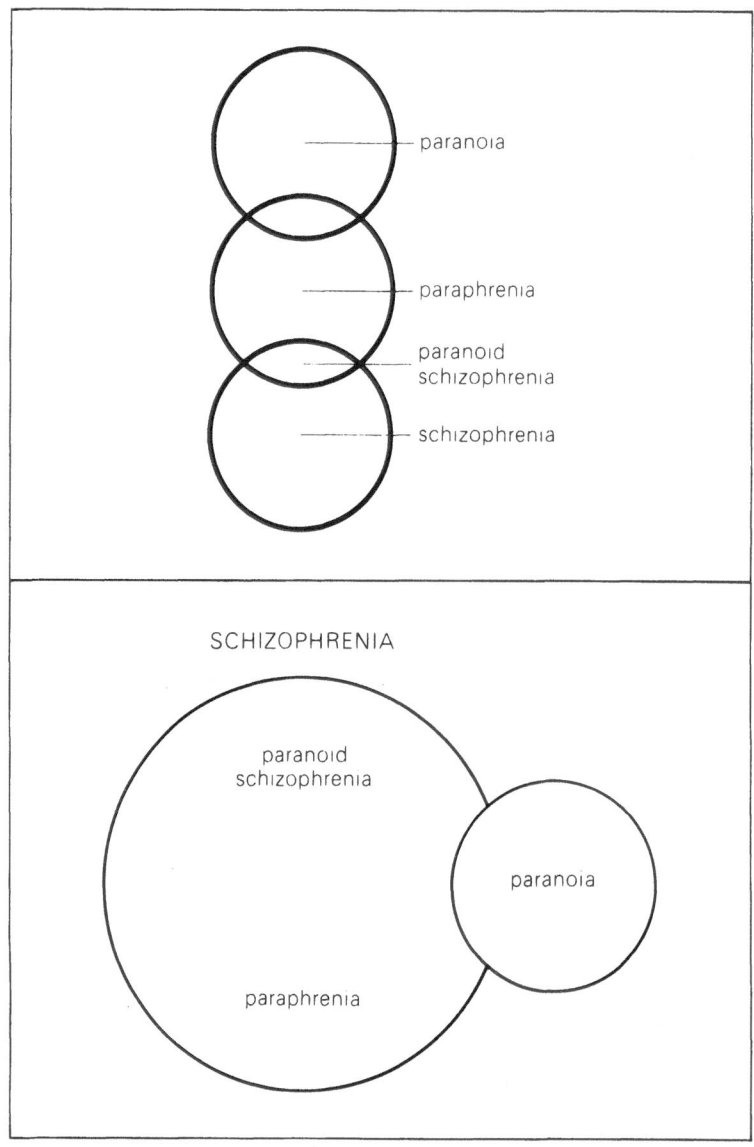

FIGURE 60 Two possible classifications of paranoid disorders showing firstly the concept of a 'paranoia–paraphrenia–schizophrenia' continuum, and secondly, the inclusion of the paranoid psychoses within the boundaries of schizophrenia itself.

likely to involve such agents as travellers from Mars, Russian spies or the Metropolitan Police, who are accredited with ingenious and involved conspiracies, influencing and manipulating the individual's thoughts by the media of television, radio telegraphy, hypnosis, X-rays or by ultrasonic vibrations.

Paranoid delusions are typically systematized so that each interlocks with its fellow delusions to form a bizarre jig-saw puzzle. By this means a fantastic sequence of Alice-in-Wonderland logic is evolved to substantiate the delusional conclusions which have already been established.

Attempts to classify paranoid disorders have in the past been fraught with difficulty and have increased rather than decreased the confusion. The tendency has been to group these disorders under the headings of three main illnesses – paranoia, paraphrenia and paranoid schizophrenia (fig. 60).

Paranoia was considered an unshakeable delusional system of internal origin which occurred in a setting of clear consciousness. Deterioration of the personality did not ensue and the presence of other psychopathological features, such as hallucinations, was by definition incompatible with this diagnosis.

Paraphrenia embraced those delusional persecutory illnesses in which hallucinations and similar pathological features occurred, yet which did not display the characteristic deterioration of the individual to a dementia of what would now be termed paranoid schizophrenia.

Paranoid schizophrenia, earlier designated with the broad grouping of 'dementia praecox', was envisaged as those illnesses which displayed hallucinations, grotesque persecutory delusions and other features of schizophrenic illness, with deterioration of the personality to a supervening dementia.

Such generalizations possessed many limitations and the situation was further complicated by a lack of agreement on nomenclature. Concepts of paranoid disorders have undergone much modification during recent times. Opinions, however, still differ widely on appropriate classification. It is interesting to note that some modern authorities dismiss the term paraphrenia as serving no useful purpose and furthermore deny the existence of a paranoid form of schizophrenic illness. They regard all cases as lying within the broad spectrum of paranoid disorder. The main distinctions which are closely drawn between the symptom complex of these three main illnesses are shown in fig. 61.

	Delusions	Hallucinations	Deterioration
Paranoia	X		
Paraphrenia	X	X	
Paranoid schizophrenia	X	X	X

FIGURE 61 A simplified aid to differentiation between the paranoid disorders.

Management

Time is the therapeutic agent of choice in the transient paranoid reactions precipitated by stress. Yet here, no less than in the more formal paranoid illnesses, much can be achieved by a sympathetic hearing and some practical counsel to contain the situation within realistic limits. Such supportive therapy in paranoid disorders may with great advantage be supplemented by an antidepressant or appropriate tranquillization. The restoration of an adequate sleep pattern is essential. Where physical disorder is responsible for a paranoid reaction the primary treatment should be directed towards the causative disease.

The prognosis in established paranoid disorder is generally unfavourable. Many cases show great resistance to treatment but patients nevertheless show a variation in the intensity of their symptoms. They may acquire the art of concealing the nature of their delusional thoughts for day-to-day purposes.

Psychiatric opinion will usually be necessary to clarify the diagnosis, but the person best able to assess the environmental factors which aggravate the disorder is frequently the patient's own physician. Adjustments of those factors is an important feature in the management of these disorders, and may well determine whether or not the patient can still lead a useful and purposeful life within the limitation imposed by his illness. It is important too for the practitioner to assess how far anxiety and/or depression are aggravating components and to apply appropriate therapy.

The best prognosis is of course to be found in the paranoid reactions in otherwise healthy people. The florid disturbed paranoid patient may require permanent hospitalization. For the less severely affected, sympathetic management by both the practitioner and relatives is an important feature of the therapy.

There is no specific drug therapy for paranoid disorders. However, depression is a powerful precipitant and should be treated appropriately. In both paranoid reactions and paranoid disorders, diazepam may be used to great effect as an anxiolytic agent in chronically disturbed psychotic patients. The previous anxious, tense, restless, aggressive and irritable paranoid patient may well become more pleasant and relaxed. Adequate sleep is essential in paranoid disorders as well as in the paranoid reaction and nitrazepam may safely be used for this purpose.

THE ORGANIC PSYCHOSES

In opposition to the functional psychoses, e.g. affective disorders, schizophrenia and paranoid states, in which organic pathology has not been demonstrated, there is a group of disorders in which the psychotic state depends directly or indirectly on present or past organic illness. This group is called either the organic psychoses or the symptomatic psychoses.

It is only rarely possible to ascribe specific mental reactions to particular ills. The reactions are usually linked far more to the underlying personality of the patient than to the physical precipitant disease. Equally the interests and work of the individual will play a considerable role in determining whether or not the particular organic disease will precipitate a psychiatric reaction. For example, arthritis may be little more than a nuisance to a sedentary worker, but for a coal miner could cause severe emotional stress with the possibility of unemployment.

Many disorders of the nervous system and those from other systems such as the cardio-vascular and uro-genital systems, may produce symptoms which mimic psychological disease. When the delicate balance of the higher centres of the brain is disturbed, in certain people profound mental disturbance may result.

Before diagnosing any psychological condition, the question must always be posed: 'Is this mental state masking and resulting from an underlying physical ailment, the effective treatment of which will restore the mental condition to normal ?'.

Among the multitude of aetiological factors can be included acute infections with delirium and confusional episodes; toxic and exhaustive states; the particular stresses of pregnancy and the puerperium; endocrine imbalance; nutrition disorders (including vitamin deficiencies) and a vast range of systemic diseases. Dramatic presentations of psychotic illness occur with general paralysis of the insane – a consequence of syphilitic infection of the brain – and in the numerous psychotic symptoms of alcoholism (alcoholic hallucinosis, delirium tremens, Wernicke's encephalopathy and Korsakow's syndrome). Psychosis may follow cerebral damage sustained by head injury. Psychotic symptoms may accompany such degenerative diseases as disseminated sclerosis; Parkinson's disease and arteriopathic conditions. Cerebrovascular accidents and arteriosclerosis are potent sources of such symptomatology in the elderly, in addition to senile dementia itself. In younger age groups, such symptoms may arise from cerebral tumours or from the pre-senile dementias, including Huntington's chorea.

In those cases where organic disorder underlies and is responsible for the psychiatric clinical picture, the symptoms may be resolved into two main groups. The first of these is the 'pathogenetic' (essential) group, dependent upon the type and pathology of the brain lesion. The second is the 'pathoplastic' (individual) group dependent upon the personality of the patient in question. A consideration of the contributions and interactions of these two groups to the psychiatric picture has been advanced as the method of 'structural analysis' of a psychosis.

There is clearly no pattern of causation in this heterogenous group of symptomatic psychoses. The fact that a multiplicity of toxic states can produce delusions and hallucinations has been considered to lend weight to a biochemical cause for schizophrenia.

THE AFFECTIVE PSYCHOSES

The affective psychoses are characterized by morbid levels of mood. In states of mania and hypomania the level will be pathologically high and in states of depression the level will be correspondingly low. In certain individuals the mood may tend to fluctuate from pathologically low to pathologically high levels, giving the classical picture of manic-depressive psychosis termed by some modern workers 'bipolar affective disorder'. Other individuals, however, may display a *forme fruste* of the pattern in one of its numerous variants. Among these, recurrent depressive episodes are extremely common.

Although types of depression may be classified as neuroses or psychoses the whole group of the depressions is considered here under the heading Affective Psychoses.

DEPRESSION

Minor fluctuations of mood, experienced by normal, healthy persons, provide an interesting feature of everyday life. Sometimes a reason can be found for the mood-swing but many are inexplicable. These minor changes, occurring from day to day, cause but little inconvenience. Mild upswings are accepted pleasurably and even thankfully, while mild downswings are dealt with by such harmless antidotes as an early night to bed or an agreeable evening with convivial company.

Whilst these commonplace fluctuations of mood are normal, certain individuals show an amplitude of the mood-swing of greater degree than average and a more delicately poised tendency to change. To this type of personality the term 'cyclothymic' is applied (p. 106). The physique of the cyclothyme favours pyknic proportions (plump, rounded body, short neck, graceful hands and feet). A strong hereditary tendency is found in cyclothymes and they are particularly prone to the numerous variants of manic-depressive psychosis.

Within the broad dimensions of normal affect, certain persons will be found whose average level of mood is set at a lower level than most. To these individuals the term 'hypothymic personality' is applied. They are the natural pessimists who pursue an existence of life-denial. Possibilities are anticipated at their worst – not infrequently as a defence against added disappointment – and events are viewed from the blacker side. Energy is frequently lacking and hypochondriacal or obsessional traits are commonly in evidence. If morose and despondent, such personalities may prove to be unwelcome colleagues at work or poor companions in leisure, yet more typically they are apt to display an engaging wry cynicism and a dry sense of humour which is not without charm and they find – in spite of themselves – they are popular and not lacking in friends.

Morbid depression

It is quite impossible to draw any hard-and-fast boundary between normal and pathological gradations of mood. In practice, depression of psychiatric significance may be said to be present whenever the intensity or duration of the downswing of mood seriously disrupts the normal function and conduct of the patient's life.

Of recent years, attempts to classify depressive illness have become increasingly more complex and controversial. No classification is entirely satisfactory.

A system which has much to commend it is the straightforward division of depressive illness into two broad groupings – 'reactive depression' and 'endogenous depression'. These two groupings, however, are by no means mutually exclusive and in some instances an illness may assume certain features of each.

Reactive depression is primarily a neurotic illness and may be viewed as but an exaggerated response to adverse external circumstance. Disaster, family tragedy, or individual misfortune may all precipitate depression of this reactive kind. Among the most common causes may be mentioned bereavement by death, a broken love affair, the failure of ambition and the parting from an adored only child.

Endogenous depression, in contradistinction, belongs more properly to the realm of the psychoses. It arises from within. The patient is frequently mystified as to its cause and at a loss to explain its onset. Alternatively, rationalization of the depressive symptoms will take place and the patient attribute them, quite erroneously but with conviction, to some fictitious origin. Endogenous depression is most closely linked with genetic endowment and, again, shows affinity with the hypothymic or cyclothymic types of personality. In many instances, the episodes of depression will represent the periodic downswings of mood of a manic-depressive psychosis.

The relevant factors and their importance in the production of reactive and endogenous types of depression are shown diagrammatically in fig. 62.

Although genetic factors are of paramount importance in the aetiology of depressive illness any precise pathology remains obscure. The fields of endocrinology and biochemistry have been fruitful though inconclusive for those seeking the origin of depression in physical terms. The greater incidence of depression among women, its increase during the pre-menstrual phase, menstruation and the menopause; its liability to appear during the puerperium and its relationship to myxoedema – all favour some elusive hormonal basis. The induction of depressive states by certain drugs, and its relief by other pharmacological agents focus

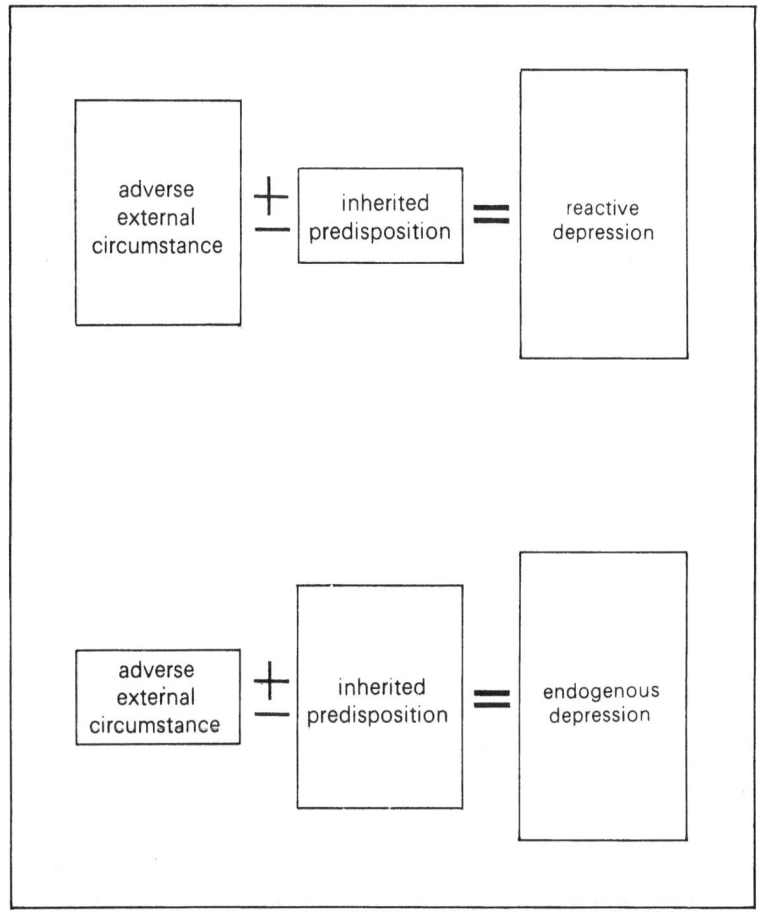

FIGURE 62 Relative factors in the production of reactive and endogenous types of depression.

attention on the possibility of an altered chemistry within the central nervous system. Nevertheless, no satisfactory explanation can today be given to account for the pathology of depressive illness.

Diagnosis

In many instances, the diagnosis of depression is possible from an initial glance at the patient and the subsequent case-history serves merely to corroborate this clinical impression. In other cases the depression will be anything but obvious even after detailed examination. It is important to appreciate that depressive illness underlies a high proportion of cases overtly presenting as morbid anxiety (see also p. 180); and is the common companion of obsessive-compulsive disorder. Moreover, the relationship between depression and schizophrenia is a highly important one. Any prolonged intense depression unresponsive to treatment, particularly in young adults, should raise the possibility of schizophrenia in the doctor's mind.

In the physical field, depression masquerades in the guise of innumerable somatic complaints and ailments – all only too familiar to the medical practitioner. Conversely, physical disorder may precipitate depression.

The psychological manifestations of depression are mirrored in the physical bearing of the patient. His facial expression is inflexible and sad, his speech slow and ponderous. His attitude is bowed and his movements clumsy and laboured. A reduced peripheral circulation accompanies a general lowering of normal metabolic function, and loss of weight soon follows upon loss of appetite. Diminished sexual interest is common to both sexes and in the female may be accompanied by the absence of menstruation.

At a more advanced level – sometimes known by the archaic name of 'melancholia' – the full devastating force of psychotic depressive illness is seen. Such depression renders the normal processes of thought impossible. Thinking becomes slowed down and cumbersome and may grind itself to a halt in a state of depressive stupor. Severe distortion is present in all aspects of thought typically showing the striking depressive guilt delusions (fig. 63). The content of these delusions is that of unworthiness, failure, self-abasement and accusation, irrevocable ruin and damnation or unpardonable sin. The intensity of the emotional turmoil frequently adds a strong paranoid component to the delusion.

In the clinical history of depressive illness, an important feature is the disturbed sleep pervaded by intensely morbid dreams. The endogenous depression shows a typical pattern of early morning awakening. The patient's sufferings tend to be at their worst on awakening, persist throughout the day but then show a characteristic but inexplicable lightening towards the evening.

In addition to these features of depression already described anxiety of varying degree frequently colours and complicates the clinical picture.

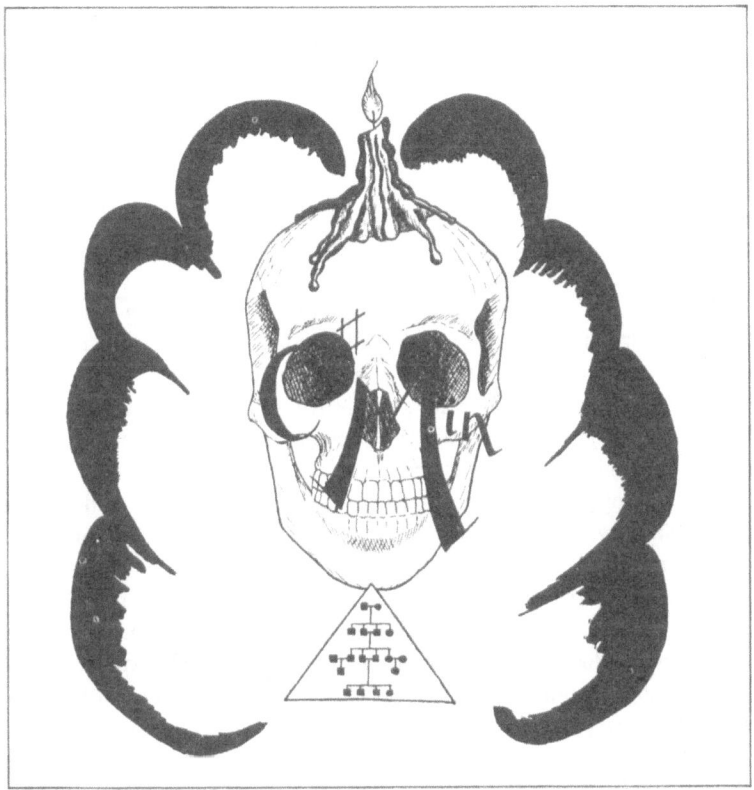

FIGURE 63 Illustration by psychotically depressed patient – a concert pianist by profession. The subject matter of death, decay and the surrounding black cloud of depression are typical. The melancholy influence of the minor musical key and the triangular impression of Mendel's Law of Heredity are extremely interesting features.

Tension, restlessness and agitation, together with marked hypochondriacal delusions, are prominent in depression of the involutional and senile periods.

Management

The management of depressive illness should combine supportive psychotherapy with medication.

For the patient to share the responsibility of the illness with his doctor eases the weight of its burden, and breaks down the feeling of isolation inflicted by the depression. The doctor should counteract the subjective distortion, prevent the taking of rash, ill-conceived emotional actions and give reassurance on the temporary nature of most depressive illnesses and on the remission that will follow in due course.

The greatest hazard of *any* depressive illness lies in the risk of suicide (p. 223). No simple formula can ever be applied to assess this possibility for any given patient, and it may prove fatally misleading to approach the problem in this manner. The practitioner is well advised to share the responsibility for assessment in any depressed patient with a psychiatric colleague.

The periods during which depressive illness is developing or receding require particular consideration and vigilance. Factors of isolation above all increase the likelihood of consummated suicide. The depressed individual who lives alone in a bed-sitting-room, without a family, friends or religious conviction, lost in the anonymity of a large city, rates very highly in terms of potential suicide.

The risk of suicide increases greatly with advancing age and suicide constitutes a very real factor in all depressive illness of the involutional and senile periods.

Because of this risk of suicide, continued surveillance of the patient during therapy is an important feature and the depressed patient who does not respond to therapy within the expected time should not be ignored. Where response is inadequate, with home care and therapy, hospital admission for closer surveillance should be considered.

Immediate medication should be directed to the restoration of a satisfactory sleep-pattern and reduction of anxiety with a safe tranquillizer. In view of their safety, even when taken in high doses, nitrazepam or flurazepam are valuable sedatives for such patients, while diazepam may be given with benefit for the anxiety. Symptomatic relief for the depression may temporarily follow the administration of amphetamine or methylphenidate, but it is now widely accepted that the use of these compounds should be avoided. Alternatively, treatment may be commenced with the more fundamental antidepressive drugs. These are of two main classes; the tri-cyclic antidepressants (p. 260) e.g. amitriptyline, imipramine and the monoamine oxidase inhibitors (p. 261) e.g. isocarboxazid. There is still no simple method of determining which patient will respond best to which class of drugs. There is a certain amount of evidence that a patient who has responded previously to one class will respond best again to that class. Equally, if a close relative of the patient has previously responded during a depressive illness to one of the two classes of drugs this should be tried first. In general terms it is probably best to start treatment with one of the tricyclic compounds, e.g. amitriptyline. They tend to cover a wider range of the depressive illnesses and give rise to far fewer side-effects than the monoamine oxidase inhibitors. These latter drugs, e.g. isocarboxazid, are often most effective in depressions occurring in patients with a previous excellent personality. Lithium carbonate is now used extensively and effectively in the management of recurrent manic-depressive psychosis. Careful control of the serum lithium levels is needed to avoid signs of toxicity (p. 262). The drugs, their dosage and problems associated with their use are given in Chapter 12 which also considers the question of drug interaction.

MANIC STATES

In disorders of mood or affect, the hypomanic and manic states represent the opposite side of the coin to that of depressive illness. But again – within that general spectrum of personality structures which collectively composes normality – healthy individuals are found whose general mood is set at a level higher than average. To these, the term 'hyperthymic personality' has been given. Cheerful and exuberant by nature, their good humour radiates infectiously around them. The moods of their more prosaic fellow creatures are correspondingly raised and, in consequence, such life-affirming personalities are popular and much sought after. They are active in their undertakings and organize their colleagues well. Their robust sense of the ridiculous provides them with an abundant fund of practical jokes and witty stories. These natural dispensers of gloom furnish the ranks of some, but by no means all, comedians. Enough of the hyperthymic personality can be highly beneficial and inspiring. Too much of the hyperthymic personality can at times be exhausting.

In both the clinical conditions of hypomania and mania, the mood is morbidly and unrealistically raised. These two conditions differ only in the degree of intensity of their symptoms and no fast line of demarcation exists between them. The condition of chronic mania, or that of acute delirious mania (Bell's mania), is but rarely found today due to the efficacy of modern treatment. Cases of mania which show lack of response to appropriate treatment must always raise the query of an alternative diagnosis of schizophrenic illness.

An acute attack of mania is usually of fairly rapid onset, most often following a day or two's prodomal features of restlessness, disturbed sleep and increased irritability. The attack itself is characterized by the inappropriate elevation of the mood and the hyperactivity displayed by the patient.

For the manic patient the whole world has now become his oyster and all schemes and attainments – no matter how grandiose – are readily within his grasp. This is life as it should be lived and no time is to be lost in the fullness of its living. The morbid degree of self-satisfaction found in the patient obscures any critical evaluation of himself, and insight into the fact that he is ill is lacking. Hence the frustration when those about him seem not to muster the same exaggerated enthusiasm for his wild and grandiose schemes. The incessant flow of talk from the manic patient indicates the pressure of the thoughts which crowd into his head. This 'flight of ideas' underlies the classical distractibility of the manic, who switches in mid-sentence from one topic to another as irrelevant external stimuli – such as a clock chiming or the passing of another person – claim his mercurial attention. His bonhomie is communicated by laughing and joking, and by the peculiar 'clang' associations of onomatopoeic origin.

In spite of its morbidly raised level, the mood of the manic is but precariously poised and its lability may induce at any moment anger, tears or depression. The quality of the mood is essentially one of 'brittleness' and the impending fragmentation is often but a short step away.

The behaviour of the manic patient is characteristically boisterous, interfering and irresponsible. 'No' cannot be taken for an answer and he above all others has the conviction of what is best. Large sums of money (if not carefully regulated by others) are liable to be squandered on a host of useless and unwanted trivia. Vast quantities of irrelevant goods may be ordered on credit and obtained, but settlement, to the distraction of the sundry retailers, is totally disregarded. The personal appearance of the manic patient will rapidly deteriorate. His manner of dress is likely to become as disorganized as will his habits of eating and sleeping. His conduct may show degraded, indecent or destructive features and his language be uninhibited and out of keeping with his normal social style.

The prognosis for the acute attack of mania is a good one, though recurrent attacks are most likely to follow unless a planned regime of medication is instigated. The dangers of a sudden swing to the depressive phase with its concomitant risk of suicide must be clearly borne in mind.

Psychosomatic disorders, hypochondriasis and neurasthenia

PSYCHOSOMATIC DISORDERS

The term psychosomatic is used at the present time in two different senses. Originally it was applied to an approach to medicine and surgery in general. It called attention to the fact that any illness produces a a change in the psyche which in its turn can accentuate the disease. It is now used more frequently to group together an apparently heterogeneous group of disorders (Table 7) which are considered to be mainly physical responses to continued emotional conflict. Any mental disturbance accompanied by stress can give rise to somatic manifestations. In consequence, since any psychiatric disorder may secondarily produce anxiety, psychosomatic disorders are not confined exclusively to any one primary mental disorder.

The stress presents as a physical illness due to an imbalance within the limbic system and diencephalic centres. These send out impulses via the autonomic system and also via the pituitary and hence the endocrine system affecting the internal organs (p. 93).

In practice there is rarely a purely psychological cause for psychosomatic disorders, for infection, allergy and other physical components are usually also present. It is therefore important for the physician or psychiatrist to assess the degree of psychological involvement. When

TABLE 7 Representative psychosomatic disorders

CARDIOVASCULAR SYSTEM
  Disordered action of the heart
  Angina pectoris
  Essential hypertension
	RESPIRATORY SYSTEM
	  Vasomotor rhinitis
	  Asthma

	SKIN
	  Urticaria
	  Neurodermatitis

GASTRO-INTESTINAL SYSTEM
  Peptic ulcer
  Colonic disorders	

	ENDOCRINES Hyperthyroidism

FEMALE GENITAL SYSTEM
  Dysmenorrhoea
  Premenstrual tension
  Menopausal disturbances
	MUSCLES AND JOINTS
	  'Fibrositis'
	  'Low Back pain'

this is great, a resolution of the stress by appropriate therapy will remove the somatic symptoms.

Since psychosomatic disorders are commonly reactions to anxiety, tranquillizers, particularly the benzodiazepines, are very effective. It is important, however, to look for and treat other primary psychiatric disorders rather than merely suppress the tension manifestations with tranquillizers.

HYPOCHONDRIASIS

By concentrating attention on a particular part of the body it is always possible to become aware of sensation in that part.

In hypochondriacal states these sensations obtain constant conscious appreciation and become a source of discomfort or even indistinguishable from symptoms of organic illness. Hypochondriasis is usually a secondary reaction to other mental disorders of an obsessional, hysterical, depressive or anxious nature, and is particularly common in persons of obsessional character.

There would appear to be a constitutional basis for hypochondriasis since it is often found in members of the same family. It is more prevalent in old age.

NEURASTHENIA

Although used in earlier days, in present-day psychiatric practice a diagnosis of pure neurasthenia is virtually unknown. Frequently, depression is the underlying disorder but nevertheless it is important to appreciate that there is a personality which even under minimal stress conditions shows itself as abnormally weak and over-sensitive, easily irritated and solitary.

Patients with such a personality are often of a special physique. They are often of small build with thin bones, flaccid muscles, small heart and generally infantile appearance.

Neurasthenia originally implied an exhaustion of the nervous system and attempts were made to differentiate such nervous exhaustion from physical exhaustion. The differentiation was however academic and both physical and mental exhaustion underlie the symptomatology which was earlier classified as neurasthenia.

Mental subnormality

For better or worse, men are not born equal. In matters of intellect – no less than in those of stature – a spectrum of gradation ranges from genius to idiot as it does from giant to dwarf.

As Stedman (p. 131) has amply demonstrated, environmental influence during the earliest years of life is of profound importance in establishing that level of intellectual functioning which any individual will display during life.

In any general population, one-half of its members will possess average degrees of intelligence and show Intelligence Quotients from 90–110. The remaining half will show, in almost equal proportions, degrees of intelligence both greater and lesser than these average values fig. 64).

Of itself, the possession of superior intelligence presents no particular medical or social problem; but within our industrialized and highly competitive society of today, a lack of intelligence in values substantially below average will at once generate problems of a formidable and at times

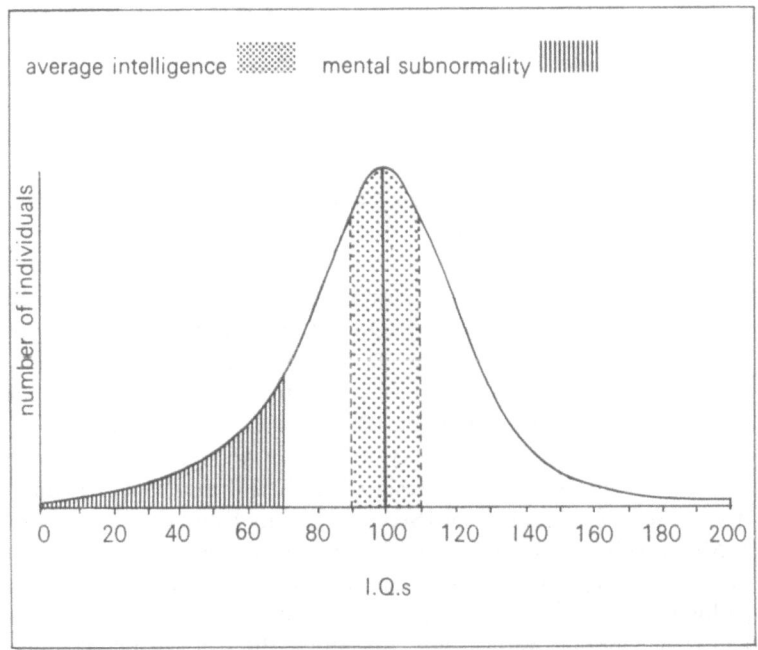

FIGURE 64 Frequency-distribution curve for intelligence. The biological distribution of intelligence throughout a random population follows the classical Gaussian curve. The asymmetry to be observed in the lower IQ range of the curve demonstrates the effects of disease in producing pathological mental subnormality.

insuperable kind. Approximately one person in every hundred is mentally subnormal – mentally deficient or mentally handicapped, to use equivalent established terms. Among such individuals a preponderance of males will be found.

For practical purposes, the mentally deficient are regarded as those persons with an Intelligence Quotient of 69 or less. The Mental Health Act 1959 divides such persons into two groupings – those showing 'subnormality' who may benefit from medical treatment or other special care or training – and those showing 'severe subnormality' who are incapable of leading an independent life or guarding themselves against serious exploitation.

An earlier tripartite classification of the mentally deficient still possesses many advantages. By this the highest grades (IQ 69–50) were termed 'feeble-minded'; the middle grades (IQ 49–25) were termed 'imbeciles'; and the lowest grades (IQ less than 25) were termed 'idiots'. (fig. 65).

Certain mental defectives may show an extraordinary dexterity for the manipulation of numbers, the memorizing of dates, the construction of miniature models and similar pursuits. To these curiously gifted defectives the name 'idiots savants' has traditionally been given.

The Intelligence Quotient is an established and convenient index for the grading of intellectual ability. It is, however, neither a simple nor a constant value, and may show considerable variation when obtained from the same individual under differing circumstances on different occasions. The limitations of the IQ must be fully appreciated and appropriate caution exercised in its determination and application. During the present century, tests for intelligence have undergone repeated modification and revision. Those scales chiefly employed in the valuation of mental subnormality today are the Stanford-Binet, the Wechsler Adult Intelligence Scale (WAIS) and the Wechsler Intelligence Scale for Children (WISC) (p. 132 and Table 5).

Mental subnormality is a state of arrested or incomplete development of mind, a condition determined *in utero* or during the early days of childhood. The factors which result in mental subnormality are complex and of an enormous variety. Pre-eminent are those of genetic influence. Considerations of the aetiology of mental subnormality may with advantage be subdivided into two broad groupings; those of subcultural and those of pathological types.

The subcultural group embodies those individuals who, apparently

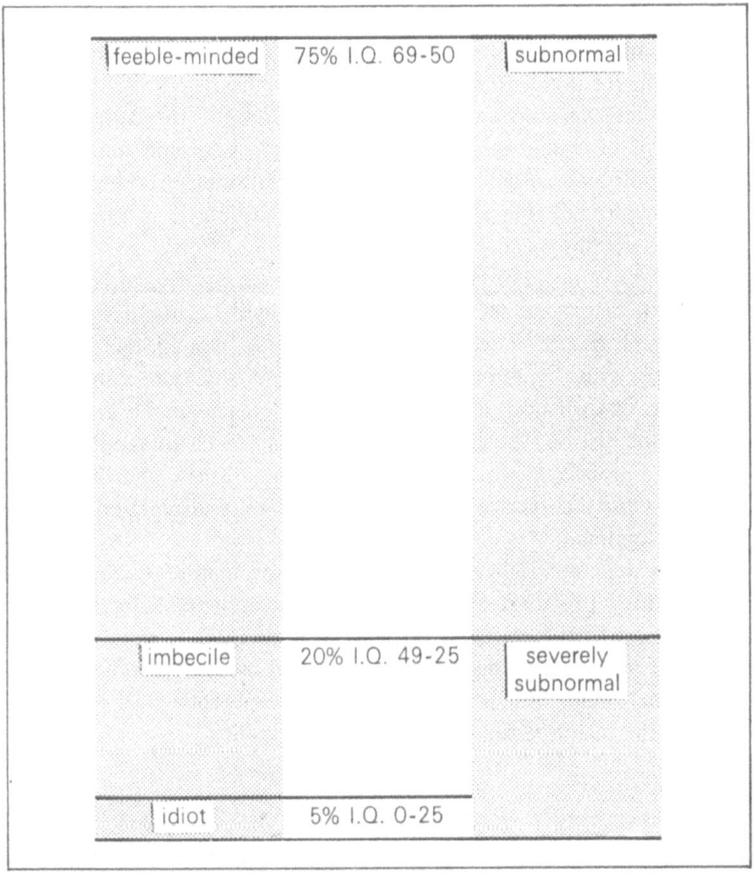

FIGURE 65 Mental Subnormality. This diagram indicates the approximate incidence among the mentally subnormal of the feeble-minded, imbeciles and idiots. It also relates these older terms to the more recent categories of subnormality and severe subnormality.

free from causative disease or injury, are merely but poorly intellectually endowed by their parents. As such they represent the lower grades of intelligence from the standard distribution of intelligence throughout the general population. The parents of defectives within this subcultural group will commonly, but by no means invariably, be of similarly restricted intellect.

The pathological group, in contrast, embodies those individuals in whom specific genetic anomaly, foetal or infantile brain damage by infection or injury, or certain physical or material deprivations are responsible for the degree of mental subnormality.

Aberrations of autosomal chromosomes underlie the conditions of mongolism (Down's syndrome), cri-du-chat syndrome and the de Lange syndrome. Anomalies of the sex chromosomes produce Kleinfelter's syndrome, Turner's syndrome, the Triple-X syndrome and associated conditions (p. 103).

An extensive range of clinical conditions, each occasioned by genetic defect and displaying mental subnormality, will be found within the pathological group. These conditions include among them cranial dysostoses with hypertelorism, microcephaly and acrocephaly; the metabolic disturbances of phenylketonuria, galactosaemia and maple syrup urine disease; the cerebral lipoidoses of amaurotic family idiocy, Gaucher's disease, gargoylism, Niemann-Pick's disease and the Hand-Schüller-Christian syndrome; the Sturge-Weber syndrome and tuberose sclerosis (epiloia),

Rhesus incompatibility, the hazards of premature birth, trauma from the birth process itself, cerebral palsy and epilepsy; infection of the pre- and post-natal periods; nutritional deficiences, toxins, acquired metabolic or endocrine disorders, sensory and social deprivations – any of these may contribute to the total range of the pathological group and produce the manifestations of mental subnormality.

Social implications

The social complications of mental subnormality, which run like some evil jinx throughout the life of the individual affected, are of the greatest importance. They ramify further in the existences of all who find themselves in close contact with the mentally deficient.

The impact of a subnormal child upon normal and unprepared parents, born as an only child or into a family of healthy siblings, is likely to engender emotional difficulties of a major kind. Family reactions may range from a frank refusal to accept the fact that the child is mentally subnormal to those of a guilt-ridden, over-indulgent solicitude, or to those of revulsion and total rejection of the unfortunate child.

Problems which emerge from the growing child's awareness of its limitations and differences from normal children, by the special arrangements necessary for care, schooling and training, by the reactions

of others to the trials of its own short-comings, these are in turn succeeded by yet further difficulties as school-leaving age is approached.
Guardianship by the local authority may be necessary, or institutional
admission may be advised. Attempts towards establishing a partially
independent life and earning a living may prove impracticable and a
poor and disappointing work record be established. Delinquency and
crime beckon invitingly to the mentally subnormal. Often retribution
follows more swiftly, from the defective's lack of resource in evading
detection. Sexual promiscuity, with its legacy of venereal disease and
illegitimate children, fosters additional social hazards. For the mental
defective marriage and parenthood may again create responsibilities for
which he or she is but poorly equipped and a common pattern of events
can be found in the sequence of desertion by the spouse, breakdown by
the defective, and the removal of any children to the care of the welfare
authorities.

Management

Specific treatment exists for certain disorders leading to mental re-
tardation, e.g. administration of thyroxin in cretinism, a milk-free diet
in galactosaemia. As the biochemical abnormalities resulting from genetically determined enzyme defects become better understood, further
specific forms of therapy will become available.

Apart from such cases, however, no specific therapy exists, but at the
same time much can be achieved by the medical practitioner. One of
the most important features in this management is an appreciation of the
difficulties which are encountered by the parents, particularly if the
child is to remain at home. Sympathetic handling and encouragement
are essential and acute anxiety in the parents should be treated appropriately. The majority of mentally retarded children will respond to
appropriate training and will improve as they get older, although never
catching up with the normal child. The training programme of the child
must be based upon a total evaluation of the child's resources, including
an appreciation of the degree of physical defect which accompanies the
brain damage. The guiding principle in all training programmes must
be patience, frequent repetition and alertness to signs of fatigue which
inhibit further benefit. Although the number of residential homes
available for training the mentally retarded is still inadequate for the
needs, most local authorities can now offer some training facilities and
with the parents' co-operation such facilities should be utilized.

It is important to assess the behaviour pattern of the child in relation to others. Many retarded children show a placid and happy disposition but where tantrums and behaviour disorders are a prominent feature, as they occasionally are, appropriate tranquillizers will often make the child more capable of benefiting from the processes.

Disorders of social behaviour

This general group embraces a wide area in which the individual indulges in aberrant behaviour which causes suffering either to himself or to society. It is often regarded as a special sub-grouping of the personality disorders.

Among the disorders of social behaviour can be included the psychopathic personality (p. 219); drug abuse (p. 220); alcoholism (p. 219) and sexual deviations (p. 221). Suicide, an important disease of society, is considered in this chapter (p. 223).

PSYCHOPATHIC PERSONALITIES

The term 'psychopathic' has recently been much overworked, abused and used to cover a multitude of sins. The psychopath's behaviour is essentially anti-social and shows no prudence or consideration for others. It is convenient to divide psychopathy into aggressive, inadequate, creative and sexual forms.

The anti-social psychopathic personality characteristically lacks normal emotional reactions and normal feelings for other people; he acts impulsively without thinking of the consequences, punishment does not deter him from his anti-social behaviour which occurs without regret, conscience or remorse. He need not necessarily conflict with the law, but often causes great pain and hardship to his relatives and friends by his thoughtless behaviour. He characteristically leaves a trail of unpaid bills. He may frequently possess a charming countenance but not one word he says should be believed easily. Often he turns to a criminal career with repeated imprisonments for fraud and false pretences. Aggressive behaviour is not uncommon in the psychopath; he may beat or rape with sadistic pleasure and on being confronted shows no evidence of regret.

Isolated claims that psychotherapy has modified the psychopathic character may be true, but the psychopath will not seek treatment unless he has to. The protection of society demands that the dangerously

218

aggressive psychopath be segregated from society and denied opportunities to do further damage.

Drug abuse is one of the major social problems of the present generation, and characteristically starts among teenagers. Initially it probably represents a process of experimenting; a desire not to be excluded from the group; a rebellion. In the majority, it is a temporary breakdown in the normal pattern because they only experiment with the 'soft' drugs. The danger lies in the contact with those who both use and peddle 'hard' drugs, for these narcotics inevitably bring the dire results of drug dependence. Almost any chemical substance can be taken in excess. Within reason therefore the accent in drug abuse should be placed on the personality of the patient rather than the substance abused, except for the narcotic group of drugs.

Whatever the legal implications of drug abuse, the physician's prime responsibility remains that of the health hazard. For the narcotics this health hazard is quite clear. A steady deterioration in the personality occurs and the sole driving force becomes restricted to the need to acquire more drugs. The management of the narcotic dependent patient is one of the most difficult problems in medicine. Special treatment centres are being established though as yet their numbers are inadequate. Whether this method will prove effective remains to be seen. The responsibility of all medical practitioners lies in trying to prevent new cases developing. The administration of narcotic analgesics for prolonged periods should be avoided and care exercised with narcotic storage, so that paramedical personnel cannot have access to them.

With the amphetamine group of drugs, there is evidence of some physical deterioration, coupled with mental and somatic disorders. Amphetamine dependence likewise requires urgent attention. In the case of abuse of the psychotomimetic compounds (e.g. LSD) there is clear evidence that they can precipitate psychotic illness, e.g. schizophrenia. Their use is however largely confined to the psychopaths and the whole problem of treatment of the underlying disorder of personality arises.

From the medical point of view the main difficulty lies with the present teenage habit of marihuana (hashish) smoking. Whereas tobacco smoking is legally acceptable but medically dangerous, the smoking of reefers is legally unacceptable even though there is at present no conclusive evidence that it is medically dangerous. In the opinion of many doctors the ultimate dangers of teenager reefer smoking are less than those of smoking cigarettes, although some believe that the habit once established may encourage a switch to other drugs.

ALCOHOLISM

Alcohol, an effective tranquillizer, has been widely used for many centuries. Limited intake is socially acceptable in most communities, and is employed to combat the stresses and strains of everyday life and to facilitate contact with strangers. Periods of increased stress in most communities lead to a general increase in the consumption of alcohol.

The excessive and compulsive intake of alcohol – alcoholism – is normally classed among psychiatric disorders, although there is still no direct evidence that all cases should be regarded in this light. Some arise in an inadequate or psychopathic personality; some represent the abuse of an effective tranquillizer during continued stress; others may indicate the recurrent incidence of depression. In many patients, however, no clear psychiatric reason for the compulsive drinking can be determined. Metabolic abnormalities (e.g. low glucose levels) suggest a somatic basis in some instances.

A distinctive feature of alcoholism is the effort made by a patient to disguise the disorder. The patient hides his drinking habits or the extent of the intake, probably because, unlike most diseases, it still carries a social stigma. Moreover, even when the diagnosis has been made there is often considerable difficulty in persuading the patient to accept treatment.

Treatment is often far from satisfactory. The patient requires to be initially 'dried out', and each expert has his own particular method of doing this. Some advise a rapid progress leading to severe abstinence symptoms, while others believe that the 'drying out' process must be taken slowly with the patient's co-operation. The 'drying out' is best undertaken in a special unit.

Once the patient is 'dried out' the general practitioner must advise the patient both directly and through responsible relatives against any further intake of alcohol. Even the single social drink can lead to a full-blown relapse into alcoholism.

The methods by which a successful improvement can be achieved will depend upon the background of the patient and reason for the alcoholism. Tranquillizers (e.g. chlordiazepoxide) have been used with success where anxiety has been a major cause. Group encouragement and psychotherapy within the framework of Alcoholics Anonymous has been successful for many, while others have achieved sufficient insight to avoid further alcoholic intake by an effort of will. The medical practitioner should be particularly vigilant with any treated alcoholic to ensure that no back-sliding occurs.

SEXUAL DEVIATIONS

It is extremely difficult, if not impossible, to define a normal pattern for sexual behaviour in terms of either frequency or style. What may be regarded as excessive sexual appetite by one partner can well prove to be frustration to the other. Difficulties most frequently occur from differences in degrees of sexual appetite.

On the behavioural side, human sexual responses provide delicately poised emotional and physical patterns. In consequence, knowledge and – even more – practice are necessary to arrive at a technique of inter-course which is gratifying and which brings satisfaction to both partners. Certain patterns of sexual behaviour have acquired a legal importance but, from the medical point of view, it is doubtful whether many of these can be regarded as true abnormalities. What is condemned as perversion in one community receives social approval in another. It is probably wise to accept that any act between willing partners which ends in normal intercourse is not a deviation.

The medical practitioner is most usually requested to advise when the pattern presents a problem for the patient or for the relatives. This may, for example, arise as the result of anxiety or guilt on the part of the patient, or may result from a brush with the police. It is usually the emotional component which is the important one for the practitioner to study. The most common problems for which advice will be sought are:

Masturbation. Self-stimulation of the genitalia will normally occur by sheer chance in the infant or young child, who, finding it pleasurable, then continues this practice to the embarrassment and worry of the mother. It is essential to reassure the mother that there are no physical consequences or permanent homosexual tendencies involved. The worried mother should provide the child with interest so that it loses the habit – but should preferably draw minimum attention to the practice. Adult masturbation, as judged by social surveys, is very common both within and outside the confines of marriage. The only danger lies in its substitution for normal sexual intercourse. Advice should be directed towards removing feelings of guilt and towards educating and enlightening the individual concerned.

Homosexual tendencies. These occur to a variable extent in different communities. It has been estimated that approximately one in twenty-five men or women is wholly homosexual and up to one in three is partly homosexual. Whilst by definition this is abnormal sexual behaviour, the current more liberal attitude has removed much of the psychiatric guilt and problems of anxiety which previously manifested themselves.

Fetishism. This is a direct association of the sexual urge with a specific object, most commonly an article of clothing. Since many styles of dress and individual pieces of wearing apparel have been designed to attract and stimulate the opposite sex, the veneration of such objects is often a question of degree. Certain odours, the texture of materials, the shape, design, proportions and colour of articles may markedly affect an individual in terms of interest, sexual pleasure, excitement or potency. One should therefore attempt to distinguish between an effect which is aphrodisiac and enhances coitus and the truer fetishistic substitution of the object for the sexual partner. Surveys show that minor fetishistic tendencies are an important feature of normal sexual behaviour. Failure to recognize this is a common cause of serious marital disharmony involving male impotence and psychological frigidity in the female.

Transvestism. This is the adopting of clothing of the opposite sex – it is a form of fetishism encountered in those who are homosexually inclined. It is usually the legal implications which lead the patient to seek advice.

Sadism and masochism. Limited degrees of sadism and masochism are again a normal feature of the behaviour of most people. They become medical problems only when the cruelty becomes excessive or there is an imbalance between the wishes of the two partners.

Exhibitionism. This is another problem which most frequently presents as a result of police action. It is likely to occur in a person previously of normal intelligence and is a sign of mental deterioration. The tendency is for repetition to occur in spite of punishment.

The management of the majority of minor deviations of sexual behaviour usually requires only reassurance and removal of the guilt feelings. To be told that they are not abnormal is frequently sufficient.

Where the deviation is marked, where it has provoked police action or where it is the sole source of sexual satisfaction, therapy is usually unsuccessful. Aversion therapy (p. 247) offers the best hope and such cases should be referred for expert opinion.

SUICIDE

In the majority of industrially developed countries suicide is found among the ten most common causes of death even though the published suicide figures underestimate the truth to a greater or lesser extent depending upon various sociological factors.

The suicide rate has, contrary to popular belief, stayed remarkably constant throughout this century in both Europe and the United States of America, if the temporary downward fluctuation during the wars and the upward move during the depression are ignored. There has certainly been no general upward trend over this century. The current published rate is about 110 per million population per year, but to this must be added a proportion of the 40 per million in which an open verdict was returned at the inquest, due to lack of evidence.

The epidemiology of suicide has been extensively studied and well documented. It is twice as common in men as women; is rare in children and increases steadily with age. It is primarily a problem of affluent societies, but is also greatly influenced by the religious beliefs which affect the published suicide rate and the method used. Thus Catholic communities have a consistently lower suicide rate than do Protestant ones, the difference not being adequately explicable on the avoidance by the authorities in such communities of a suicide verdict. Urban areas have higher suicide rates than rural ones, but in the urban areas the highest rate is not seen in the areas of poor housing and overcrowding, but in places where there is a moving population. The suicide rate rises to a maximum in the spring and early summer and is also most likely to occur in the early hours after midnight. All these points suggest that social isolation is a major contributory cause.

The major precipitating cause of suicide is depression (p. 208), for about 50 per cent of suicides are suffering from depressive illness. Indeed it is calculated that about one in seven manic-depressives eventually take their own lives. Alcoholism (p. 220) comes second among the disorders leading to suicide. Among the elderly there is a relatively high proportion of physical illness, particularly Parkinsonism and neoplasms. Only a very small proportion (under 10 per cent) can be regarded as having been psychiatrically normal, that is to say, have had no history of psychiatric illness and are thought normal by relatives and friends.

While depression is the underlying disorder in a major proportion of the cases, the mental state at the time of the suicidal act can usually be inferred as primarily being 'useless and unwanted', and it is for this reason that social isolation appears to be a major precipitating cause. The majority of suicides indeed take their lives when they are alone, the only exception being the occasional exhibitionist desire even in death or the intent to stir up public feeling for a particular cause (e.g. the self-cremation of Buddhist monks in South Vietnam).

There are a few bizarre methods of suicide often ritual in form (e.g. Hari-kiri in Japan; swimming out to be eaten by sharks in Tikopian women), but the majority of suicides employ a limited number of typical methods. The method chosen depends particularly upon the availability factor. In the United States of America, possession of firearms is more frequent than it is in Europe and suicide from firearms is equally much more common. In the United Kingdom poisoning by either coal gas or barbiturates (often with alcohol) is the preferred method.

Violent forms of suicide have declined over the years in most countries as 'more pleasant' methods have become available, and this has coincided with an increase in the proportion of female suicides. Probably because of the ready availability of easy methods, the rate is l gh among doctors and medical auxiliaries.

The group of attempted suicides differs in great measure from those in the successful group. It contains a large proportion of people who really have no intention of dying. While more men than women commit suicide, the number of women in the 'unsuccessful' group far exceeds the number of men. Attempted suicide is in fact frequently nothing more than a form of blackmail to achieve a purpose. This purpose is most likely to be an attempt to coerce love from a consort or from parents.

The methods used in attempted suicide differ from those used in a serious attempt to end the life. The risks involved are usually low, and as might be expected the really efficiently lethal methods are avoided. In Britain it has been estimated that some 30,000 to 40,000 people attempt suicide each year, and of these about half require hospital resuscitation. The main tragedy with attempted suicide is that a proportion albeit small will succeed by mistake.

The management of an unsuccessful suicide, whether it arises from a genuine attempt or not, involves hospitalization for at least a period. Blood transfusion or surgery may be required, but the greatest group are those who have poisoned themselves, particularly with barbiturates. Aspiration is almost certain to be required, gastric lavage, treatment for shock and mechanical ventilation may also be necessary, together with an assessment of the electrolyte balance. Dialysis is required in very few cases, and analeptic therapy with bemegride is now rarely used. For the majority supportive treatment is all that is necessary. On the other hand all unsuccessful suicides must be seen and fully assessed by a psychiatrist, for a significant proportion subsequently die by their own hand and they are therefore a group which is at particular risk.

The prevention of suicide depends upon the accurate recognition of the potential risk. Various factors are particularly associated with a high suicide rate, e.g. broken homes, particularly when coupled with social upsets later in life (unemployment, marital disharmony or bereavement) and then social isolation. This risk is increased in the emotionally unstable and particularly in depressive illness, alcoholism and hysteria. Such mental disorders should be vigorously treated, though treatment of the retarded depressive often produces a temporary increase in the suicide risk. The second aspect of suicide prevention is the reduction of availability of easy methods. The determined suicide will always find the means, but such obvious opportunities as a high-rise flat or a month's prescription of a powerful barbiturate should be avoided if possible.

Many areas are now establishing suicide prevention centres. Some are run by federal authorities (e.g. Los Angeles); others are based upon voluntary or religious groups (e.g. the Samaritans). The majority of such groups consist of psychiatric social workers or psychiatrists, who organize a twenty-four-hour service. Whilst the value of their work cannot be doubted, the percentage of those about to commit suicide who seek and accept the advice is very small and a high proportion of suicides arise as an impulsive act.

Suicide preventative measures have not been very effective. Indeed over 50 per cent of suicides were either currently or recently attending a doctor – in a high proportion under psychiatric care. This is, however, no justification for failing to make strenuous efforts in the individual patient at risk.

10
CRITICAL AGES OF MAN

The child is father of the man and is, moreover, at one and the same time, heir to such intellectual eminence or mental derangement as together constitute the psychological heritage of humanity.

No two children can ever be alike nor is the metamorphosis from infant to child, or from child to adult, in any way standardized. Enormous individual variations are superimposed on the broad principles of any general schema. For this reason, the range of normal childhood behaviour must be vast. Many apparent discrepancies or deviations from concepts of normality will, furthermore, prove transient since time with its twin processes of development and maturation lends a dynamic dimension to any attempted assay of suspected childhood abnormality.

How far then can such individual variance extend yet still remain within the limits of normality? In practice, this must always prove a matter of conjecture. In instances of fairly gross psychological disturbance, little room will usually be left for doubt; but in the identification of minor degrees of abnormality, opinions will differ and as such may be disputed between parent, teacher, general practitioner and psychiatrist.

The origins of childhood disorders
The origins of childhood disorders may with advantage be resolved into two broad groups – those aetiological factors operating before

birth and those which exert their influence after birth (fig. 66). The first of these groups concerns itself predominantly with considerations of heredity, the second with considerations of environment. The relative importance of each of these groups and their interaction in the genesis of psychiatric disorder is frequently in doubt. It differs from one community to another, from one disease to another and from one individual to another. A broad spectrum exists, with at its one end purely hereditary influences, at the other purely environmental and between the two the complex interaction of both.

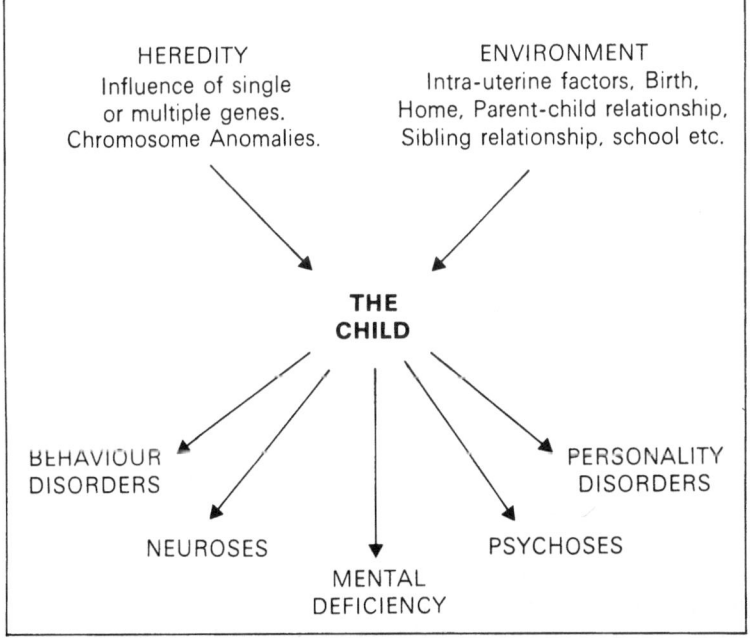

FIGURE 66 Factors in the genesis of psychological disorders of childhood.

The fœtus *in utero* is already equipped with its own highly specific genetic pattern – the units of which may well prove the harbingers of mental illness. A single dominant gene, for example, will determine the dementia of Huntington's chorea, appearing in youth or early middle age. Other single genes may induce the occurrence of manic-depressive psychosis or of schizophrenia. The additive influence of a number of genes may promote the emergence of neurotic illness or predispose to the psychopathic personality.

The hazards of intra-uterine life and of the birth process itself may result in damage to the infant's brain or interfere with normal cerebral development. Misfortune of this kind is likely to bequeath a legacy of mental defect of varying degree. Such intellectual deficit, in turn, creates its own behaviour problems. Children so handicapped experience difficulty in the formation of normal personal relationships; they learn but poorly from experience; their emotional responses show exaggeration; and, unable to keep pace with the normal requirements of life, they may opt out of these, turning their attention to substituted activities.

During infancy and the early years of life, it is the factors of social environment which emerge pre-eminent in the genesis of childhood disorders. Of paramount importance among these is the parent-child relationship. Parental faults of over-solicitude, over-indulgence and over-protection; of indifference and neglect; of hostility and rejection; of excessive ambition for the child; and of loading excessive responsibility upon the child, all predispose to the production of childhood disorders.

The environment of the young child is exclusively its home. Here the prevailing atmosphere, emotional tone and attitudes of those that dwell therein – parents, siblings and possibly grandparents – mould and determine the emotional reactions and behaviour of the child. It is here that an absence of love, of the demonstration of affection, of happiness, of attention or of security, can wreak such havoc upon the emotional development of the child and create severe conflict between the child and its environment. At a later age, the environment of the child is extended to include also the school. It is far from uncommon, in the special environment of the school, for the behaviour of a disordered child to contrast strikingly with its behaviour at home – often to the astonishment of the parents concerned.

A hitherto only child may resent intensely the birth of a sibling into the family and refuse to share parental attention and affection with the new rival. The emotional displeasure, jealousy and frustration of such a child is expressed frequently as temper tantrums, attention-seeking and manipulative behaviour, or at times as overt cruelty to the new-born infant. Similar resentment may be demonstrated along these same lines towards a recently acquired step-father or step-mother.

The broken home is a potent source of habit disorders, conduct disorders and of frank delinquency. Occasioned by the death of one or both parents; by divorce, desertion or separation; by prevailing drunkenness or severe economic distress, its host of deprivations deny to the developing child those requisite essentials of a healthy and stable social environment.

The nature of childhood disorders

Organic disease of the brain, injuries and infections most commonly underlie the grosser forms of childhood mental illness – with or without an accompanying epilepsy.

For the majority of mental disturbances in childhood observed by the Medical Practitioner, no physical basis will be demonstrable and the disorder will be psychologically determined. Within these psychological disturbances is included the group generically known as the behaviour disorders and further sub-divided into habit disorders and conduct disorders.

Habit disorders, observable particularly in younger children, are exemplified by disorders of food intake (refusal of food, food fads, aerophagy, rumination and pica); disorders of sleeping (difficulty in getting to sleep, restless sleep, sleepwalking, nightmares and night terrors); disorders of elimination (enuresis, encopresis, diarrhoea and constipation); disorders of speech (stammering and stuttering); motor disorders (tics, fidgetiness, head-rolling and body-rocking); and manipulation of parts of the body (thumb-sucking, nail-biting and masturbation).

Conduct disorders, observable particularly in older children, are exemplified by lying, stealing, wandering, truancy, destructiveness, aggressiveness, cruelty, sexual misdemeanours and other forms of anti-social conduct.

Personality disturbances displayed during childhood show normal childish traits to excessive degree and in exaggerated form. Such traits include shyness, timidity, hyperconscientiousness, hysterical manipulative behaviour, moroseness, pugnacity and also paranoid or schizoid tendencies. It is, of course, essential that any disturbance of personality should be judged within its childhood setting and not be evaluated by measures of adult standards. Such disturbances prove frequently but a passing phase in the phenomenon of development and maturation of the personality and do not, of themselves, prognosticate for permanent personality defects. Neurosis and psychosis are each encountered during childhood. The psychoses of childhood are, however, rare.

Neuroses and psychoses of childhood

Anxiety and fear are normal emotional responses of childhood and even when present in major degree may still fall well within the accepted limits of normal psychology. Much childhood anxiety is extremely purposive and serves as an efficient early warning system to compensate for the helplessness of the infant and the vulnerability of the child.

Morbid anxiety in the child is a very common result of morbid anxiety in a parent and here, factors of inherited constitution may combine with the principles of indoctrination. In children, such morbid anxiety is typically encountered as any of the multitude of designated phobias. Fears of the dark, of crowds, of open and closed spaces, of solitude, of heights and of many types of animal (fig. 67) are

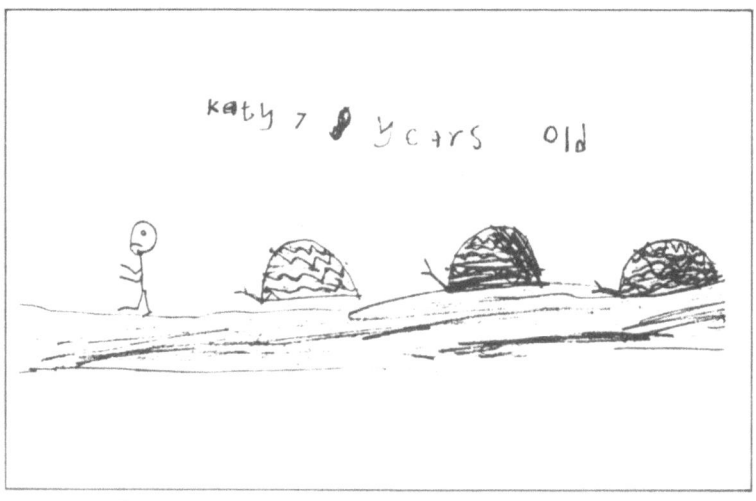

FIGURE 67 Drawing by a girl of 7 years, who displayed severe morbid anxiety directed to snails and slugs.

common. It is important to appreciate that a high proportion of so-called 'school phobias' do not in fact indicate primarily a fear of school. These frequently are representative of 'separation anxiety' (fig. 68) related to the security of home and to the parents, rather than fear of the conditions and situation prevailing at school. Should, however, the child's difficulties become known and talked about by the other children

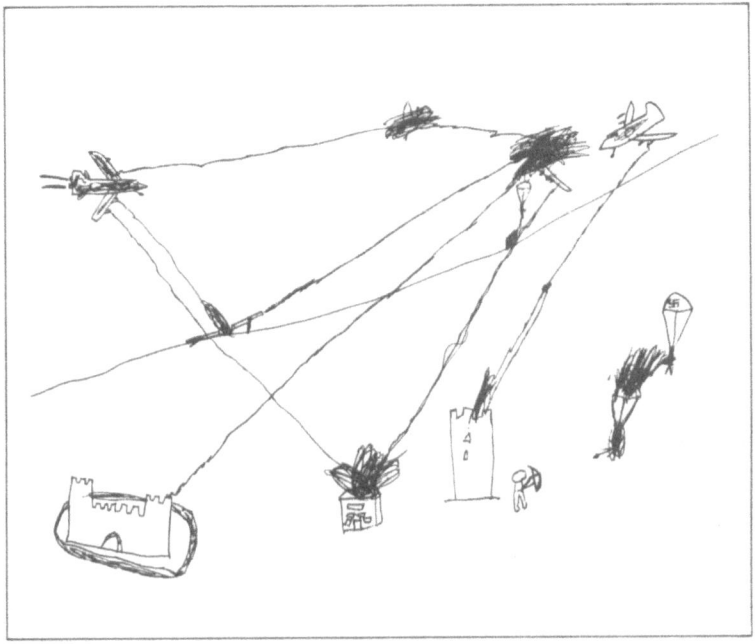

FIGURE 68 Drawing by a boy of 8 years, whose father was a bomber pilot in the Royal Air Force. The child's illness presented as a 'school phobia'. It was in fact an overwhelming separation anxiety, engendered by an intense concern for his father's safety when flying. This concern, with its accompanying morbid fear, is very well depicted.

at school, secondary anxieties of the school situation may well be superimposed upon the fears of leaving home. Anxiety may beset the child as periodic attacks in which marked somatic symptoms can be seen, or again, it may pervade the hours of sleeping as anxiety dreams, nightmares and night terrors.

The immaturity of the child's personality lends itself readily to hysterical reactions and to the symptoms of hysterical illness. Fainting, vomiting, aphonia, blindness, anaesthesia and paralysis are but few of the many symptoms counterfeited. The object of such symptomatology is not difficult to detect and the *modus operandi* of child hysteria is relatively unsophisticated.

Obsessive-compulsive features are observable in many aspects of quite normal childhood behaviour and play. These features must not be confused with symptoms of childhood obsessive-compulsive illness which can declare itself at almost any stage of the child's life – often within the setting of parental pressure to excel.

Manic-depressive psychosis has little place among the mental illnesses of childhood – though morbid states of depression and elation may occur. In this latter case, an important differentiation must be made between the hyperactivity of a child in manic and hypomanic states and that which occurs in the condition of hyperkinesis, when major degrees of fidgetiness, restlessness and distractibility occur in many cases as a sequel to cerebral damage.

The incidence of schizophrenia in childhood is a low one – though numerous psychotic illnesses of childhood have in the past been erroneously labelled as this. Of recent years the condition of infantile autism has received much interesting attention. Though some symptoms can be present from birth, the autistic condition is characterized by the child who has undergone normal development during the first year or years of life and then displays the striking features of withdrawal into an isolated and lonely world of its own. A further important feature is the delay in speech development, and in addition, the peculiarities of attempted communication. Such difficulties, of course, increase and accentuate the child's overwhelming problems of isolation. The onset of infantile autism may coincide with some critical event in the developing child's life such as serious illness or the birth of a sibling. In other instances, no obvious precipitating event can be found.

Management

The freshness and malleability of the growing child's mind permit extensive modification of its mental processes. Herein lies the fundamental difference in approach between the therapy of childhood psychological disorders and the corresponding treatment of psychiatric illness in the adult.

Treatment of the disordered child will, however, most advantageously commence with treatment of the parent. A careful case-history should be taken – in which due allowance must be made for parental emotional bias – and be followed by a physical examination of the child to exclude any obvious underlying organic disease – including such important factors as deafness or visual defects. In minor disorders, therapy is best begun with explanatory guidance to the parents on the nature of the disorder and should include enlightenment on those aetiological factors responsible for the symptoms. Practical advice should be given on possible modifications within the home or school environment. It is in such matters that the highly specialized knowledge of the family by the medical practitioner will prove invaluable, and his professional counsel, together with some periodic supervision combining encouragement and reassurance of both child and parents, will in many cases of minor disorder prove to be all that is required.

The behaviour disorders and anxiety reactions of childhood may be greatly relieved by appropriate medication. Sedation or tranquillization may not only render a difficult situation accessible to therapy but can effectively forestall the formation of conditioned patterns of morbid behaviour. Amphetamine may prove useful in the treatment of enuresis and, paradoxically enough, in the hyperkinetic child.

In all but the minor disorders of childhood, the medical practitioner would be well advised to call for the special investigation of the child by a Child Guidance Clinic. Here psychiatric examination of the child will be made together with any specialized testing that may be necessary. Furthermore, the services of a trained psychiatric social worker are available for additional investigation of domestic problems and for assistance in the resolution of those difficulties which present themselves in the social environment.

ADOLESCENCE

The age of adolescence is the age of adjustment from childhood to adult life, of discovery of a new identity, of a change from a school environment to the carving out of a career and of the first experience of the sexual urge.

Rapid mood fluctuations are the rule, with violent swings from childhood to adult behaviour within minutes, while the conflicts between parents and child which stem from the need for each to adjust to the new relationship present as rebellious behaviour of greater or lesser degree. A certain amount of rebellion should be regarded as a necessity of normal development at that stage.

Rebellion is only serious when encountered in the extreme, i.e. when it becomes both destructive to the adolescent and to the people around him. When present to this extent, a psychopathic personality is probably involved. Rebellion against social convention in the form of 'beatniks' or 'hippies' is a harmless form of exhibitionism which like any other fashion passes. The less publicity given to any rebel group the more chance there is of the fashion dying quickly. If attention is drawn to them then generally they go further with their 'shock' tactics.

Drug taking is in its early stages an experiment. The adolescent takes drugs for 'kicks' and where the 'soft' drugs are concerned, it is relatively harmless. Unfortunately, it does not always stop there, and progression is made from the 'soft' drugs to the 'hard' drugs. This progression usually follows contact with 'hard' drug pushers who are callous when encouraging young people to take them.

Management

Where the *adolescent* has understanding parents the problems which arise during adolescence are usually far less than in the adolescent who has received very little guidance. Parents can help to solve the problems by trying to be understanding and sympathetic towards the various situations which arise.

It is important for parents to separate in their own minds what is just a fashion, for fashions matter very little, from that which is likely to be. harmful on a long-term basis and which may affect others. If parents employ a sensible set of rules, most adolescents will readily accept these. It is only when they appear to be completely unreasonable that serious problems arise.

If there are any serious problems these are sometimes difficult for the parents to treat alone, but it is important that rapport is established with the patient, on the part of both the doctor and the parents – but this does not mean succumbing to the patient's whims.

THE MENOPAUSE

The end of the child-bearing period is marked irrevocably by the menopause. No normal healthy woman could but regret the passing of these years but the effect of this new phase of life will vary enormously from woman to woman. The smoothness of the psychological adjustment will depend to a large degree upon the personality and it is estimated that some 15 per cent of women experience no untoward menopausal symptomatology at all. Many approach this time of life ambivalently and while still regretting the passing of the fertile years none the less look forward to a future unhampered by a monthly inconvenience. In many the general health may show a surprising improvement.

The smoothness of the physical adjustment which contributes substantially to the individual variation in the psychological adjustment depends most frequently upon the vagaries of a readjusting system of hormonal control. This adjustment includes not only those within the ovaries but also the general imbalance within the total endocrine system. The extent of the somatic manifestations, affecting both the autonomic nervous system and endocrine system, demonstrates that an important component of this change results from diencephalic (probably hypothalamic) alterations. It is important to appreciate that the required compensation is a dual one to the interaction which exists between these physical and psychological changes.

Regret is a normal reaction to the natural process of ageing, and such regret will show itself even before the menopause; the misgivings about birthdays, the search for the additional wrinkles; the visit to the bathroom scales; the anxious search for grey hairs. Already by this time attempts will have been made to restore the situation to the *status quo ante* by artificial measures. The menopause, constituting a definite milestone, accentuates this feeling of ageing. Evidence suggests that the average age at which these changes take place is increasing. They may occur with a surprising steadiness or be spread gradually over a lengthy period of time. Whichever form they may take, they demand from the woman a physical and psychological adjustment to the new circumstances.

The presentation of psychiatric disorders

Psychologically most women experience a temporary emotional lability. In the majority, any such personality changes occurring at this time reflect the underlying hormonal dysfunction and will revert to their normal proportions as adjustment to the new endocrine equilibrium is made.

For three out of every twenty, these psychological changes are so minimal as to be totally unrecognized. For the rest, the extent of the manifestations and their presentation will vary widely although fortunately they are usually of a transient nature.

Degrees of depression are fairly common, with typical features of weeping, guilt and distortion of thought. Irritability may be very marked and cause special distress in the patient's daily dealings with the family.

Anxiety too is liable to be very much in evidence at this time. It can attach itself to any of a number of specific concepts or objects and take the form of well-defined phobias, or it may be experienced as the less definite but equally distressing 'free-floating' anxiety. The fear of insanity, as might be expected, occurs with an unfailing frequency. A morbid preoccupation for the future health of the husband or acute concern for other close members of the family or personal friends is again very typical. In those so predisposed, obsessive-compulsive symptoms may emerge. Irrational behaviour may occur, not infrequently with undertones of sexual excitement, and can lead to impulsive actions, including the onset of kleptomania. Sometimes hysterical features may predominate. Such features, in typical fashion, will conceal some 'secondary gain' and may thrive in a setting of feigned self-sacrifice and exquisite martyrdom.

Paranoid reactions may occur as the characteristic ridiculous jealousies directed to young and attractive women, or again may take the form – to the acute distress of the innocent spouse – of intense suspicions of the husband's infidelity with acrimonious denunciations of his moral conduct.

Schizophrenic illness is likely to show exacerbation at the menopause or, in the case of its paranoid form, may declare itself for the first time at this period. The onset of a pre-senile dementia or of involutional melancholia will coincide with this time of life. A marked increase in sexual desire can make itself felt at the menopause and these feelings of the day can be translated into disturbing, erotic dreams of the night. The psychological impact of these circumstances upon the single woman may cause considerable distress.

While we are primarily concerned with psychological disorders, in these particular circumstances it is impossible to dissociate the psychological changes from the physical, Indeed the breadth of the physiological changes is such that an imbalance within the diencephalon must be postulated – an imbalance which is itself frequently associated with emotional disturbances.

The physical manifestations of the menopause, in terms of their underlying causes, divide themselves chiefly between a temporary disturbance of autonomic function and endocrine imbalance. To these, however, additional physical features are contributed on a basis of psychosomatic pathology. The main autonomic features consist of vasomotor instability, manifested by 'hot flushes', accompanying sweating, or at other times 'pallor and chilling'. Deficient ovarian function accounts for changes which occur both in the vagina and in the skin leading to local or general irritation.

Some or all of the other endocrine glands may also be affected. For example, thyroid imbalance may occur giving signs of hyperthyroidism or hypothyroidism. Adrenal medulla instability may play a part in the cardiovascular symptomatology, while androgens from the adrenal cortex may cause an increased growth of hair on the female face.

Among the psychosomatic symptoms which present with greatest frequency are giddiness, digestive and bowel disturbances, muscle aches, headaches, fatigue and lethargy.

Management

Where menopausal symptoms can be attributed to a substantial endocrine deficiency or excess, the treatment will include a supplementation or reduction of the hormones in question. In practice, this will most usually mean the administration of thyroid or its antagonists, or the prescribing of synthetic oestrogens.

The percentage of patients requiring such hormonal treatment should not be large, whereas many of the patients are likely to benefit from some simple sedation or appropriate tranquillizer (e.g. diazepam). Whenever psychological symptoms are evident, it is particularly important to secure a normal pattern of sleep. Care should be exercised in the selection of an appropriate hypnotic to avoid dangers of suicide. In this respect some of the more recent and safer non-barbiturate hypnotics (e.g. nitrazepam or flurazepam) are to be preferred to the older barbiturates.

Since so many of the difficulties encountered at the menopause reflect an attitude of mind, psychotherapy of a superficial kind, incorporating both explanation and reassurance, will prove of great value and will do much to dispel the apprehension and fears which so frequently aggravate the situation. The patient should understand quite clearly that though the capacity for child-bearing is lost at the menopause, this need in no way detract from the continued enjoyment of normal sexual practice for many years. Advice may be given on dietary adjustment for weight problems, on adequate rest and exercise and on the need to consider new interests and activities. Accent should be placed on the maximum enjoyment which can be anticipated in terms of both health and activity.

THE AGED

The plight of the elderly is not an enviable one. The problems of ageing, both mental and physical, for society no less than for the individual, increase in number and complexity with each ensuing year.

As life becomes longer the years take an increasing toll of the body reactions. The span of ageing is inconsistently wide, one person is already old at 60 whilst another remains unbelievably young at 90. The reason for this variation in the rate of ageing is still unknown.

The psychological needs of the aged – though somewhat less obvious than the somatic – proceed *pari passu* with increasing physical infirmity. The sense of not belonging, of no longer being wanted, of an absence of daily purpose, of an inability to contribute to life, are all felt keenly by a great number of the elderly.

The prevailing attitude of society is of fundamental importance in affecting the mental health of the aged. Those communities where the care of the aged is still regarded as a natural responsibility of the young usually show a smaller extent of mental abnormality than societies which rely upon the provision of impersonal social services.

A normal process of mental ageing can be recognized. A diminished power of adaptability is shown by the inability to keep pace with changing events and circumstances which fosters an attitude of phlegmatic conservatism. Selective memory defects aggravate the situation and difficulty in recalling names and recent happenings contrasts with a retained ability to recall events of long ago. An increasing failure to cope with the present day leads to a retreat into the remote days of the past.

The progressive physical infirmity necessitates greater, but reluctant, dependence upon others which automatically removes the self-reliance and earlier authority. This leads in turn to feelings of resentment which may show themselves as self-assertive manœuvres, e.g. obstinacy, cantankerousness, hostility or frank aggression. Moreover, the feeling of insecurity created by this dependence causes compensatory psychological mechanisms, for example, the hoarding of useless articles, or suspicions which, coupled with the increasing defects of memory, lead to false accusations and ideas of persecution.

With the intellectual deterioration, interests become more narrow and egocentric and hypochondriacal features may predominate. Moreover the loss of some of the higher brain centres leads to a blunting of finer feelings and degrees of coarseness may appear, which are particularly distressing to relatives.

The presentation of psychiatric disorders in the aged
The aetiological factors involved and the presentation of mental disorders in the aged are shown in fig. 69.

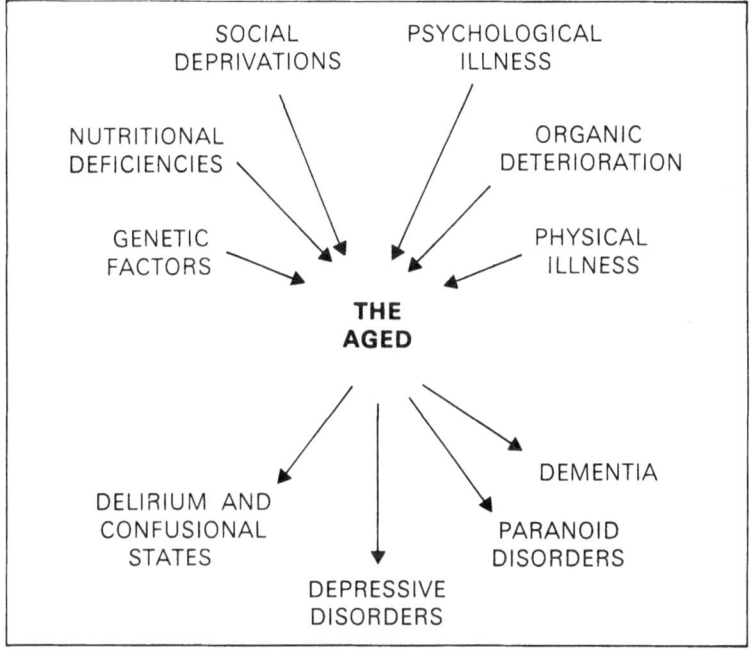

FIGURE 69 Aetiological factors in the presentation of mental disorders of the aged.

Among the aged, depression is common and of special importance. The extent of the tension, agitation, restlessness and paranoid delusions is greater at that period than earlier. Moreover there is a far greater risk of consummated suicide. The depression is commonly reactive, following personal misfortune, bereavement or adverse circumstance, but endogenous depression can also be seen. This latter may signify an extension of a previous manic-depressive psychosis. Mania and hypomania are occasionally seen in the elderly and are liable to make great demands on the limited physical resources.

In addition to the psychological causes of depression, somatic illnesses may themselves precipitate an attack. These illnesses include cerebral arteriosclerosis, Parkinson's disease, general paralysis and neoplasms, no less than severe deficiencies of the vitamin B group.

The second main group of disorders encountered in the elderly is provided by dementia, commonly divided into two types, arteriosclerotic and senile, which show many features in common. Arteriosclerotic psychosis occurs at an earlier age than senile psychosis and is seen more frequently in men. Other signs of arteriosclerosis are also present, e.g. hypertension, or a history of previous cerebrovascular accident. In the early stages the symptoms are frequently subjective and indefinite, with headaches and dizziness, an impairment of memory for names, and insomnia. Minor intellectual deterioration follows but the progress of the dementia is slow (fig. 70). Insight remains good and

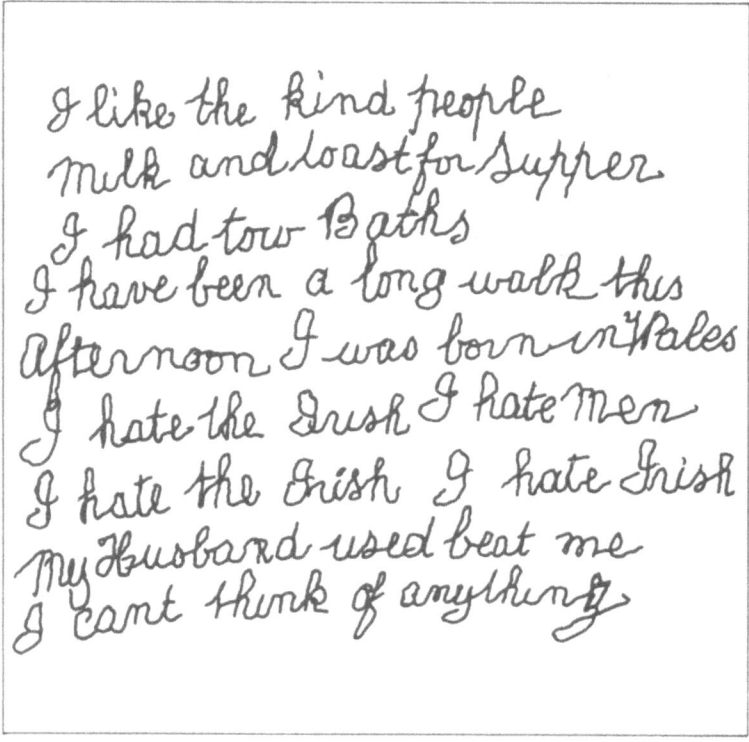

FIGURE 70 Specimen of handwriting from woman aged 73 years. Note perseveration, missing words, omissions in dotting i's and crossing t's and the tremor.

the patient's personality remains normal until late in the course of the illness. Depressive features are common and there is marked emotional lability and emotional incontinence with incongruous responses of laughing and weeping. Delusions and hallucinations may occur together with episodes of acute delirium. A troublesome feature is the nocturnal wandering. As the progression takes place other signs of central nervous system damage, e.g. aphasia, agnosia, apraxia may also become evident. In senile dementia, the features initially develop insidiously with the early indefinite symptoms resembling those found in the arteriosclerotic form. The disease is rarely encountered before the age of 70 and rapidly progresses through severe dementia to death within a few years. The downhill course may be accentuated by additional stress, e.g. infections. Memory changes are a prominent feature and there is a rapid disintegration of the personality. The conjoined defects of intellect and memory lead to disorientation and misunderstanding and foster endless confusion. Delusions of grandeur, of melancholia or of persecution readily occur and belligerence is a fairly constant feature. The terminal stages are characterized by complete and unqualified destruction of the psyche.

Management in medical practice

The medical practitioner's management of the aged person displaying symptoms of mental disease may for practical purposes be described in three basic principles.

Firstly, adjustment or restoration must be made of those social factors which play an essential role in maintaining the mental health of the aged. Among these measures will be included advice to the relatives how best the daily management and general supervision of the patient may be conducted. Many local authorities now provide day facilities for the care and welfare of the aged and these will frequently help relieve the burden of the relatives. If necessary, hospital admission can be contemplated and for those who live alone this may produce considerable benefit. On the other hand, removal to hospital from the family environment frequently leads to a more rapid deterioration.

Secondly, effective treatment should be given for any physical condition which of itself may be precipitating or accentuating the mental problems. Important among these must be considered the effects of cerebral anoxia and uraemia.

Thirdly, specific treatment will be required for the symptomatology of the mental illness itself. Here both tranquillizers and sedatives will be found extremely helpful in reducing agitation, restlessness and nocturnal wandering and also in ensuring a good night's sleep, not only for the patient but for the relatives.

In the elderly, however, a greater variation in response to individual drugs and dosage will be encountered and the most effective drug and dose level must usually be found on a basis of trial and error. The dose used in the elderly is usually smaller than that which would be effective in a young person showing the same symptom complex. Intensive vitamin therapy will sometimes be followed by a dramatic resolution of acute confusional episodes, when these result from chronic nutritional defect and greater emphasis is now placed upon the need for an adequate vitamin level in the elderly.

Depression in the aged, with its greatly increased suicide risk, should always be treated energetically and with adequate supervision of the patient. Amitriptyline is usually the drug of choice for depression in the elderly.

It is important, when considering the aetiology and therapy of mental illness in the elderly, always to consider what other drugs are being administered. Certain of the modern drugs greatly favoured for the treatment of both psychological and somatic conditions in the aged may if the dosage is not carefully adjusted produce a symptomatology suggestive of a classical mental illness. Appropriate adjustment of drug and dosage can then produce a dramatic response.

11

THERAPY FOR
PSYCHIATRIC DISORDERS

The origins of almost all psychiatric disorders remain obscure to us. It is for this reason that so much controversy and bewildering speculation arise whenever attempts are made to discuss the aetiology of mental illnesses. Disorders of cerebral biochemistry, genetic endowment, social and environmental factors, repressed conflicts from the years of infantile development, all have their protagonists, and in like fashion – all have their violent antagonists.

It is quite clear that in a small and restricted number of cases a specific chemical defect is the causative factor (e.g. the inherited disorders of galactosaemia or phenylketonuria). It seems likely that in some cases an unfavourable and stressful environment may be sufficient to generate mental illness in those constitutionally vulnerable. But in the overwhelming majority of all psychiatric patients it will be a combination of both intrinsic and extrinsic factors which are responsible for the appearance and the course of their particular illness.

With so many conflicting theories of causation, it is scarcely surprising that equally controversial views are held on the question of therapy. Most patients are likely to receive a composite form of therapy, that is to say one which employs the most advantageous features of a number of differing types of therapy. Preferably this should not be based merely on the prejudices of the clinician-in-charge but as far as is at all possible on such established scientific principles as can exist in this elusive sphere.

The following aspects and forms of therapy are considered: Psychotherapy (below); Behaviour therapy (p. 246); Occupational therapy (p. 247); Physical methods of treatment (p. 247); Hospitalization (p. 250); Community care (p. 252).

PSYCHOTHERAPY

This may take various forms, but the fundamental feature throughout is the communication which exists between the patient and the therapist.

In its simplest form – *supportive psychotherapy* – the current difficulties are investigated and the patient helped to cope with the problems of life both in the present and in the future. It is this form of psychotherapy that is practised by all doctors daily. For the patient to share the responsibility of the illness with his doctor eases the weight of its burden, breaks down the feeling of isolation in a depression or of the tension in an anxious state, and by this simple means aids the relief of the disorder.

The psychotherapy of many mental illnesses effectively commences at the initial interview. Both the manner and conduct of this consultation are of paramount importance. The patient's narrative must be heard in full, uncritically and – an important feature if the practitioner's time will permit – unhurriedly. Reassurance should be given on individual issues as each arises, together with any practical counsel which may be indicated for their solution. It is important to reassure the patient by an explanation of the symptoms and by enlightenment on their mode of origin.

When there are somatic complaints, a full physical examination should be made to dispel authoritatively the patient's concern for his somatic symptomatology.

An alternative method of supportive psychotherapy is covered by the grandiose term – *environmental modification*. The doctor, acting on the assumption that present factors in the environment are important in the maintenance of the disorder, seeks to change this environment, e.g. by interviewing and counselling the spouse, arranging for rehousing via the local authorities, advising a change of occupation etc.

Two important aspects of even the most simple psychotherapy are *suggestion* and *persuasion*. In suggestion the doctor's comments and views are accepted even in the absence of adequate grounds. Suggestion forms a part of the therapeutic armamentarium of all good practitioners, whether they are psychiatrists, physicians or surgeons. Suggestion plays a part in the effectiveness of physical methods of treatment in medicine, e.g. massage, radiant heat etc., and even more plays an important part in pharmacotherapy, e.g. colour of the medicine.

In persuasion the patient is encouraged to play an active part in his own rehabilitation by a different approach to his life and environment.

All these methods of simple psychotherapy depend on a good doctor-patient relationship. The patient must feel that the doctor is intensely interested in him, and the patient must respect and accept the doctor's views if success is to be achieved.

Intensive and prolonged analytical psychotherapy may follow the Freudian or associated schools (p. 153). This involves multiple ana-lytical sessions over weeks, months or years, during which attempts are made to pinpoint those repressed primitive conflicts which are held to be the precipitation of the illness. This is done by the examination of both past experiences and current dreams. The analyst must have considerable experience to achieve success.

Among the specific techniques used in analytical psychotherapy are *hypnosis* and *abreaction*. In hypnosis a state of artificially increased suggestibility is induced, concentrated on the hypnotist alone. The level of hypnosis can vary from a low state to a deep trance. Hypnosis induction should only be undertaken by those with previous training and experience, for it is not devoid of dangers. The term abreaction was originally used by Freud for the emotional release when previously repressed material was brought to the surface and described. An abreaction response can be facilitated by various drugs including intravenous barbiturates, methedrine, halucinogenic substances (e.g. lysergic acid diethylamide – LSD) and inhalation anaesthetic sub-stances. None of these techniques is suitable for non-specialist use, and even in the hands of experts dangers and difficulties exist.

Group psychotherapy originally developed from individual psycho-therapy as a time-saving expedient. Experience, however, suggested that interactions within the group of patients had their own intrinsic merits and group methods have recently increased in popularity. The number in each group is usually about 6–10. Although the process grew originally from the analytical school, group therapy is now con-ducted not only for analytical purposes, but also for re-education, socialization, abreaction and character modification *inter alia* depending on the background and ideas of the leader and the needs of the group.

One specific form of group psychotherapy is *psychodrama*, which involves structured, directed and dramatized acting-out of the patient's personal and emotional problems, in addition to his problems of interaction with the group.

In children *play therapy* may be regarded as the equivalent of group psychotherapy in the adult. The permissive environment of the therapeutic play room helps to demonstrate the emotional attitudes which exist.

There is general agreement that the psychiatric disorders which are most likely to benefit from psychotherapeutic methods are anxiety states, reactive depressions, psychosomatic disorders and addictions, though ardent protagonists claim benefit in a broader range of mental disorders.

BEHAVIOUR THERAPIES

Behaviour therapies, regarded by many as a particular form of psychotherapy, may be defined as procedures based on modern learning theories that lead to a change in the behaviour of the patient. They have their greatest value in the treatment of neurotic symptoms, i.e. a previously learned maladjusted response to an environmental stress. Thus behaviour therapy employs various procedures to unlearn the maladjusted response and relearn an appropriate one.

Negative learning has its greatest value in involuntary movements, e.g. tics. The patient rigidly adheres to a regular fixed and frequent voluntary repetition of the tic movement. A state of inhibition is set up which aborts the involuntary tic.

Reciprocal inhibition has its greatest value in phobic anxieties. It consists of a gradually increasing exposure to the stimuli that provoke the anxiety but at each stage only to a level which produces no tension state. This can be achieved by varying the time of exposure or by the use of anti-anxiety therapy concomitantly – e.g. tranquillizers, hypnosis. In a more recent technique called flooding or implosion the patient is confronted in imagination or reality with massive exposure to the phobic stimuli and encouraged to remain in contact with that situation until the resulting anxiety subsides. It is used most commonly in animal phobias and is made more acceptable by the administration of anxiolytic drugs during the first one or two stages.

Operant conditioning follows the classical learning procedures whereby a reward is given for a correct response or a punishment for the

246

undesirable one. It has its greatest value in childhood behaviour disorders lies, stammering etc.

Another form of positive operant conditioning used in the hospital environment is token economy. In this system the patients earn tokens by an appropriate desirable behaviour, the tokens being used to 'buy' rewarding activities such as time out of the hospital, or in a recreational centre environment.

One form of regular operant conditioning is the most commonly used type of behaviour therapy, viz. aversion therapy. It is widely used in the treatment of addictions and sexual perversions, i.e. when the abnormal behaviour is pleasurable to the patient. Therapy consists of associating the behaviour or stimuli that are pleasurable to the patient with a noxious response. For alcoholism this may be the nausea and vomiting that occurs when apomorphine and alcohol are taken simultaneously; for sexual deviations it is usually the simultaneous administration of an electric shock. The coupling of the pleasurable stimuli with a noxious response reduces the pleasure and in a proportion of patients cures the abnormality.

OCCUPATIONAL THERAPY

The standard form of occupational therapy until recently has been the provision of handicraft activities primarily designed to act as a diversion for the patients.

Now with the general accent on returning patients to a useful life in the community the accent has been placed on active rehabilitation. For men industrial training has become the main form of occupational therapy, within either a closed training centre or even in open industry under the care of a psychiatric nurse. The patients are paid for the results they achieve and the intention is that they shall gradually become self-supporting back in the community.

Women on the other hand may either receive training in the general sphere of light industry with a like intention, or are trained in home care. The choice depends upon the determination of which is more appropriate for the individual.

Thus occupational therapy is now a particularly important aspect of rehabilitation of the mentally ill.

PHYSICAL METHODS OF TREATMENT

The rationale for physical methods of treatment in psychiatry as opposed to psychotherapeutic methods is that there is a biochemical abnormality in the brain associated with the disorder. This chemical abnormality may be primary and causative, and those diseases in which there is such a chemical abnormality will show the best responses to the physical methods of treatment. It is important to realize, however, that even in such disorders specific curative therapy for the basic abnormality is not currently available.

Where the reactive factor is marked or there is a fundamental personality disorder physical methods are likely to give at best only modest improvement. However, even in such patients they may sometimes be combined with psychotherapeutic procedures to the patient's benefit. In neurotic patients in particular the primary aim of physical treatment is symptom relief. Neurotic patients develop symptoms when they can no longer cope with the stresses to which they are exposed. The insomnia or ill health that results leads in its turn to a vicious circle of sustained and increased inadequacy. For such patients the relief of the symptoms by physical methods may break the vicious circle, help the patients to face up to their problems, to get back to their work and social activities. This in its turn helps to improve the personal function. It is important to realize, however, that in such patients physical methods must be regarded as adjunctive therapy with the accent placed on techniques that are designed to overcome the real problem. Indeed it is important to accept that for most patients physical methods represent only one facet of the total therapeutic regimen. To have to continue physical methods of treatment indefinitely for symptom relief is to admit failure in the treatment of the underlying disorder. For some disorders this may be necessary at the present state of our medical art. Thus, for example, the maintenance approach to drug therapy is important in most schizophrenic patients in whom the cessation of treatment would lead to permanent deterioration in the mental health.

There are four different forms of physical treatment, narcosis: psychosurgery, electroconvulsive therapy and pharmacotherapy.

Continuous narcosis was one of the most popular treatments for psychiatric disorders in the earlier part of this century. Heavy and continuous sedation by paraldehyde or barbiturates was maintained for twenty hours a day and for several weeks at a time. Without expert medical and nursing care bronchopneumonia, cardiovascular collapse and renal failure lead to mortality rates of up to 5 per cent. Though continuous narcosis was therapeutically effective, the advent of safer but equally effective forms of therapy lead to classical continuous narcosis being abandoned.

However, a modified form of continuous narcosis, in which a state of drowsiness is maintained each day and deep sleep each night for 5–7 nights, is very effective in severe and acute anxiety states, particularly those that stem from a well defined and limited stress situation. The marked though temporary improvement that results enables other forms of therapy to be instituted, while the patient is still receptive and before relapse occurs.

While classical continuous narcosis could only be undertaken in hospital, the modified short form can be undertaken at home in an otherwise fit person if there are sensible relatives available. The exact choice of drugs and dosage varies with the doctor, but most techniques depend on the use of large doses of a tranquillizer during the day and a short acting hypnotic at night. This short acting hypnotic may sometimes be given as a supplement after lunch to ensure a very drowsy afternoon. The greatest danger lies in the patient experiencing bronchial obstruction from falling asleep while eating, and nurses or relatives must be warned that constant attention is necessary during mealtimes.

Psychosurgery is the use of brain surgery for the relief of psychiatric disorders. The standard operation of leucotomy was effective for the relief of intolerable states of anxiety but the side effects were incapacitating. Various modifications have been made, and the most popular operation now is a bimedial leucotomy with orbital undercutting. The operation is indicated in intractable anxiety of long standing, but only where there is a stable basic personality, for the operation may itself reduce the patient's self-control.

Electroconvulsive therapy is an empirical form of therapy, the popularity of which varies from time to time depending largely on the success of other methods of treatment. At the present time it is used for certain patients selected from two groups of disorders – schizophrenia and depression.

In schizophrenia the combination of electroconvulsive therapy with a neuroleptic can be used with effect not only in catatonic states, but in acute onset cases with a pronounced affective component and in chronic paranoid schizophrenics that have proved resistant to drug therapy alone.

The main indication for electroconvulsive therapy is endogenous depression with marked agitation, excluding those of the neurotic type.

Since the antidepressant drugs are usually effective and are easier to handle in mild to moderate cases, electroconvulsive therapy should be reserved for the severe case where it should probably be used without a prior trial of antidepressant drugs, for the results of drug therapy are rarely good in this group. This also holds for patients with suicidal tendencies. Nowadays in such patients it is common practice to give antidepressant drugs concomitantly with electroconvulsive therapy to avoid the relapse which may occur later. Electroconvulsive therapy is now always given under an anaesthetic in combination with a muscle relaxant, and with an experienced team the procedure is no more dangerous than is the anaesthetic itself. The only absolute contra-indication is a recent cardiac infarct; for other diseases the assessment of whether to use electroconvulsive therapy is the assessment of the dangers of a short anaesthetic.

Electroconvulsive therapy is usually given two or three times a week for the first and second week. Many patients begin to show improvement after the third or fourth treatment, and in such patients six or seven treatments will probably be sufficient for the first course, though it may be necessary to give one or two more later at weekly intervals to maintain the improvement. When no improvement is found after about six treatments it is unlikely that electroconvulsive therapy will be successful and it should be abandoned.

With classical electroconvulsive therapy amnesia is the rule, particularly in the elderly. It is usually transient, but may last for several weeks on some patients and be a source of annoyance.

Recently electroconvulsive therapy has been given only in the non-dominant hemisphere, and this has led to a reduced incidence and severity of amnesia.

Pharmacotherapy is the use of the central nervous system active drugs for the relief of psychiatric illness. The use of some drugs (even if only a sedative) at some stage is almost universal and since there is now a very wide range of drugs available, this whole subject is considered in a separate chapter (p. 254).

considered in a separate chapter (p. 254).

HOSPITALIZATION

Current psychiatric opinion favours the treatment of the patient within his own home and environment rather than in hospital, and reduction of the length of the hospital stay to the minimum. Hospital administration is usually confined to the diagnosis and therapeutic control of schizophrenics, care of potentially suicidal depressives, care of the mentally subnormal and to an ever increasing extent care of senile dementias whose relatives either cannot or will not stand the strain of home care any longer. Such hospital admissions as are required should be arranged as far as possible on a voluntary basis (p. 273).

In many cases of schizophrenia hospitalization is desirable for a period once the disorder is suspected, though this hospital care with its specialized techniques and nursing is still indicated for all acute exacerbations. The duration of such temporary periods of hospitalization has become progressively shorter. This is due to the rapid control of symptoms which is now possible by the use of neuroleptic drugs, by the use of active rehabilitation and the policy of social care of the schizophrenic patient within the community.

While most depressives can be treated within the home environment, when there is any suicidal risk the continued surveillance of the patient during therapy is an important feature and in such patients hospital admission is desirable. Unfortunately it is not always possible to assess the suicidal danger in the individual patient, and if in doubt any medical practitioner should seek a second opinion.

While it is accepted that mental defectives should, as far as possible, be cared for within the home and family, social problems may make this impossible for some. Training based upon a total evaluation of the child's resources is an important aspect of the medical care, but unfortunately the number of residential hospitals available for training the mentally retarded is still inadequate for the needs.

It was always difficult to determine whether hospitalization is the optimum choice for the care of a patient suffering from senile dementia and many local authorities and community groups now provide day facilities for the care and welfare of the aged. This helps to relieve the burden on the relatives. For those who live alone hospital admission may produce considerable benefit, but on the other hand removal to hospital from a good family environment frequently leads to a more rapid deterioration.

The responsibility of the practitioner does not end when the patient enters hospital for treatment of a mental illness. Indeed wherever possible the practitioner should try to maintain contact during the period of hospitalization so that the patient may have confidence of continued support in the period after his discharge from hospital. Whatever the mental disorder, it is important that the practitioner maintains constant regular contact with the patient for several months or even years afterwards, until it can be firmly established that the patient requires no further medical attention. In many mental disorders, continued support is required for some considerable time and the patient must not get the impression that the doctor is 'losing interest'. The frequency of relapse can be significantly reduced by periodic routine consultation with the practitioner and it is the duty of the practitioner to make sure that such regular visits are made. These obviously should be at increasing intervals until ultimately the patient can be discharged from medical care happy in his own mind that he will be given further support and treatment if there is a recurrence.

The practitioner has a further responsibility towards the patient over his employment. Although we are emerging from the dark ages of prejudice against the mentally ill, there is still a great tendency on the part of many employers to avoid employing those candidates who have suffered from mental illnesses. Indeed relapses in mental illness are not uncommon in mental patients as a direct result of their failure to secure appropriate employment due to their previous history. It is therefore the responsibility of the practitioner to present the medical picture of the patient in as favourable a light as possible relative to their ability to undertake the work. To this end, the phrasing of the certificate of health which is called for should be considered carefully. When there is difficulty the practitioner should consider a telephone call to the employers where this will benefit. Any medical report must be honest and helpful not only to the employer but to the patient, whose permission will of course be sought before any approach is made to third parties.

COMMUNITY CARE

Current practice in psychiatry is placing more emphasis on the care of the patient within his own community and removal as soon as possible from the hospital environment. This development stemmed from the 'open door' policy which began about 25 years ago and has become possible due to the rapid strides that have been made in therapeutics over this period, particularly in the field of physical methods.

Effort has been devoted to the prevention of permanent institutionalization and to the development of community care as a viable alternative to hospitalization. Such community care requires the coordination of the health and welfare services concerned with the support, treatment and after-care of psychiatric patients.

Among the important facilities that must be integrated are:

(a) *General social and medical care* – Support and encouragement from tolerant and enlightened relatives, general practitioners and social workers.

(b) *Therapeutic regimens* – Controlled use of appropriate physical and psychotherapeutic methods which will abolish symptoms and facilitate stable adjustment within the community. In essence the patients' care is undertaken in smaller organizations tailored to their particular needs. These include *inter alia* day hospitals, night hospitals, special units in general hospitals, occupation centres, special workshops. These must all be linked to the general medical facilities involving both medical practitioners and social workers.

The details of the administrative arrangements differ from one country to another. In Great Britain steps are currently being undertaken to integrate the medical and social services so that community care may become a practical reality. This situation is discussed in further detail in the Appendix (p. 280).

12

PSYCHOTROPIC DRUGS

The last 20 years has seen major advances in the treatment of psychiatric disorders and to a great extent their progress is the result of the remarkable achievements in the field of psychotropic drugs. Before 1950 the number of drugs available for the treatment of the mentally ill was small and even among these, efficacy was not great. At the present time the medical practitioner is provided with an immense and bewildering range of compounds with a varying range of activity.

The psychotropic drugs are now one of the most widely used classes of medicine. This is in fact not surprising when it is considered that approximately 30 per cent of patients attending a doctor have some mild or moderately severe mental disorder. Whether this wide incidence of psychiatric illness may be attributed to the greater stresses of modern life, or to the more open approach to mental illness or to better diagnostic skills, is a matter for dispute.

It is important to stress that the psychotropic drugs have little if any effect on the basic pathology of mental disease. Their primary activity consists in suppressing the symptoms and signs, particularly those associated with the emotions. They are, therefore, most valued as adjuvant therapy. It is essential that other therapy should be used in addition, whether this is rehabilitation or psychotherapy. The psychotropics make the patient more accessible to other forms of therapy.

There is, however, no doubt that they have been a major cause of the change that has been possible over the past few years in the mental institutions. The open-door policy would not have been possible without them. Nevertheless the use of these drugs at the present time would appear to be rather more widespread than can be medically justified. It may in fact be indicative of the pressure under which most medical practitioners now work.

The psychotropic drugs fall into one or the other of two broad pharmacological classes: 'higher nervous system' stimulants or 'higher nervous system' depressants. These two classes coincide broadly with the clinical use of the drugs.

Many further attempts have been made to classify psychotropic drugs but all suffer from disadvantages. Among the better ones was that proposed by the study group of the World Health Organization in 1958. Over the following fifteen years some of the drugs then included have fallen into disuse and other chemical classes have been developed.

A simplified working classification based on that of the WHO is given in Table 8.

Function	Group	Classes
Psycho-sedatives	Neuroleptics	Phenothiazine type Thioxanthine type Reserpine type Butyrophenones
	Tranquillizers (Anxiolytics)	Some phenothiazines Propanediols Hypnosedatives Benzodiazepines
Psycho-stimulants	Euphoriants	Amphetamine type
	Thymoleptics	Imipramine group Amitriptyline group
	Lithium carbonate	—
	MAOI's	—
Psycho-tominetic		LSD Mescaline, etc.

Table 8 Practical therapeutic classification of psychotropic drugs

While it is useful to accept a rather stereotyped classification like this for description purposes it is important to realize that there is considerable overlap in the pharmacological and clinical effects of different members of the groups. This is shown diagrammatically in fig. 71.

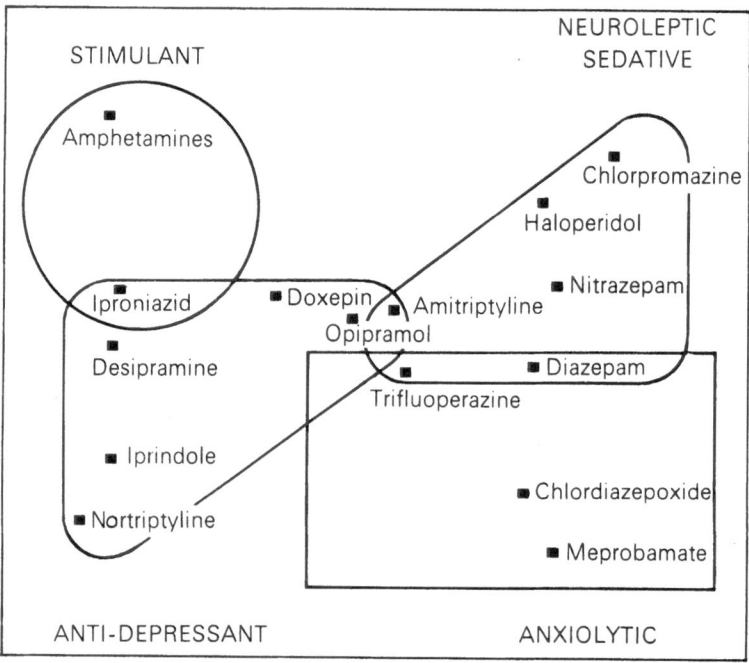

FIGURE 71 The diversity of clinical effect of drugs showing that rigid chemical or pharmacological classification is difficult.

COMMONLY USED REPRESENTATIVE DRUGS

It is difficult if not impossible to keep one's knowledge apace with the large number of psychotropic drugs that have become available over the past few years. A selection of representative drugs has therefore been made, covering the main chemical classes. Those selected are mainly the original compound in the class together with more recent derivatives that either are widely used or appear to show some distinct advantages.

Psychotropic Drugs

Neuroleptics

Compounds in this class (previously called major tranquillizers) suppress psychomotor activity and counteract behavioural restlessness in sufficiently powerful a fashion that they are effective in the psychoses (e.g. mania, schizophrenia). At present the main active drugs fall chemically into four classes: phenothiazines, thioxanthines, Rauwolfia alkaloids and their derivatives and the butyrophenones.

Phenothiazine derivatives are effective in many psychiatric disorders, including manic and overactive psychoses, schizophrenia, senile agitation and in anxiety states. The first member of the phenothiazine series was chlorpromazine. This drug was, and is, a valuable adjunct to analgesics; it is an anti-emetic, as are certain other members of the series. While chlorpromazine is effective in the hyperactive psychoses, its effects have not been encouraging in the neuroses. In the treatment of the psychoses, chlorpromazine is usually administered in doses around 25–50 mg tds.

Many related compounds are now available which show gradation in activity per dose unit and a varying frequency of side-effects. The most active compounds usually show less sedation, autonomic side-effects, jaundice, agranulocytosis and skin rashes, but more extrapyramidal side-effects than do the less active compounds. The more powerful compounds have their greatest use in the major psychoses although small doses of most of the more active compounds or larger doses of the milder members of the series may be used in the neuroses. An interesting recent development has been depot fluphenazine enanthate which enables maintenance phenothiazine therapy by injections at one to four week intervals. Unfortunately this often leads to increased side-effects. The *thioxanthines* are structurally related to the phenothiazines and resemble them in pharmacological experiments. The main product in this series is chloprothixene. In the clinic, chlorprothixene at a high dose schedule (50–150 mg per day) is effective in the hyperactive psychoses, while in lower dosage (5–30 mg per day) it has been used with some benefit in anxiety states. Some psychiatrists believe that there is a mild antidepressant activity, which though not so powerful as the thymoleptics is sometimes useful where depressive and anxiety symptoms are present in the same patient.

The alkaloids of Rauwolfia including reserpine have become less popular recently in the treatment of mental illness. Similar therapeutic

257

effects can be obtained more quickly and with less side-effects by using phenothiazine derivatives. The onset of action of reserpine is slow (up to 14 days) and in the meantime an increase in tension is likely to occur. Extrapyramidal side-effects are common and there is the danger of severe depression which may persist for a long time. The dose of reserpine as a neuroleptic is usually 1–2 mg tds. The benzoquinolizines are related to reserpine and have similar actions. Though seldom used now as a neuroleptic, one drug in this group – tetrabenazine is valuable in the treatment of Huntington's chorea.

Many compounds in the *butyrophenone class* have been synthesized. The best known compounds are haloperidol and trifluoperidol. Their pharmacological actions bear a general resemblance to the phenothiazines and their clinical actions also resemble this class of compound. The butyrophenones are successful in the treatment of certain affective disorders, particularly manic states, and of some schizophrenics. Extrapyramidal side-effects occur frequently though hypotensive and sensitivity reactions are encountered less with the butyrophenones than with the phenothiazines, and they are virtually free of autonomic side-effects.

Of the butyrophenones the parent compound – haloperidol – has much to commend it. The daily dose range for the treatment of psychotics is about 3–9 mg. Smaller doses have been advocated for mild tension states.

Whether a phenothiazine or a butyrophenone should be used first in a previously untreated psychosis is still a matter of controversy.

Tranquillizers

This class embraces the groups described in the WHO classification as minor tranquillizers and tranquillosedatives. Although from the theoretical point of view there is a clear distinction, from the practical point of view small doses of hypnosedatives should also be considered in this class. The tranquillizers are distinguished from the neuroleptics by the improved symptomatic relief which they produce in the broad range of anxiety states, but with only a minimal behavioural effect in the psychoses.

Certain phenothiazines and butyrophenones (see above) have been used as tranquillizers but the main chemical classes in this group are the diphenylmethane series, the propanediols and the benzodiazepines.

The hypnosedative group comprises both the barbiturates and the non-barbiturates.

The best known members of the *diphenylmethane* series are benactyzine and hydroxyzine. Though side-effects were infrequent and mild the diphenylmethanes have been superseded by more effective newer compounds.

The drugs of the *propanediol group* are muscle relaxants and depressants of polysynaptic reflexes. Meprobamate, the main member of the group, has very little action in the psychoses but is used in anxiety and tension states. The side-effects are less frequent and less troublesome than those encountered with the phenothiazines at equivalent therapeutic dosage. Meprobamate is usually administered at a daily dosage of 400–800 mg. The propanediol group has also been largely superseded by the benzodiazepines.

Benzodiazepine derivatives are a rapidly developing group, used very extensively in the treatment of anxiety. Pharmacologically they all show tranquillization, mild sedative properties and inhibition of polysynaptic reflexes. Different members of the class show considerable variation in their relative potencies for these various pharmacological actions and these differences have been used clinically.

Chlordiazepoxide was the first member of the series which now includes among the commercially available drugs diazepam and nitrazepam. Their greatest value lies in the relief of anxiety occurring as a single entity or as a component of other disease states, e.g. psychosomatic disorders. In addition, diazepam is a good central muscle relaxant which can be used in muscle spasms, even those as severe as tetanus. Nitrazepam, which has a greater sedative component, is valuable in the induction of sleep. The main side-effects which are usually dose-related are ataxia and sedation. Freedom from side-effects is an important feature of the benzodiazepines. It is said to be almost impossible to commit suicide with any of these benzodiazepines used alone. The normal daily dose for chlordiazepoxide is 15–60 mg; and that for diazepam 6–20 mg, while the sedative dose for nitrazepam is 5–10 mg. In view of the slight sedative effects with all the current benzodiazepines it is usual to split the daily dose such that the evening dose is higher. Their large margin of safety is a valuable point when a suicide risk exists.

The *barbiturate hypnotics* are not tranquillizers as defined strictly, but they are used in small doses as psychosedatives. They are reasonably effective in this respect. They suffer, however, from three disadvantages. Firstly, they tend to produce excessive sedation at a therapeutic level, secondly, they show habituation and convulsions on withdrawal and thirdly, since the lethal dose is low relative to the therapeutic dose they should not be given to patients where there is any suicide risk. Many medical practitioners indeed consider that the barbiturates have no place in therapy, with the more effective and safer compounds that are now available. Most of the above comments also apply to many *non-barbiturate hypnotics*. Their use in small doses as tranquillizers is now very limited.

Antidepressants

These have also been termed psychostimulants but this is not a very appropriate name and is best avoided. Four main groups of antidepressants are used for the treatment of mental disorders. These are the direct euphoriants (of amphetamine type), the thymoleptics (chemically embracing the imipramine and amitriptyline series), the monoamine oxidase inhibitors and lithium carbonate.

Euphoriants of the amphetamine class have been widely used for the treatment of mild depression, either alone or in combination with a sedative. Initial improvement can be rapid and though the combination of sedative with stimulant may appear paradoxical in theory, in practice it is found to be effective. When administered for some length of time, less effect may be seen and drug habituation is a very real danger. They should be used with caution, indeed it can be argued that their therapeutic value is inadequate to justify their use at all.

The daily dose of amphetamine is about 10–15 mg per day preferably given in the forenoon.

Paradoxically, although they are central nervous system stimulants, good therapeutic results have been obtained by their use in hyperkinetic children.

The term *thymoleptics* has been coined to describe one type of antidepressant compound. The thymoleptics in use are all iminodibenzyl derivatives and are also known as tricyclic antidepressants from their chemical structure. The parent compound is imipramine. These compounds are not euphoriants and act best in endogenous depression. Some patients with depression respond best to the thymoleptics, some to monoamine oxidase inhibitors. Unfortunately, there is at present no clear method of distinguishing between them although there is evidence that this response pattern may be genetically determined. However, the thymoleptics have a wider spectrum of activity and should probably be regarded as the drug of choice for initial trial in most depressives, unless there are clear indications (e.g. previous good response) for the monoamine oxidase inhibitors.

Although these compounds act clinically as 'psychostimulants' their pharmacological activity is mainly depressant and similar to the chemically related phenothiazines. They show a latent period (10–14 days) before clinical effect is seen and, with the suicide risk for any depressed patient, this lag period is a distinct disadvantage. The main side-effects encountered with the thymoleptics are hypotension and parasympathetic nervous system suppression.

Amitriptyline has similar but more powerful pharmacological actions than imipramine. This increase in activity is also observed in the clinic. Amitriptyline may have less risk of producing side-effects when used in combination with certain other drugs. The initial daily dosage for amitriptyline is usually 100–150 mg but once improvement is seen this can often be reduced to about 50 mg. The sedative component of amitriptyline is valuable for improving the sleep pattern particularly if a larger dose is given at night.

Recently a number of new antidepressants have been introduced, not all of which are tricyclics though they show clinical similarity. They show a spectrum of varying sedative potency at equiactive antidepressant dosage. They may be considered in three groups for convenience, viz:

Activating	*Neutral*	*Sedative*
Desipramine	Nortriptyline	Amitriptyline
Imipramine	Dibenzepin	Trimipramine
Protriptyline	Iprindole	Doxepine
	Clomipramine	Opipramol
	Prothiaden	

The other established group of antidepressants is the *monoamine oxidase inhibitors* (*MAOIs*) which are found in many chemical groups – though most widely used compounds are hydrazine derivatives. The original compound of this group, iproniazid, and the later isocarboxazid show anti-tubercular activity. These compounds show few central nervous system effects in animals, and these only when administered with other substances. They exert their effect by inhibiting one of the enzymes responsible for the breakdown of brain amines (p. 39).

Clinically, the MAOIs appear to show their best activity in the more reactive or atypical depressions although there are no clear distinctions between those patients who respond best to MAOIs and those who respond best to the thymoleptics (see above). Like the thymoleptics, a lag period of ten days or more precedes any therapeutic effect. Many of these drugs are hepatotoxic and can cause hypotension. They are liable to create further problems by their potentiation of other chemicals (p. 269). Their troublesome side-effects and the dietary precautions that are necessary reduce their use.

Although iproniazid (daily dose 150 mg) is the most active compound, it is also the most toxic and should be reserved for patients who fail to respond to less active members of the group. Isocarboxazid at a daily dose of 30 mg is an appropriate drug for initial therapy.

Lithium Carbonate. The use of this substance as a prophylactic in depression and mania has now been established for it reduces the mood swings, particularly in those with marked manic manifestations. It should be reserved for use under the direct control of a hospital for the dose must be based upon blood-level determinations, the effective serum level being 0·6–1·2 m.eq./litre. Side-effects (e.g. fine tremor and diarrhoea) occur at higher blood levels and the toxic manifestations of vomiting, drowsiness, ataxia and convulsions may occur at levels above 2·0 m.eq./litre.

Psychotomimetic Drugs

Several drugs are now known which produce a change in affect, normally a euphoria (psychedelics). Some, in addition, produce hallucinations, with a clinical picture resembling a toxic psychosis rather than schizophrenia. Although several synthetic compounds are known, most of these drugs are naturally occurring substances, used for centuries in tribal rites.

The most widely studied compounds are marihuana, mescaline and lysergic acid diethylamide (LSD). Other drugs with psychotomimetic effects are bufotenin, harmine, yohimbine, psilocybin and dimethyl tryptamine.

Drugs of this type are used occasionally for therapeutic purposes and are claimed to render certain psychiatric patients more accessible to psychotherapy. Unfortunately, several drugs of this group and the drugs of the euphoriant group (e.g. the amphetamines) have been abused, usually by adolescents with inadequate personalities. There is no absolute evidence that these drugs are capable of producing physical dependence but their abuse is dangerous and to be deprecated.

CHOICE OF DRUGS TO USE

With the wide range of compounds from which the medical practitioner may make his choice there is obvious difficulty in selecting the appropriate therapy for the individual case. To describe in detail the choice of appropriate therapy is beyond the scope of this book, however, an outline of the principles of selection appears appropriate. A guide to drug selection is shown in fig. 72. It must, however, be stressed that there is considerable individual variation in response to many of these drugs and that fig. 72 only gives a broad view of the group of compounds most likely to be effective.

MODE OF ACTION OF PSYCHOTROPIC DRUGS

Existing psychotropic drugs all have a symptomatic effect; they relieve the symptoms of mental illness but have little or no effect on the underlying cause of the disease. Final conclusions on their mode of action must await further experiments but tentative theories are now possible.

The psychotropic drugs act mainly at diencephalic and mid-brain levels and on centres concerned with emotional responses (p. 122). The action of psychotropic drugs can be considered at either a pharmacological or a biochemical level of cell interaction. Methods of study include EEG recordings from different sites, electrical stimulation or extirpation of different centres and determination of the effects on various forms of conditioned changes within separate areas of the brain. Most of these studies have been undertaken in animals but there is some confirmatory work in man.

The majority of the known facts on the pharmacology and therapeutic activity of the psychotropic drugs can be explained on the basis of differential effects on the following systems:

(1) Various parts of the reticular formation, including the wake mechanism (p. 89).

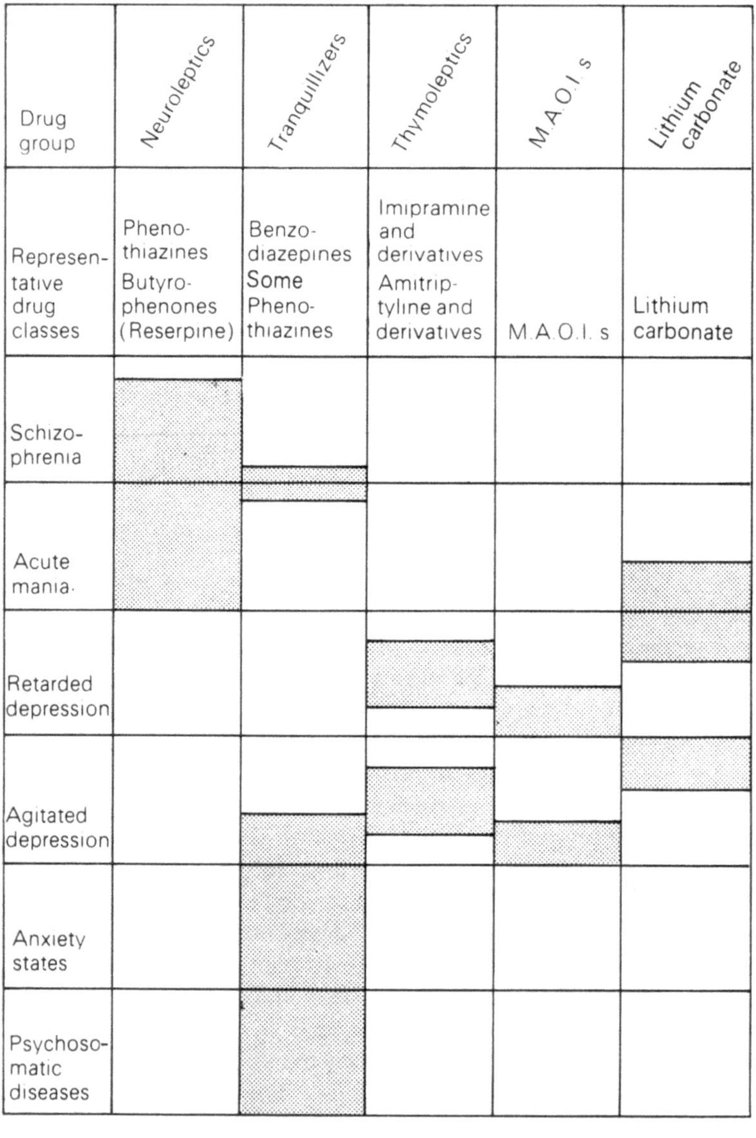

Drug group	Neuroleptics	Tranquillizers	Thymoleptics	M.A.O.I.s	Lithium carbonate
Representative drug classes	Pheno-thiazines Butyro-phenones (Reserpine)	Benzo-diazepines Some Pheno-thiazines	Imipramine and derivatives Amitrip-tyline and derivatives	M.A.O.I.s	Lithium carbonate
Schizo-phrenia					
Acute mania.					
Retarded depression					
Agitated depression					
Anxiety states					
Psychoso-matic diseases					

FIGURE 72 Representation of the drug group which is likely to be effective in the main psychiatric disorders

(2) The centres of the reticular formation and corpus striatum for muscle tone control (p. 87).

(3) The limbic system, and probably specifically the amygdaloid nuclei and the hippocampus (p. 123).

(4) The thalamus and thence the cortex (p. 73).

(5) The hypothalamus and thence the effector mechanism of the autonomic nervous system and the endocrine system (p. 89).

(6) Polysynaptic reflexes in the spinal cord (p. 78).

From the data presented, it may be concluded that a compound which produces sleep must be blocking the wake component of the reticular formation; a compound which produces extrapyramidal nervous system side-effects must be acting on the tone-modifying component of the reticular formation or on the corpus striatum; a compound which produces autonomic side-effects as a major feature must have an activity on the hypothalamus or lower structures; a compound which shows a marked taming effect in animals must be acting within the limbic system, or on structures that affect the limbic system.

Meprobamate and chlordiazepoxide both depress principally – though not exclusively – the limbic system (probably the amygdaloid nucleus), the thalamus and polysynaptic reflexes in the spinal cord. Chlorpromazine, on the other hand, does not depress and may even stimulate the thalamus and amygdaloid nucleus. It exerts its main action within the reticular formation and in hypothalamic areas. Rauwolfia alkaloids also tend to stimulate the limbic system, to depress the reticular formation and to depress sympathetic and stimulate parasympathetic centres in the hypothalamus. Barbiturates, on the other hand, generally depress all these sites. The anatomical site of action of psychostimulants is far less clear.

At a cellular biochemical level, the liberation of acetylcholine or interference with its transportation has been claimed as a primary mechanism of the psychotropic drugs. So, too, have the suppression of energy release from the citric acid cycle, action upon its enzymes and those of the electron transport system and the release of energy from energy-rich phosphates. Though these may play a part, the effect of many but not all psychotropic drugs may be explained on the basis of interchanges occurring within the amine pool (p. 41). This probably applies in particular to drugs that act on the hypothalamus, corpus striatum and other areas that are amine rich.

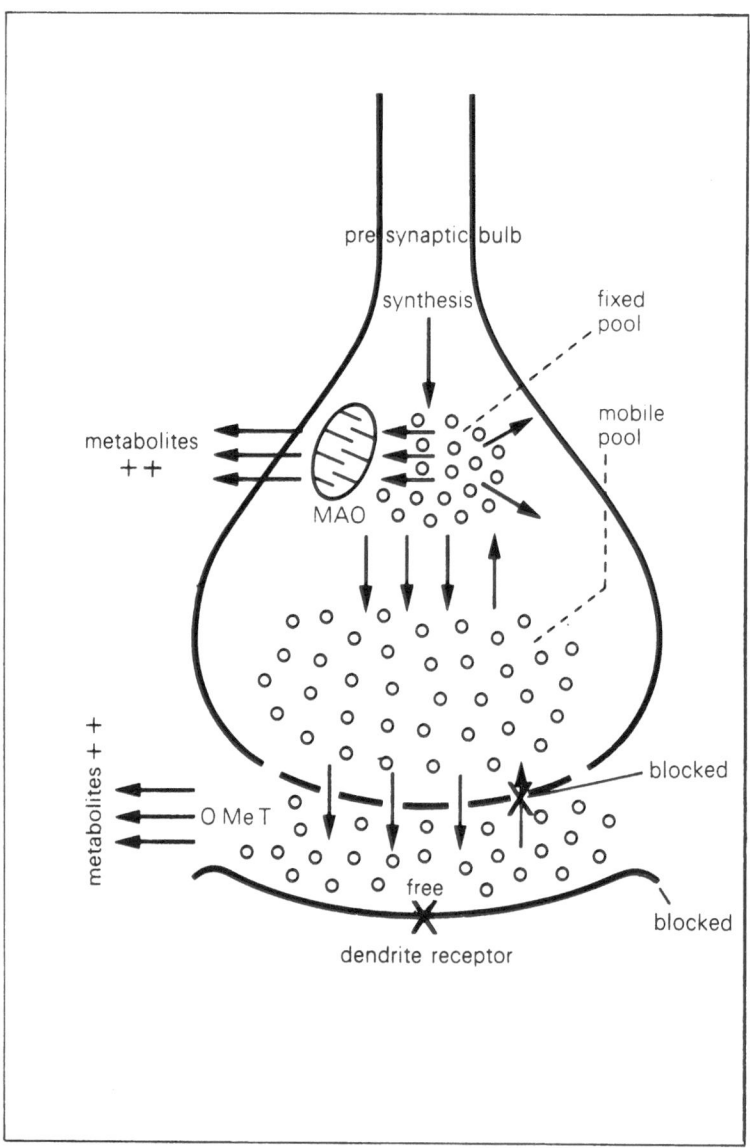

FIGURE 73 Biochemical change in adrenergic cells which may explain the action of chlorpromazine.

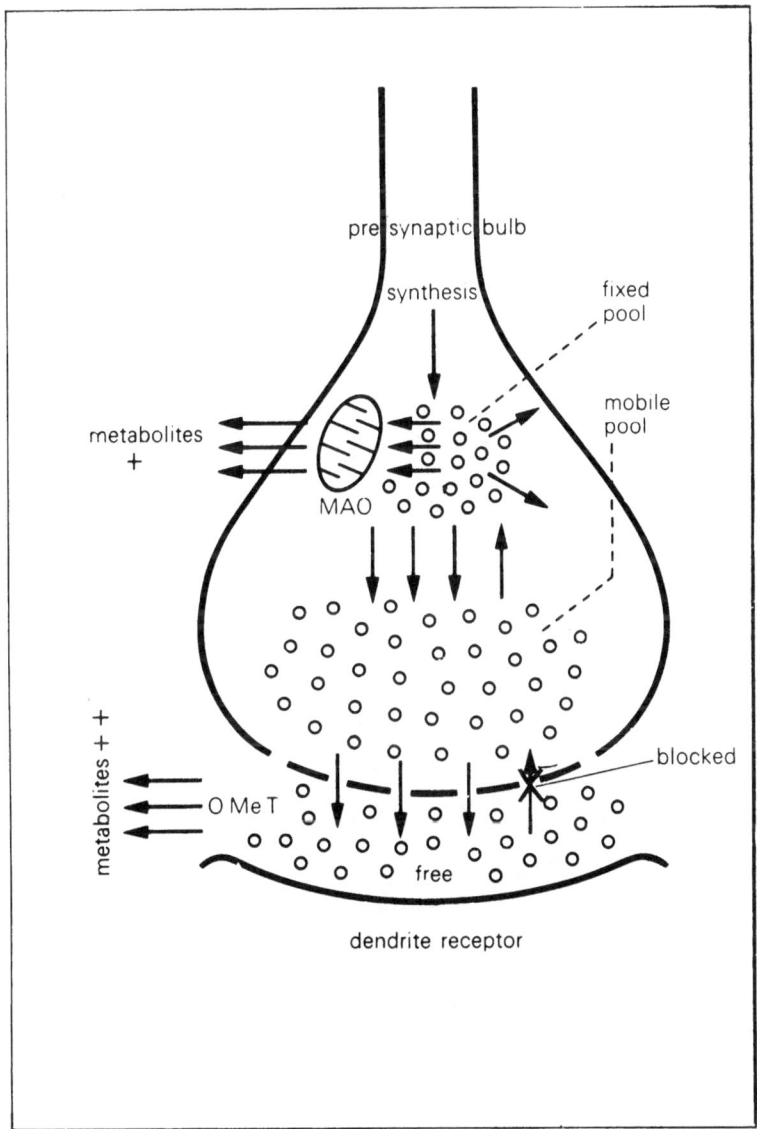

FIGURE 74 Biochemical changes in adrenergic cells which may explain the action of thymoleptic drugs.

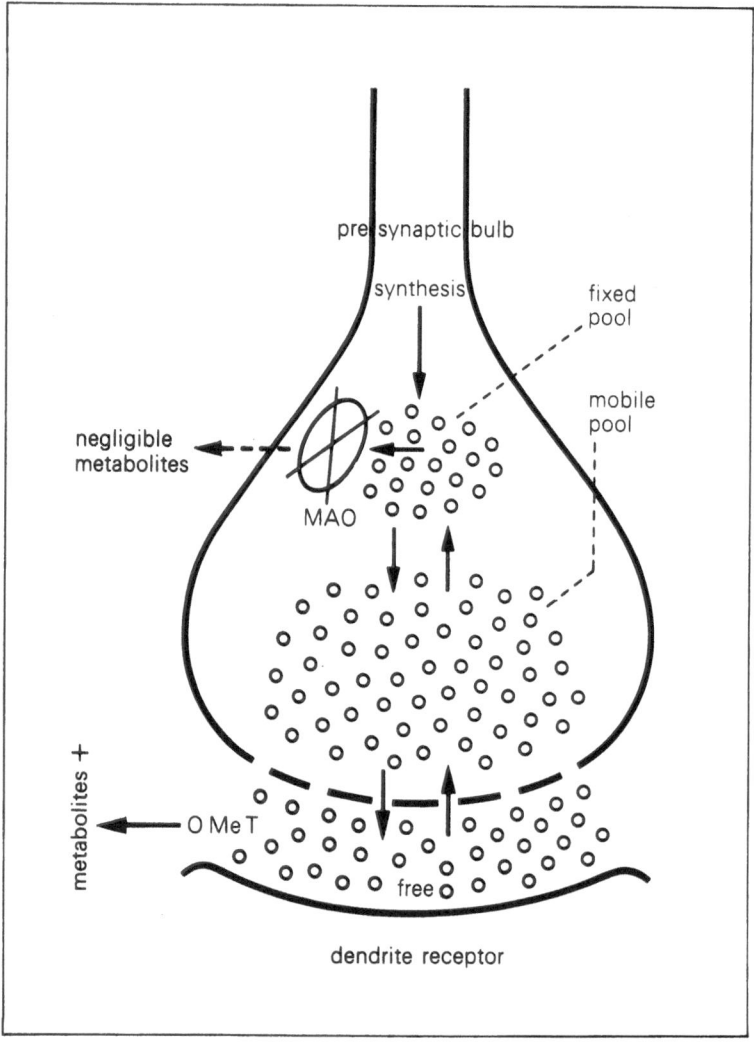

FIGURE 75 Biochemical changes in adrenergic cells which may explain the action of monoamine oxidase inhibitors.

Many brain centres contain primary amines, which exist within the brain in two forms – 'bound' and 'free'. The brain is stimulated when the proportion of free to bound amine is increased and is retarded when the majority of the amine is in the bound form. Within the frame-

268

work of this theory, changes in mood could be caused by releasing the bound amine, by preventing transport across the membrane between the bound and free forms and by releasing the amine and preventing its subsequent breakdown.

Reserpine releases the bound amine to produce a high free level which produces initial excitation (p. 257). The free form is rapidly metabolized, leaving a retarded state due to low levels of free and bound amines. Chlorpromazine increases outward flow of amines from the presynaptic membrane and reduces reuptake. However, it blocks the receptor site and no excitation results (fig. 73). Biochemically, thymoleptics resemble chlorpromazine. Release from the presynaptic membrane is facilitated and reuptake is inhibited. The resulting higher levels with unblocked receptor sites gives a stimulant effect (fig. 74). Monoamine oxidase inhibitors block the enzyme (MAO) and stimulation results (fig. 75). A frequent side-effect with reserpine, phenothiazines and the butyrophenones is Parkinsonism, almost certainly due to the interruption of dopaminergic pathways in the corpus striatum.

INTERACTIONS INVOLVING PSYCHOTROPIC DRUGS

Since patients are frequently polysymptomatic, various combinations of psychotropic drugs are used. Psychotropic drugs may also be given with drugs for entirely different medical conditions. Such combinations are liable to produce additive side-effects. Food, also, contains substances with which some psychotropic drugs can interact.

Such interaction of the psychotropic drugs can be divided into three classes :

(a) Simple summation of known effects (e.g. two weak, hypotensive compounds producing additive orthostatic hypotension; two parasympatheticolytic compounds producing paralytic ileus).

(b) Specific interaction (e.g. monoamine oxidase inhibitors potentiate the action of certain amines and produce hypomania and hypertensive crises. Such reactions may occur with dopa (broad bean), tyramines (certain cheeses, Marmite, Bovril), amphetamines, thymoleptic compounds (imipramine and less commonly amitriptyline).

(c) Indirect action (e.g. certain monoamine oxidase inhibitors also inhibit non-specific oxidases – a liver enzyme responsible for the metabolism). Barbiturate, alcohol and narcotic potentiation occurs.

Appendix

LEGAL AND SOCIAL ASPECTS OF MENTAL ILLNESS

Legal aspects

The mentally ill – no less than those who are mentally well – are rightly subject to the laws of the country in which they find themselves. Nevertheless, the ability to observe those laws (which exists as a basic presumption in all healthy persons) is liable to be diminished and may be absent in those suffering from mental illness or from the handicap of mental subnormality.

It is for this reason that all civilized countries extend to such persons an acknowledgement of lessened responsibility for their acts when these are answerable at civil or criminal law. Periodically, the laws relating to mental disorders are revised and updated in pursuance of the medical advances in psychiatry and in conformation with the more enlightened knowledge available. But in such progress, legal change will always be notoriously slow. The enactment of new legislation will follow progressive thought but will rarely, if ever, lead such change. Typically a frustrating time-lag intervenes between the social acceptance of such updated principles and their official establishment as law. This more secure if snail-like process of advancement is not devoid of civil and social advantages. Nevertheless, where human suffering or the welfare of the sick are at stake judicial and administrative delay may sometimes prove intolerable in the practice of modern medical advances.

Much room still exists for further progressive legislation throughout the world in the interests of those suffering from mental illnesses. The attitudes prevalent in many countries towards such patients – as mirrored in their current legislation – still vary enormously. In certain countries themselves, as for example the United States of America, the laws themselves may vary greatly in content from State to State. Yet for all this, the continuing trend must be towards an ultimate goal of greater uniformity as more and more enlightened knowledge is made available.

For validity at law, and therefore to qualify for the special privileges extended by the judiciary to mental disorder, such disorder must first be established as existing in the person under consideration. In all individuals the presumption of mental health must be made until the contrary can be established.

Whilst offering degrees of protection to the mentally sick against the normal legal consequences their acts might incur, so too must the law consider the protection of society. At times the seriously disturbed mental patient will constitute a dangerous threat to society. In these and in other circumstances, where it is clearly in the interests of the patient's own health, the individual may be temporarily deprived of his liberty and committed to a mental hospital. When this occurs, elaborate safeguards are written into the relevant legislation to ensure the preservation of the patient's best interests. The compulsory admission of a patient to hospital in contradiction to his wishes is an exact procedure in most countries. For England and Wales, the pattern of modern psychiatric legislation can be found in the Mental Health Act of 1959. This Act emerged from the 'Royal Commission on the Law relating to Mental Illness and Mental Deficiency' set up by the British Government and which published its findings in 1957.

THE MENTAL HEALTH ACT (1959)

The Mental Health Act of 1959 repealed all previous legislation dealing with mental illness and mental deficiency. In so doing, it established an entirely new basis for our attitudes, approaches and administration for patients in need of psychiatric help. The passing of the Act marked the curtailment of an outdated era in psychological medicine and the commencement of a new, modern and forward-looking period, the key-word to which was informality in both treatment and care of the mental patient.

Gone now was the authority vested in the Lunacy and Mental Treatment Acts (1890–1930), in the Mental Deficiency Acts (1913–1938) and in the relevant sections of the National Health Service Act (1946). In its stead had arrived a simplified yet comprehensive substitute for all such psychiatric legislation. The Board of Control, formally responsible for the liberty of the individual, was now dissolved and its responsibilities passed to the Minister of Health, in conjunction with the Mental Health Review Tribunals. A Mental Health Review Tribunal was appointed for each of the 15 Regional Hospital Boards in England and Wales.

The essential principles of the Mental Health Act may be summarized:

(a) Informality. Both inside and outside hospital, psychiatric treatment should be given, whenever possible, on a completely informal basis.
(b) Compulsory admission. Proper provision should still be made for the residual category of case, where compulsory admission to hospital is necessary in the interests of the patient or of society.
(c) Community care. So far as is possible, the emphasis in mental cases shall be shifted from institutional care to care within the community.

The Act itself consists of 154 Sections, arranged as nine Parts. To this main body of the Act eight Schedules are appended.

Much of the Act's substance has a limited application to the routine, practical problems of everyday psychiatry and tends therefore to be of somewhat academic worth.

Certain sections, however, have a vital application to the daily problems of the psychiatrist and General Practitioner alike and it is with these that each must be familiar. Among them Sections 25–29. dealing essentially with compulsory admission of patients to hospital, are of particular importance.

The Act concerns itself with persons suffering from 'mental disorder'. This all-embracing term has been chosen to include 'mental illness, mental subnormality, severe mental subnormality, psychopathic disorder and any other disorder or disability of mind'.

The Act made medical history by legally defining the highly controversial term 'psychopathic disorder'. According to the Act 'psychopathic disorder' is a persistent disorder or disability of mind (whether

272

or not including subnormality of intelligence) which results in abnormally aggressive or seriously irresponsible conduct on the part of the patient and requires or is susceptible to medical treatment.

Although great emphasis throughout the Act is placed upon the informality of treatment for the mental patient, both inside and outside hospital, occasions must none the less arise where a patient clearly needs to be in hospital yet cannot be persuaded to enter hospital of his own volition, or perhaps is already in hospital on an informal basis and gives notice of leaving in circumstances which medically are completely inadvisable. For such occasions the compulsory procedures to admit or detain a patient in hospital exist and these concern themselves with safeguarding the patient's interests, health and safety and also with the protection of other persons.

To admit compulsorily a patient to hospital, two simple, though essential, requirements must be met. Firstly, an application must be made by the nearest relative (or social worker deputizing for the nearest relative) to the hospital to receive the patient. Secondly, this application must be accompanied by the medical recommendations of two appropriate doctors (only one doctor in the case of the Emergency Admission: Section 29).

The Act is specific in its attempts throughout to safeguard the interests of the patient and prevent any wrongful detention. It is most important to realize that the onus of applying to a hospital for the admission of a patient is NOT that of the medical practitioner but is vested in the nearest relative (or Social Worker deputizing for the nearest relative). The doctors give their opinion on the desirability of admission in support of the application. The nearest relative, in furnishing the application to the hospital, will normally be assisted by the Social Worker who will explain the technicalities involved.

Such Compulsory Admission may be for Observation (Section 25); for Treatment (Section 26); or for Observation in Emergency (Section 29). The periods for which patients may be compulsorily detained under these procedures are 28 days (Observation); one year (Treatment); and 72 hours (Observation in Emergency). It should be noted that, in the case of compulsory admission for Treatment (Section 26), authorization may be made on the grounds of subnormality and psychopathic disorder only if the patient is under the age of 21. On the ground of mental illness or severe subnormality, compulsory admission for Treatment (Section 26) may be authorized for patients of any age.

273

After one year the compulsory admission for Treatment (Section 26) may be renewed for a further year and thereafter at two-yearly intervals. The essential principles of compulsory admission are summarized in Table 9.

Type	Duration	Application	Medical Recommendations
OBSERVATION (Section 25)	28 days	Nearest relative or Social Worker	1. Doctor approved by Local Authority
			2. Another doctor (if possible, patient's GP)
TREATMENT (Section 26)	1 year	Nearest relative or Social Worker	1. Doctor approved by Local Authority
			2. Another doctor (if possible, patient's GP)
OBSERVATION IN EMERGENCY (Section 29)	72 hours	Any relative or Social Worker	1. Any doctor (if possible, patient's GP)

TABLE 9 Summary of the regulations covering compulsory admission

A Justice of the Peace, on information from a Social Worker, has powers to order the removal of a patient to a place of safety if his suspicions that the patient may be ill-treated, neglected or not kept under proper control or is living alone and unable to care for himself, are confirmed by a visit from a medical practitioner, a Social Worker and a police constable. Furthermore, any police constable finding an apparently mentally disordered patient in need of care or control in a public place may again remove him to a place of safety and detain him there for not more than 72 hours.

The Act provides for power to discharge a patient compulsorily detained in hospital and delegates this authority to the nearest relative, to the hospital and to the Mental Health Tribunal.

The courts are empowered to admit compulsorily patients to hospitals willing to receive them by making a Hospital Order (Section 60) or Hospital Order with Restrictions (Section 65). In the latter case, authorization for discharge lies with the Home Secretary and the duration of the patient's detention in hospital is stipulated.

The Mental Health Act directed that a comprehensive community care service should be established by all local health authorities for those mentally disordered patients who did not require treatment in hospital. Such community care service is required to provide residential accommodation for such persons as the educationally subnormal, maladjusted young persons in employment, elderly mentally infirm persons, who do not need the service and resources of a hospital and patients discharged from mental hospitals who need some support on re-entering community life. The community care service is further required to provide centres or other facilities for training and occupation to meet the needs of children who are unsuitable for education at school, and for adults (Adult Training Centres) who need a considerable amount of supervision to perform the simplest operations or who, unable to be trained for normal or sheltered employment elsewhere, can obtain useful occupation in a local authority workshop or industrial centre. The Adult Training Centres should, where necessary, offer residential accommodation and, in addition to the foregoing, should assist those needing industrial training or who require some social stabilization as a preliminary to entering ordinary or sheltered employment.

It is regrettable that nearly two decades after the passing of the Mental Health Act, much of the comprehensive community care service in certain areas remains at a most rudimentary level. A major factor in the delays involved has always been the matter of finance.

Disparity has been found between the provisions of the Act and the reality situation of those persons who are psychiatrically incurable and legally criminal. More security hospitals, other than such hospitals as Broadmoor, Moss Side and Rampton, have been advocated as an urgent necessity.

In cases of Compulsory Admission to Hospital, it is the Social Worker who will advise and assist the relatives with arrangements for the application for admission. He may be responsible for returning a patient to hospital who has absented himself or herself without leave; he may enter and inspect premises if he has cause to believe that a mentally ill patient is not under proper care. He is protected by law in his duties provided he acts in good faith and with reasonable care. The

Social Worker works closely with the courts in matters of admission to hospitals and security hospitals of mental patients under Section 60 (Hospital Order) or Section 65 (Hospital Order with Restrictions) of the Mental Health Act (1959). Local authorities maintain a 24-hour duty rota of Social Workers. In times of doubt and difficulty, when dealing with any mental crisis occurring among his patients, a general practitioner is always well advised to seek the counsel of his responsible Social Worker. One problem that is encountered in a number of areas is that due to the considerable demands for the Social Worker's services, he or she is very overworked and may consequently be difficult on occasion to contact.

Both Scotland (1960) and Northern Ireland (1961) introduced their own Acts for Mental Health. Although these correspond most closely to the Mental Health Act (England and Wales) 1959, nevertheless each shows its own individual variation. In Scottish law, the Mental Welfare Commission corresponds to the Mental Health Review Tribunal of the English Act. This Commission consists of 7–9 members of whom 3 are doctors, 1 is a lawyer, and 1 is a woman. Apart from their role in investigating complaints of wrongful detention of patients, the Mental Welfare Commission is concerned with the protection of mentally disordered persons who are incapable of looking after themselves.

The Act for Northern Ireland – like that for Scotland – avoids addressing itself to 'psychopathic disorder'. Nevertheless it provides for the compulsory admission to hospital of patients who are aggressive and/or irresponsible, if requiring or are susceptible to medical treatment. Mentally subnormal (mentally handicapped) persons in this Act are designated 'persons requiring special care'.

It will be appreciated that the Sections of both the Scottish and Irish Acts will differ appreciably in their numbering from the Sections to be found in the Mental Health Act (England and Wales) 1959.

CIVIL RESPONSIBILITY

Voting

A person who is mentally ill is entitled to vote, providing he is of appropriate age and appears on the electoral roll of his district. Residence in a mental hospital does not confer the right for inclusion in the electoral roll of that district though In-patients may still vote in their own home districts provided they appear in their particular electoral roll.

Persons suffering mental defect amounting to severe subnormality may not vote, nor may persons convicted of felony by the courts and committed to hospital by Hospital Order.

Testamentary capacity

A person suffering from mental illness can make a valid will but must be *of sound disposing mind*. To establish this, he should appreciate the nature and extent of his property, be satisfactorily aware of those who might reasonably expect to have a claim on the estate, and be sufficiently unclouded in judgement and will-power as to evaluate the relative importance of such claims.

Problems of testamentary capacity arise most frequently in elderly senile patients. Where difficulty exists the Court of Protection may appoint a Receiver to supervise the control and management of the patient's property.

Contracts

Contracts made before the occurrence of mental illness are binding for the patient. Thereafter, a person of unsound mind is held responsible in contracting for the necessities of life, the clarification of which may be left to the court.

(a) *Marriage*. A mentally disordered person can contract a valid marriage providing he (or she) is of appropriate age and both parties know what they are doing. If it can be proved that at the time of the ceremony, one of the partners was incapacitated by mental illness to the extent that he or she could not appreciate the nature of the contract or the concomitant obligations, then that marriage would not be valid and any children would be illegitimate.

(b) *Annulment*. The Matrimonial Causes Act (1950) rules that a marriage contract may be invalid if at the time of the ceremony either partner was suffering from a mental disorder to render him or her unfit for marriage and the production of children, or was subject to recurrent attacks of epilepsy or insanity. The partner petitioning must have been ignorant of the facts when marrying and must start proceedings within one year of the marriage date. Furthermore, sexual intercourse must not have occurred with the petitioner's consent since discovering these facts.

(c) *Divorce*. Divorce on the grounds of mental illness can be sought if the respondent has been continuously under care and treatment for a period of five years immediately preceding the petition. This does not mean that a patient must be compulsorily detained in hospital for this period and informal care and treatment during this time, demonstrated to the satisfaction of the court, would be successful grounds for divorce.

CRIMINAL RESPONSIBILITY

Forensic psychiatry is that special division of psychological medicine which is primarily concerned with matters relevant to the criminal courts of law. It applies the principles of general psychiatry to those in conflict with the criminal law, giving specialist advice to the courts and concerns itself, in addition, with the treatment of offenders as defined by the courts. Any crime may fall within the range of forensic psychiatry from murder, rape and arson to the battering of babies, habitual drunkenness and shoplifting, for forensic psychiatry is concerned with the mental state of the criminal rather than the crime *per se*. Problems of psychopathy and other personality disorders, together with those of alcoholism, sexual offences and drug addiction, recur frequently and commonly in the practice of forensic psychiatry. The extent of these social problems within our current society is substantial. Their treatment is problematical, controversial and in many instances, obscure.

Appointments in the specialized field of forensic psychiatry are normally joint ones to a prison and mental hospital. Unless special facilities exist for the treatment of psychopaths within their hospital organization, most mental hospitals are uneasy at accepting patients with marked anti-social tendencies or criminal records. There are good reasons for this, for most local mental hospitals cannot assume custodianship of their patients. Special hospitals, such as Broadmoor, Rampton, Moss Side and Carstairs State Mental Hospital, exist as security institutions. Equally within the Prison Service, Grendon Underwood near Aylesbury, is run on the lines of a therapeutic community and offers all normal forms of psychiatric treatment.

The McNaghten Rules

It was the case of Daniel McNaghten which led in 1843 to the establishment of the historic McNaghten Rules in law, whereby a verdict of 'guilty but insane' could be returned with detention of the patient as a criminal lunatic during Her Majesty's pleasure (Trial of Lunatics Act 1883) .McNaghten, suffering from intense paranoid delusions, set out to murder the Prime Minister of the time – Sir Robert

278

Peel. But mistaking the Prime Minister's identity, McNaghten shot and killed a Mr. Drummond, Sir Robert Peel's secretary, instead. At his trial for murder McNaghten was found to be insane and was acquitted. To establish defence by the McNaghten Rules it must be proved that at the time of committing the offence, the accused did not know the nature and quality of the act he was doing or, alternatively, did not know that what he was doing was wrong.

In addition to this general principle governing the question of responsibility for an offence, several specific English Acts have relevance to the practitioner and psychiatrist, viz.:

(a) *The Homicide Act (1957)*. This act differentiated capital murder from non-capital murder and allowed new grounds for reduction of a conviction to the lesser form of criminal homicide, namely manslaughter. The Homicide Act (1957) allows the concept of 'diminished responsibility' and in Section 2 states that 'where a person kills or is party to killing another, he shall not be convicted of murder if he was suffering from such abnormality of mind (whether arising from a condition of arrested or retarded development of mind or any inherent cause or induced by disease or injury) as substantially impaired his mental responsibility for his acts and omissions in doing or being a party to the killing'.

A successful defence on the grounds of diminished responsibility under the Homicide Act (1957) would be likely to be followed by Hospital Order with Restrictions (Section 65) (p. 275). Since most prisoners would prefer a fixed term of imprisonment rather than a Hospital Order which could involve loss of liberty for a longer period – this plea has little application beyond the charge of murder.

(b) *Abortion Act (1967)*. Contrary to popular belief, abortion remains a criminal act. The Abortion Act (1967) does, however, create certain legal exceptions. Pregnancy may be terminated if two registered medical practitioners are of the opinion that the continuance of pregnancy would endanger the life of the pregnant woman or pose a serious threat to the physical or mental health of that woman or to any existing children of her family; or equally, if a substantial risk exists that the child, if born, would suffer from serious mental or physical handicap. It is not necessary for either of the two medical practitioners concerned to be a psychiatrist. Termination of the pregnancy must be made in a place approved by the Department of Health and Social Security.

(c) *Sexual Offences Act (1967)*. This Act, which followed the work of

279

a Royal Commission, legally permits homosexual practice between two consenting adults over the age of 21 years provided this activity takes place in private. The crews of merchant ships of the United Kingdom abroad cannot claim the protection against prosecution which this Act affords homosexuals.

(d) *Suicide Act (1961)*. In England, the taking of one's own life or attempts at this have been traditionally crimes against both State and Church. Until the nineteenth century, burial of a consummated suicide was precluded from consecrated ground and such patients were interred at the meeting point of four crossroads and with a stake driven through them into the ground. Though such barbarous practices by society were removed, it remained illegal to take, or attempt to take, one's life until the passing of the Suicide Act (1961). Within this Act, there still remains provision for proceedings against surviving members of suicide pacts, who can be accused of aiding, abetting, counselling or procuring the suicide of another or an attempt by another to commit suicide. In past years, considerate coroners have circumnavigated the felony of suicide and its subsequent stigmata by a verdict when possible that the deceased person was of unsound mind, or the balance of mind was disturbed when the act of suicide was committed.

The social services

In Great Britain, the social services have recently undergone a most drastic and far-reaching reorganization. It is too early to assess the wisdom of all that has been attempted, or indeed whether the new arrangements will result in an improvement in patient community care. Indeed since the current period is a transitional one, and calls for far more experience and special training of the very large numbers of social workers involved, no valid assessment of its improved service will be possible for some years to come. Whilst impressive plans and imposing arrangements can be drawn with ease in Ministerial or Local Authority offices, the critical evaluation of such reorganization can only be based on the ultimate ease, efficiency and effectiveness which the patients themselves experience as community care.

Whereas some of the planning of these Social Services for Great Britain must inevitably carry about it a domestic quality, it is none the less true that the social problems of all modern societies are now showing a remarkable similarity in the specific needs of their peoples. These needs must include effective arrangements during pregnancy and for the birth of children (including civilized facilities for the unmarried mother); the subsequent care of children (where the efforts of the parents need supplementation, or in certain cases substituting for the parents); the complicated problems of the adoption of children; care for the physically sick and disabled (including the blind, deaf and spastic); care for the mentally ill and those who are mentally defective; care for the aged; and welfare arrangements for the homeless.

Any comprehensive social organization adopted by one particular country will be of more than passing interest to many others – if only perhaps to take advantage with hindsight of its proven assets and to avoid its pitfalls and liabilities. On this basis, the recent reorganization of social services within Great Britain has special interest to similar countries overseas.

In England and Wales, the Mental Health Act of 1959 (p. 271) had already charged the Local Authorities with providing a system of care for the mentally sick within their respective communities. Similar responsibility had been placed upon the Local Authorities for the care and welfare of the mentally deficient.

The recommendations of the Seebohm Committee (on Local Authority and Allied Personal services), which were given the force of law in 1970, brought about the drastic and far-reaching changes in the social services which are now being implemented.

Previously, social workers had been employed by various different authorities and were given appropriate titles such as Mental Welfare Officer; Children's Officer, etc. These heterogeneous social facilities have now been unified under the Local Authority responsible in the form of one comprehensive system of social service. Old titles disappeared and the generic terms 'social worker' and 'client' were adopted.

The social workers are responsible to a Director of Social Services for each Local Authority. Whilst they provide essentially a community service, it is encouraging to find that the new system has been effective in the establishment of some joint appointments for its social workers, making these responsible for both Hospital and Community patients.

This liaison not only breaks down with great advantage the false division between hospital care and community care, but also allows a much smoother passage of the patient in his transition from one type of care to the other, thus safeguarding the patient's interests and welfare to a much higher degree.

The efficient functioning of this new system of social services will depend critically upon the nature of the relationship which can be established and maintained with the medical profession. The clients of the social workers have long since been the patients of the doctors. By tradition and training, medical men are sensitive to any apparent interference with their patient from outside sources – particularly from a seemingly para-medical source.

A number of the new social services arrangements, if insensitively or tactlessly applied, could be seen or misinterpreted as providing a threat or substitution for the personal doctor–patient relationship and an erosion of the patient's rights. An important point in question arises when information divulged to the doctor, under the seal of professional secrecy which governs any consultation, should with very good reason be made available on request from the social worker. Though to do so would clearly be in the patient's best interests, the doctor has no choice in this matter. The approval of the patient must first be obtained and his permission freely given before any information or notes are passed.

In spite of an inherent conservatism which is inevitable with any learned profession, doctors are not narrow-minded in the pursuit of their patients' interests nor where advantage for their patients can be gained. With courtesy on both sides, with a conscious desire to co-operate and a willingness to appreciate the difficulties experienced by the alternate profession, there seems little reason why doctor and social worker should not work in excellent harmony together, each conducting his own specialized work to the great advantage of their mutual interest, be this semantically designated by the term of patient or client.

INDEX